Hot Topics in Acute Care Surgery and Trauma

Series Editors

Federico Coccolini
Pisa, Italy

Raul Coimbra
Riverside, USA

Andrew W. Kirkpatrick
Calgary, Canada

Salomone Di Saverio
Cambridge, UK

Editorial Board

This series covers the most debated issues in acute care and trauma surgery, from perioperative management to organizational and health policy issues. Since 2011, the founder members of the World Society of Emergency Surgery's (WSES) Acute Care and Trauma Surgeons group, who endorse the series, realized the need to provide more educational tools for young surgeons in training and for general physicians and other specialists new to this discipline: WSES is currently developing a systematic scientific and educational program founded on evidence-based medicine and objective experience. Covering the complex management of acute trauma and non-trauma surgical patients, this series makes a significant contribution to this program and is a valuable resource for both trainees and practitioners in acute care surgery.

More information about this series at http://www.springer.com/series/15718

Federico Coccolini • Manu L. N. G. Malbrain
Andrew W. Kirkpatrick • Emiliano Gamberini
Editors

Compartment Syndrome

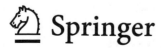 Springer

Editors
Federico Coccolini
General, Emergency and Trauma Surgery
Department
Pisa University Hospital
Pisa, Italy

Andrew W. Kirkpatrick
Regional Trauma Services
Foothills Medical Centre
Calgary, AB
Canada

Manu L. N. G. Malbrain
Intensive Care Unit
Ziekenhuisnetwerk Antwerpen Stuivenberg
Antwerpen, Belgium

Emiliano Gamberini
Chief Physician in Intensive Care Unit and
Trauma Management in Level-1
Trauma Center
"M. Bufalini" Hospital
CESENA, Forli/Cesana, Italy

ISSN 2520-8284   ISSN 2520-8292   (electronic)
Hot Topics in Acute Care Surgery and Trauma
ISBN 978-3-030-55380-7   ISBN 978-3-030-55378-4   (eBook)
https://doi.org/10.1007/978-3-030-55378-4

The logo of the WSES and the one of the AAST will be printed on the volume cover.

This Springer imprint is published by the registered company Springer Nature Switzerland AG
The registered company address is: Gewerbestrasse 11, 6330 Cham, Switzerland

Foreword

More than 150 years ago, Marey and Braune first studied the physiology of intra-abdominal pressure. In the last four decades, elevated intra-abdominal pressure (intra-abdominal hypertension, IAH) and the sinister upshot of untreated IAH (the abdominal compartment syndrome, ACS) have become menacing problems in all aspects of intensive care, transcending specialties and age groups. The critical issues surrounding pressure and perfusion in the ubiquitous rigid compartments in the human body have become frequent and challenging as we began to care for the massively injured and seriously ill patients on the very edge of survival. The need to understand these phenomena, anticipate them, attempt prevention, diagnose promptly, and institute therapy effectively has never been more acute.

The World Society of the Abdominal Compartment Syndrome (WSACS) recently expanded to the WSAC or World Society of the Abdominal Compartment, an international group of interested scientists toiled hard to review the entire existing literature and formulate evidence-based guidelines. The commendable work of this society defined clinical terms and recommended management precepts by consensus. These advances culminated in organ-sparing and life-saving critical care. The society even revisited, in 2013, their original statements to provide concise, updated guidelines. The results have been spectacular. Surgical and trauma critical care units began to talk a common language in terms of bladder pressure (intra-abdominal pressure), abdominal decompression for IAH, and "open abdomen" management. Not unexpectedly, ACS began to fade away. The prospect of eliminating the morbid ACS was suddenly on the horizon!

Despite this rosy outlook, awareness of the pathophysiology of compartment syndromes, unfortunately, seems to be patchy at best and nonexistent at worst. The intransigent attitudes of nonsurgical intensivists in refusing to acknowledge the phenomenon of compartmental hypertension are repeatedly documented by survey after survey. Even among the surgeons in the northern hemisphere, who have to be familiar with the story of IAH and ACS, monitoring of compartmental pressures and early decompression to reduce the pressure has not been universal. Many critical care physicians and nurses are still ignorant of the consensus guidelines. The sole solution to this recalcitrant attitude is recurring, repeated, and reproducible reinforcement by respected educators. That is exactly what the present work, *Compartment Syndrome* is bound to accomplish. The editors need no introduction. They are leaders in the societies of WSACS and WSES and pioneers of best practices in the fields of critical care and emergency surgery. The assembled list of international contributors are experienced clinicians and instructors. The topics are exhaustive with all facets of compartment syndromes covered in a format easy to read and assimilate.

This book is a valuable contribution that will promulgate crucial concepts of pressure–perfusion phenomena and realize optimal outcomes in saving life and limb. It is recommended for all involved in the care of critically ill and injured patients.

Rao R. Ivatury, MD, FACS
Department of Surgery
Virginia Commonwealth University
Richmond, VA, USA

Foreword

The book *Compartment Syndrome* comes at a perfect time. The concept and understanding of the subject has evolved and improved over the last few years. This set gathered here by Coccolini, Malbrain, Kirkpatrick, and Gamberini is simply remarkable since they have managed in a very special way to agglomerate and expose all the current aspects of the *Compartment Syndrome* from its basic concepts to future perspectives, passing through a fascinating way, by organs and systems, diagnostics and treatments.

Compartment syndrome is a condition in which increasing pressure within one of the body's anatomical compartments results in insufficient blood supply to the tissue. In the past, this concept was attributed to the extremities and little was known about abdominal compartmental or thoracic syndrome and neither polycompartmental syndrome. It is at this moment that this book will serve you in a grand way. If you seek to study extensively about compartment syndrome, this is your book.

In a humble attempt to further sharpen your expectations about this work, I would like to emphasize that the keyword here is "perfusion."

Under normal physiological conditions in our body, arterial blood flow to the venous system requires a gradient or difference of pressure. When this pressure gradient is decreased, the blood flow from the artery into the vein is in turn reduced. This causes a pool of excess blood and fluid to escape from the capillary into the interstitium, leading to fluid accumulation in the extracellular space and an increase in intracompartmental pressure. Soft tissue edema around blood vessels further compresses blood and lymphatic vessels, causing more fluid to accumulate in the extracellular spaces, leading to the vicious cycle of local hypertension. This cycle of aggravation decreases the tissue perfusion and finally leads to tissue death. With this last paragraph, I hope you keep in mind the value of the compartment syndrome and its influence on physiology. The real core of this enormous condition silently deteriorates the health of our critically ill patients.

While reading this book, keep in mind the essential physiology and perfusion process in different pathological states. This will certainly make your reading even more exciting.

Enjoy your reading!

Bruno M. Pereira, MD, MSc, PhD
World Society of the Abdominal Compartment
Campinas, SP, Brazil

Contents

History of Compartment Syndrome

Ari Leppäniemi

1.1 Introduction

Compartment syndrome is a condition where increased pressure within one or more confined spaces in the body results in insufficient blood supply to tissue within that space threatening the viability of tissue and organs. There are four major compartments in the human body, namely the head, chest, abdomen, and the extremities.

A compartment syndrome can develop in any of these compartments or even in multiple compartments. External compression such as caused by extensive burn scar can create a compartment syndrome in the affected area. Burn injury causes accumulation of tissue fluid that together with external compression of the burn tissue results in high pressures in a closed fascial space leading to impaired perfusion and subsequent vascular compromise. In addition, burns in the torso area can cause severe constricting effects with impaired respiration unless released with timely escharotomy.

Furthermore, there can be isolated compartment syndromes within those four major compartments, for example, in the chest where pericardial tamponade represents a form of compartment syndrome of the heart even though the pressure in the pericardial sac caused by blood or pericardial fluid initially threatens the function of the heart, not its intrinsic blood supply.

This historical review highlights some of the landmark observations on different types of compartment syndromes in various parts of the body.

A. Leppäniemi (✉)
Meilahti Hospital, Helsinki, Finland
e-mail: Ari.Leppaniemi@hus.fi

© Springer Nature Switzerland AG 2021
F. Coccolini et al. (eds.), *Compartment Syndrome*, Hot Topics in Acute Care
Surgery and Trauma, https://doi.org/10.1007/978-3-030-55378-4_1

1.2   Compartment Syndrome in the Extremities

In 1881, Richard von Volkmann (1830–1889) suggested that interruption of blood supply to the extremity muscles resulted in paralysis and contracture, later known as Volkmann's contracture [1]. It occurred more commonly in upper limb and was thought to be caused by application of tight bandages to the injured limb. The importance of obstructed venous circulation was considered important by Murphy in 1914 who advocated a prophylactic fasciotomy of the forearm [2].

The role of spasm in arterial injuries was thought to be important when during the First World War unexplained contractures associated with arterial injuries directed the treatment toward interrupting the sympathetic reflex arc with sympathectomy or arterial stripping [2].

Dr. Edward Wilson was one of party of five that reached the South Pole with Captain Scott in 1912. After a day's march of 22 miles, his left leg became swollen and painful with edematous red skin. The condition continued for about 3 weeks, and his meticulous daily entries to his diary probably consist of the first clinical description of an anterior tibial compartment syndrome [3].

Subsequent discoveries of the role of tissue edema hindering normal fluid exchange through capillaries in the muscle leading to first to venous and eventually capillary and arteriolar occlusion lead to the recommendation of prompt and generous fasciotomy to disrupt the vicious microcirculatory circle [2].

Following the discovery of the role of increased intracompartmental pressure in causing compartment syndrome, the actual clinical measurement of compartment pressure was introduced in the 1970s, and a threshold for fasciotomy was established at that time being a difference between the intracompartmental pressure and the diastolic blood pressure of less than 30 mmHg [2].

1.3   Intracranial Hypertension

In 1893, A German Physician Heinrich Quincke described the first report on idiopathic intracranial hypertension [4], and in 1904 the term "pseudotumor cerebri" was coined by Max Nonne [5]. Many reports of increased intracranial pressure caused by different underlying conditions were reported thereafter, and the diagnostic criteria for idiopathic intracranial hypertension were developed by Walter Dandy, a Baltimore neurosurgeon, in 1937 [6]. He also introduced the technique of subtemporal decompressive surgery to treat this condition.

Although trepanation to manage traumatic brain injuries was already practiced in ancient times, the importance of intracranial pressure rather than skull damage being the main cause for pathology was first suggested in the eighteenth century and confirmed in the nineteenth century [7]. The introduction of intracranial pressure monitoring in the 1950s and modern imaging techniques from the 1970s onward (CT in 1972) paved the way to modern treatment of traumatic brain injuries.

1.4 Pneumothorax, Cardiac Tamponade, and Thoracic Compartment Syndrome

The idea of draining substances (fluid, pus, blood) from the thoracic cavity has been known for thousands of years, but the oldest reference is from Hippocrates (c. 460–370 B.C.) in whose texts "empyemas" are described as abscesses in the thoracic cavity. If conservative management with medications and physiotherapy failed, open evacuation of the empyema was performed [8]. The first description of a tube thoracostomy was probably mentioned in the Parzival by Wolfram von Eschenbach in the thirteenth century [9], but it was Guy de Chauliac, the leading physician-surgeon of medieval France, who in 1395 in his Chirurgia Magna described the approach to the management of penetrating thoracic wounds that included thoracic drainage [10].

Traumatic pneumothorax secondary to rib fractures was described by a Turkish surgeon Serafeddin Sabuncuoglu (1385–1468) who suggested simple aspiration as treatment method [11]. Pneumothorax was described in 1803 by Jean Marcc Gaspard Itard, a student of Rene Laennec [12]. The Heimlich valve was designed by Henry Heimlich, an American thoracic surgeon in 1968 [13]. He was also the first to describe the Heimlich maneuver.

Avicenna (980–1037) was one of the first physicians to describe cardiac tamponade [14]. Although it is commonly believed that the French Royal Surgeon Ambroise Pare (1510–1590) provided the first report of delayed death due to an acute traumatic hemopericardium, Haly Abbas (930–994 AD), a predecessor of Avicenna, actually reported such a phenomenon in the tenth century [14]. Claude Beck (1894–1971), a pioneer American cardiac surgeon, famous for performing the first defibrillation in 1947, described the physiological basis for the signs of acute cardiac tamponade, collectively known as the Beck's triad [15].

Thoracic compartment syndrome was described in adult and pediatric patients undergoing cardiac surgical procedures where sternal closure in patients with substantial myocardial edema, acute ventricular dilatation, or non-cardiogenic pulmonary edema could precipitate cardiac tamponade [16]. The first case of thoracic compartment syndrome associated with a thoracic gunshot wound was described in 1996 [17].

1.5 Abdominal Compartment Syndrome

Although ascites was recognized as a pathological entity requiring interventional treatment already in the thirteenth century, the physiological effects that increased intra-abdominal pressure (IAP) especially on respiration were first described by the Frenchman Etienne-Jules Marey in 1863 [18]. Christian Wilhelm Braune from Germany was probably the first to measure IAP though the rectum in 1865 [19].

Several papers on IAP measurements were published in the late nineteenth century, but the truly ground-breaking paper was published in 1911 by the Harvard educated physician Haven Emerson [20]. He showed the connection between high

IAP and cardiovascular collapse, and that evacuation of ascites was followed by cardiac recovery. In 1939, Bellis and Wangensteen demonstrated vascular impairment caused by raised IAP [21].

The progress in our understanding the consequences of raised IAP was slow until 1951, when MG Baggot, an anesthesiologist from Dublin suggested that forcing distended bowel back into the abdominal cavity of limited size could kill the patient [22]. He advised leaving the abdomen open with dressings.

With the introduction of laparoscopy in the 1970s, a better understanding of the effects of increased IAP ensued. Sönderberg and Westin correlated IAP directly measured via laparoscope to that measured through the urinary bladder [23], and Ivancovich and colleagues described cardiovascular collapse during gynecological laparoscopy [24].

Although the cardiovascular, renal, and endocrinological effects of raised IAP were described by various authors in the early 1980s, it was the landmark paper from Kron, Harman, and Nolan in 1984, where IAP was measured after aortic repair and was used that to determine the cutoff values for abdominal re-exploration and decompression in surgical patients [25]. The term Abdominal Compartment syndrome was probably first mentioned in 1989 by Fietsam and colleagues [26].

Finally, the surgical and critical care pioneers in this field, Moshe Schein, Gene Moore and the Denver group, Rao Ivatury, Mike Cheatham, Manu Malbrain, and Michael Sugrue together with the World Society of Abdominal Compartment Syndrome formalized, categorized, and brought our understanding of elevated IAP to its current level [27–29].

1.6 Polycompartment Syndrome

In 2007, Tom Scalea and colleagues from Shock Trauma in Baltimore described the interactions of multiple compartments in a study of 102 blunt trauma patients [30]. The management of a polytrauma patient with fluid therapy may increase IAP and intrathoracic pressure and in a patient with traumatic brain injury may lead to elevated intracranial pressure creating a cycle that ultimately produces multiple compartment syndrome requiring sequential use of decompressive craniectomy and decompressive laparotomy. To avoid confusion with multiple extremity compartment syndrome, the term polycompartment syndrome was created to better describe the interconnected relationships of the various body compartments [31].

References

1. Volkmann R. Die ischämischen Muskellähmungen und Kontracturen. Centralblatt fur Chirurgie. 1881;8:801–3.
2. Klenerman L. The evolution of the compartment syndrome since 1948 as recorded in the JBJS (B). J Bone Joint Surg. 2007;89:1280–2.
3. Freedman BJ. Dr. Edward Wilson of the Antarctic. Proc R Soc Med. 1953;47:183–9.
4. Quincke HI. Meningitis serosa. Sammlung Klinischer Vorträge. 1893;67:655.

5. Nonne M. Ueber Falle vom Symptomkomplex "Tumor Cerebri" mit Ausgang in Heilung ("Pseudotumor Cerebri"). Deutche Zeitschrift fur Nrevenheilkunde. 1904;27:169–216.
6. Dandy WE. Intracranial pressure without brain tumor—diagnosis and treatment. Ann Surg. 1937;106:492–513.
7. Granacher RA. Traumatic brain injury: methods for clinical & forensic neuropsychiatric assessment. 2nd ed. Boca Raton: CRC; 2007. ISBN 978-0-8493-8138-6.
8. Christopoulou-Aletra H, Papvramidou N. "Empyemas" of the thoracic cavity in the Hippocratic corpus. Ann Thorac Surg. 2008;85:1132–4.
9. Hughes J. Battlefield medicine in Wolfram's Parzival. J Medieval Mil Hist. 2010;8:119–30.
10. Lindskog GE. Some historical aspects of thoracic trauma. J Thorac Cardiovasc Surg. 1961;42:1–11.
11. Kaya SO, Karatepe M, Tok T, Onem G, Dursunoglu N, Goksin I. Were pneumothorax and its management known to 15th century Anatolia? Tex Heart Inst J. 2009;36:152–3.
12. Laennec RTH. Traite de l'auscultation mediate et les maladies des poumons et du Coeur—part II. Paris: Brosson & Chaude; 1918.
13. Heimlich HJ. Valve drainage of the pleural cavity. Dis Chest. 1968;53:282–7.
14. Dalfardi B, Mahmoudi Nezhad GS, Ghanizadeh A. Avicenna's description of cardiac tamponade. Int J Cardiol. 2014;172:e145–6.
15. Stembach G. Claude Beck: cardiac compression triads. J Emerg Med. 1988;6:417–9.
16. Milgater E, Uretsky G, Shimon DV, et al. Delayed sternal closure following cardiac operations. J Cardiovasc Surg. 1986;27:328.
17. Kaplan LJ, Trooskin SZ, Santora TA. Thoracic compartment syndrome. J Trauma Injury Infect Crit Care. 1996;40:291–3.
18. Marey EJ. Physiologie medicale de la circulation du sang, base sur l'etude graphique des mouvements du coeur et du pouls arteriel avec application aux maladies de l'appareil circulatoire. Paris: A. Delahaye; 1863.
19. Braune W. Messungen uber die Kraft der peristaltischen Bewegungen des Dickdarms und der Bauchpresse. Centralblatt fur die medizinische Wissenschaften. 1865;3:9134.
20. Emerson H. Intra-abdominal pressures. Arch Intern Med. 1911;7:754–84.
21. Bellis CJ, Wangensteen OH. Venous circulatory changes in the abdomen and lower extremities attending abdominal detention. Proc Soc Exp Biol Med. 1939;4:490–8.
22. Baggot MG. Abdominal blow-out: a concept. Curr Res Anesth Analg. 1951;30:295–8.
23. Sönderberg G, Westin B. Transmission of rapid pressure increase from the peritoneal cavity to the bladder. Scand J Urol Nephrol. 1970;4:155–65.
24. Ivankovich AS, Albrect RF, Zahed B, et al. Cardiovascular collapse during gynaecological laparoscopy. Ill Med J. 1974;145:58–61.
25. Kron IL, Harman PK, Nolan SP. The measurement of intra-abdominal pressures as a criterion for abdominal re-exploration. Ann Surg. 1984;199:28–30.
26. Fietsam R Jr, Villalba M, Glover JL, et al. Intra-abdominal compartment syndrome as a complication of ruptured aortic aneurysm repair. Am Surg. 1989;55:396–402.
27. Schein M, Wittman DH, Aprahamian CC, Condon RE. The abdominal compartment syndrome: the physiological and clinical consequences of elevated intra-abdominal pressure. J Am Coll Surg. 1995;180:745–53.
28. Burch JM, Moore EE, Moore FA, et al. The abdominal compartment syndrome. Surg Clin North Am. 1996;76:833–42.
29. Ivatury RR, Cheatham ML, Malbrain MLNG, Sugrue M. Abdominal compartment syndrome. Georgetown: Landes Bioscience; 2006.
30. Scalea TM, Bochiccio GV, Habashi N, et al. Increased intra-abdominal, intrathoracic, and intracranial pressure after severe brain injury: multiple compartment syndrome. J Trauma. 2007;62:647–56.
31. Malbrain ML, Wilmer A. The polycompartment syndrome: towards an understanding of the interactions between different compartments! Intensive Care Med. 2007;33:1869–72.

Definition and Pathomechanism of the Intracranial Compartment Syndrome

Tommaso Tonetti, Susanna Biondini, Francesco Minardi, Sandra Rossi, and Edoardo Picetti

2.1 Definition

A compartment syndrome is, by definition, a clinical syndrome characterized by a severe increase of pressure in an enclosed body district (compartment) and subsequent hypoperfusion and tissue damage due to compression of vital structures such as vessels and nerves [1]. The prerequisite for a compartment syndrome to develop is that the compartment must be non-extensible above a certain limit, i.e., its compliance must be close to zero after a critical level of stretching of its structures has been reached. Some compartments in the body, due to their physical and physiological characteristics, are more prone than others to develop a compartment syndrome.

The intracranial compartment, completely surrounded by a rigid, noncompliant bony case, can be intuitively considered the ideal environment for a compartment syndrome to occur since slight increases in volume of the enclosed structures translate into wide increases in compartment pressure. A quick rise in intracranial pressure (ICP) can displace the brainstem, which can suffer from possibly irreversible ischemia, leading to rapid death. Slower (though acute) rises in ICP can result in brain tissue compression, hypoperfusion, and diffuse ischemic damage, leading to severe and irreversible neurologic damage [2].

The intracranial compartment syndrome (ICS) has been known and studied for the last two centuries, but it has usually been referred to as intracranial hypertension (IH). Depending on different classifications, some forms of IH can develop slowly (e.g., growing cerebral tumors), others can be chronic or even benign. In this chapter, we will consider ICS a synonym of IH caused by an acute brain injury (ABI).

T. Tonetti · S. Biondini · F. Minardi · S. Rossi · E. Picetti (✉)
Department of Anesthesia and Intensive Care, Parma University Hospital, Parma, Italy

© Springer Nature Switzerland AG 2021
F. Coccolini et al. (eds.), *Compartment Syndrome*, Hot Topics in Acute Care Surgery and Trauma, https://doi.org/10.1007/978-3-030-55378-4_2

2.1.1 Clinical Definition

A comprehensive dissertation about the clinical aspects of IH is outside the scope of this chapter. However, in order to define IH and ICS operatively, we need to introduce the concept of ICP monitoring, which is often applied in patients with ABI. Whichever the technology adopted (e.g., intraparenchymal probe, intraventricular catheter), the measure of ICP allows the clinician to react adequately if the patient reaches a critical threshold level, which defines IH [3]. Historically, the most frequently adopted ICP cutoff to define IH has been 20 mmHg, which is derived from the seminal Lundberg study [4]. More recent research tend to confirm this cutoff, showing that an ICP above 20 mmHg correlates with mortality and poor outcomes [5, 6]. However, the latest Guidelines for the Management of Severe Traumatic Brain Injury recommend treating ICP values above 22 mmHg [7], thus implying that lower values should not be considered as IH and suggesting that below that level the patient should not be at risk of ICS. This new threshold fired the debate since many experts do not agree with such strict limits and recommend that the diagnosis of IH (and of ICS) be based not only on a mere number but on a complete clinical picture of the patient [3, 8, 9]. IH should be considered in terms of insult severity and duration possibly with the aid of multimodal neuromonitoring [3, 8, 9].

2.2 Pathomechanism of the Intracranial Compartment Syndrome

2.2.1 The Monro-Kellie Doctrine

As stated above, IH leads to ICS, but what leads to IH in the first place? The basic concept of ICP is described by the Monro-Kellie Doctrine, which is based on separate studies by the Scottish physician Alexander Monroe *secundus* (1733–1817) and the surgeon George Kellie (1770–1829). Essentially, the doctrine states that total intracranial volume is constant and fixed although the relationships between its components may vary. Total intracranial volume is determined by the sum of the volumes of cerebrospinal fluid (CSF), blood, and brain tissue. We can roughly estimate that CSF and blood occupy each 10% of the volume, leaving to the brain tissue the remaining 80% (near 1900 mL in adults) [2].

ICP is normally below 10 mmHg, and it is relatively constant through all the brain regions. The introduction of an additional volume in one of the three components must be compensated by changes in the other two components; however, a volume increase of more than 10% leads inevitably to the upper limit of the system's compliance and so to an increase in ICP. Since the skull is rigid, from this point on, minimal increases in intracranial volume translate into wide increases in ICP (exponential relationship, see Fig. 2.1).

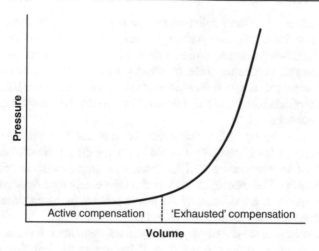

Fig. 2.1   Cerebral pressure–volume curve

2.2.2   Compensatory Mechanisms

As stated before, the limit of compliance of the intracranial compartment is an increase in volume of about 10%. This means that the brain is not normally able to swell more than 10% of its volume and the same is true for the CSF and the blood component. According to the Monro-Kellie Doctrine, these changes modify the total volume and must be counterbalanced by a correspondent reduction of the other components. Namely, both the CSF and the blood components are able to shift outside the intracranial compartment as explained below. Displacement of CSF and blood explains the horizontal part of the pressure–volume curve represented in Fig. 2.1. Of course, individual patients may show better compensation than others, for example, due to cerebral atrophy, which warrants higher volume reserve by shifting the pressure–volume curve to the right.

2.2.2.1   Shifts of CSF
The CSF is able to shift from the ventricular or subarachnoid space to the spinal compartment. However, the spinal compartment has limited distensibility and may be insufficient to compensate for pathologic changes in intracranial volume.

Moreover, in case of increasing intracranial volume, CSF outflow and resorption may be forced through the low-resistance arachnoid villi.

2.2.2.2   Shifts of Cerebral Blood Volume (CBV)
Most of the blood (about two thirds) in the intracranial compartment is contained in the dural sinuses and venules, while the remaining one-third is in the arteriolar system. Cerebral blood volume (CBV) in the intracranial compartment is regulated both on the arteriolar side (inflow) and on the venous side (outflow). The blood-based compensation mechanism is based on the reduction in volume of the venules

and dural sinuses (up to their collapse) and on the vasoconstriction/vasodilation of the arterioles and other vessels. Although it may seem a rather ineffective mechanism, especially when compared to fast shifts of CSF between the intracranial and the intraspinal compartments, shifts in intracranial blood content are in fact ample enough to compensate for wide variations in intracranial volume: intracranial blood volume can oscillate between 15 and 70 mL, thus making it a really important compensation mechanism [2, 3].

Cerebral blood flow (CBF) in the healthy brain is strictly regulated according to the autoregulation mechanism, that is able to maintain a physiologic blood flow (~750 mL/min in a normal adult) in a wide range of mean arterial pressures (~50–150 mmHg). The mechanism is based on the continuous fine-tuning of cerebrovascular resistances, mediated by myogenic reflexes in the endothelium and by vasodilating agents released by the tissues [2].

On the contrary, in the acutely injured brain, autoregulation is often impaired (in a variable manner, according to the type of lesion and its site). Brain injury can disrupt cerebral autoregulation (the degree of the disruption is generally directly proportional to the degree of brain injury), and this translates in a pathologically linear relationship between CBF and cerebral perfusion pressure (CPP).

Other factors influencing CBF are the arterial partial pressures of oxygen (PaO_2) and carbon dioxide ($PaCO_2$). In particular, hypercapnia (and, to a lesser extent, hypoxemia) increases CBF through vasodilation and may lower the upper limit of autoregulation. Reactivity to CO_2 is continuous up to partial pressures of about 80 mmHg, for which cerebral vasodilation is about 100% of the baseline value; above 80 mmHg, no further vasodilation occurs. Reactivity to hypoxemia is much less pronounced and is significant only below 50 mmHg of PaO_2 [2].

Drugs may also significantly alter CBF. Most notably, barbiturates act as potent cerebral vasoconstrictors, but their effect on CBF is only partly explained by their effect on the cerebral circulation. In fact, they also reduce CBF by reducing neuronal metabolism. Inhalational anesthetics can instead induce cerebral vasodilation and increase CBF.

Other acute conditions, such as fever and seizures, are associated with CBF augmentation, which often translates in IH in patients with ABI and impaired autoregulation.

Chronic arterial hypertension significantly modifies cerebral autoregulation, resulting in a rightward shift of the pressure–CBF curve (meaning that constant CBF is maintained at higher arterial pressures).

2.2.3 Intracranial Causes of IH

Intracranial causes of IH are summarized in Table 2.1.

2.2.3.1 Brain-Related Causes of IH
The most important brain-related causes of IH are expansive processes inside the brain or between the brain and the meninges. Excluding neoplasms, which normally

Table 2.1 Causes of IH

Component	Possible cause of increased volume
Brain	• Expansive processes • Cytotoxic edema • Vasogenic edema
CSF	• Increased production • Decreased absorption • Obstructed outflow
Blood	• Vasodilation • Obstructed outflow (venous side)

IH intracranial hypertension, *CSF* cerebrospinal fluid

cause a slow and chronic increase in ICP, hemorrhages are the most frequent expansive processes. They are usually classified according to their location into the following: epidural, subdural, subarachnoid, and intraparenchymal. Regardless of the site of the hemorrhage, their effect on the ICP is mediated by the mass effect they produce on the brain and the other intracranial structures.

The other common cause of acute increase in brain volume is brain edema, which can be classified into two major pathologic entities: vasogenic and cytotoxic [2].

The origin of vasogenic edema lies in a disruption of the blood–brain barrier (BBB). This causes swelling and subsequent breakdown of the myelin. CBF and cellular functions tend to remain mostly unaltered since edema is mostly extracellular. This type of edema is usually caused by inflammatory/infective processes.

On the other hand, cytotoxic edema is intracellular and mostly localized in the astrocytes. Thus, it involves the gray matter more than the white matter and is typically observed in ischemic/anoxic injury and in serum electrolytes imbalances (see below).

2.2.3.2 CSF-Related Causes of IH

Increases in CSF volume may be due to increased CSF production, decreased CSF absorption, and/or obstructed outflow of CSF toward the spinal subarachnoid space (see above). In ABI, and especially in subarachnoid hemorrhage (SAH), obstructive hydrocephalus is a common condition, due to blood accumulation into the ventricular system; in this situation, a decreased CSF absorption can also be observed due to an involvement of the arachnoid granulations [10, 11]. Another typical mechanism of acute obstructive hydrocephalus is the fourth ventricle compression, for example, due to a posterior fossa hematoma.

2.2.3.3 Blood-Related Causes of IH

Increased in CBV has been previously described. The main mechanism is arteriolar vasodilation, most commonly caused by hypercapnia and/or hypoxemia. Fever and seizures can cause wide increases in CBF and CBV especially when they are associated to an impaired CBF autoregulation.

On the other hand, an increase in CBV can be determined by an obstructed venous outflow; this is often iatrogenic and due to jugular veins compression (erroneous head positioning, cervical compression) or to elevated intrathoracic/intraabdominal pressures (see below).

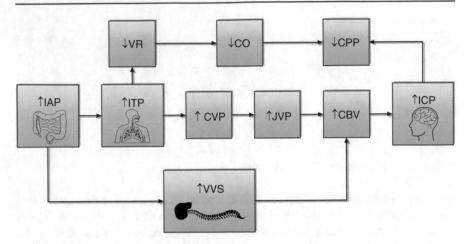

Fig. 2.2 Extracranial organs and ICP. *ICP* intracranial pressure, *IAP* intra-abdominal pressure, *ITP* intrathoracic pressure, *VR* venous return, *CO* cardiac output, *CPP* cerebral perfusion pressure, *JVP* jugular venous pressure, *VVS* vertebral venous system, *CBV* cerebral blood volume

2.2.4 Extracranial Causes of IH

In Fig. 2.2, we summarize the complex network of extracranial organs that can possibly influence and increase the ICP.

2.2.4.1 Intrathoracic Pressure (ITP)
The interaction between ITP and ICP is fundamentally based on one mechanism: venous outflow obstruction. Indeed, an increase in ITP directly translates to an increase in central venous pressure (CVP) and so in jugular and intracerebral venous pressure. This in turn expands CBV and impairs CSF absorption (see above). Moreover, the increased ITP can also lower the CPP by impairing venous return and lowering cardiac output (CO).

In the setting of ABI, the most common cause of increased ITP is mechanical ventilation, and in particular the application of positive end-expiratory pressure (PEEP). Mechanical ventilation is also responsible for other transient, but significantly high surges in ITP, during lung recruitment maneuvers or during coughing in patients who are poorly adapted to mechanical ventilation. The third most important cause of increase of ITB is the increase in intra-abdominal pressure (IAP), which will be discussed in the next paragraph.

The use of PEEP in ABI patients has been debated for a long time [12]. Adequate levels of PEEP keep lung units open during expiration and avoid the so-called atelectrauma (lung injury due to cyclic opening and closing of lung units), thus improving oxygenation and, according to some authors, helping to protect the lung from further damage ("open lung approach"). Accordingly, many patients with ABI may theoretically benefit from the use of PEEP, given that lung damage is often present (due to direct trauma, aspiration, infection, etc.), but some concerns still exist as for the safety of PEEP in patients with IH. Many studies show that PEEP has minimal effects on ICP, especially if it is titrated to be lower than ICP itself [13–15]. A recent retrospective study (reflecting the current trends in ventilatory settings) on 341 patients and 28,644 paired PEEP and ICP measurements confirms no significant relation between PEEP and ICP or CPP, except in the subgroup of severely lung-injured patients. However, even in those patients with highly impaired lung compliance (in whom airway pressure increases are more easily transmitted to the vessels and so to the brain), the direct relation between PEEP and ICP appears to be statistically significant but not very relevant from a clinical point of view. Indeed, this retrospective study shows that on average a 5 cmH_2O increase in PEEP translates in modest 1.6 mmHg increase in ICP and 4.3 mmHg decrease in CPP, and the authors conclude that PEEP can be safely applied in most of the ABI patients [16].

To date, only a very small number of studies have investigated the relationship between lung recruitment maneuvers and ICP increase. In 11 patients with ABI and acute lung injury, Bein and colleagues showed that aggressive recruitment maneuvers (sustained pressures up to 60 cmH_2O for 30 s) have detrimental effects on cerebral hemodynamics and metabolism [17]. Another study on 16 patients with SAH and acute respiratory distress syndrome (ARDS) compared recruitment maneuvers in pressure control mode from PEEP 15 cmH_2O up to an inspiratory pressure of 50 cmH_2O for 120 s with recruitment maneuvers at a constant positive airway pressure of 35 cmH_2O for 40 s. The results of this study show that recruitment in pressure control mode has a much smaller impact on ICP and CPP and much higher impact on oxygenation [18]. Nevertheless, larger studies are certainly needed to better define the "pros and cons" of lung recruitment maneuvers in patients with ABI.

2.2.4.2 Intra-abdominal Pressure (IAP)

The anatomical foundation of the complex interplay between IAP and ICP lies in the vertebral venous system (VVS). This system was firstly described almost two centuries ago, but it has continued to be thoroughly studied even in the last decade although under different names [19, 20]. The VVS is constituted by valveless veins that allow free flow of blood between the head and the distal end of the spinal canal [19]. It has been described as a large and valveless "venous lake," where blood can move freely, and its flow direction is strongly influenced by the pressures in the different body compartments [21]. Indeed, the VVS is widely anastomosed with the inferior and superior caval system (through the azygos and lumbar veins) and to other cranial, cervical, thoracic, abdominal, and sacral venous plexuses [22]. Consequently, two main mechanisms explain the interplay between IAP and ICP: according to the first, an increase in IAP produces a blood shift into the VVS, which directly translates into a blood shift into the intracranial compartment. The second mechanism involves a transfer of IAP to the ITP through the diaphragm muscle, thus producing a back pressure on the jugular system, as already described in the previous paragraph [22].

Whichever the mechanism involved (normally both of them), the interaction between IAP and ICP has been studied in animal models and in human patients, and it has shown that increases in IAP invariably translate into raises in ICP by increasing the volume of intracranial venous blood [23].

Some of the most important clinical studies on the interaction between IAP and ICP have been conducted in traumatic brain injury (TBI) patients. In an elegant physiologic study in 2001, Citerio and colleagues externally increased IAP (by positioning a 15-L water bag on the abdomen) in 15 TBI patients after stabilization and resolution of IH. This acute rise in IAP translated almost immediately in concomitant and rapid increases of CVP, internal jugular pressure, and finally ICP, which rose significantly from an average of 12 mmHg to an average of 15.5 mmHg [24]. In a retrospective study on 102 patients with severe TBI who underwent decompressive craniotomy (DC) or decompressive laparotomy or both, Scalea and colleagues found statistically significant decreases in ICP after DC and laparotomy, regardless of whether laparotomy was done before or after craniotomy. In addition, they found that decompressive laparotomy was successful in reducing ITP regardless of whether it was done before or after DC [25].

2.2.4.3 Fluids and Electrolytes
Plasma osmolarity is a key determinant of ICP. The BBB acts as a real barrier to the entry of molecules and solutes into the brain. An intact BBB is completely impermeable to sodium [26] and so any water flow across the barrier is sodium-free [27]. The concept of osmolarity and its relationship to ICP is important in the normal brain but has the utmost importance in the setting of ABI, when the BBB loses, at least partially, its function. When the function of the BBB is disrupted, hydraulic permeability and conductivity to solutes increase, raising the flow of water (accompanied by proteins) across the capillary membranes. This increase in water is the vasogenic edema, which was already described in a previous paragraph [28, 29]. This is especially important for fluid management in ABI patients and is the foundation of osmotherapy for increased ICP.

2.3   Conclusions

The ICS has a complex pathogenesis, which is often influenced by the presence of other coexisting compartment syndromes. The understanding of brain physiology and of the compensatory mechanisms to IH may help the physician in making the right choices for protecting the brain from secondary injuries and avoiding iatrogenic damage.

References

1. Merriam-Webster. Compartment syndrome. Merriam-Webster's Med. Dict. 2016.
2. Wijdicks EFM. The practice of emergency and critical care neurology. 2nd ed. New York: Oxford University Press; 2016.
3. Chesnut RM. Intracranial pressure. In: Le Roux PD, Levine JM, Kofke WA, editors. Monitoring in neurocritical care. Philadelphia: Elsevier Saunders; 2013. p. 338–47.
4. Lundberg N. Continuous recording and control of ventricular fluid pressure in neurosurgical practice. Acta Psychiatr Scand Suppl. 1960;36:1–193.

5. Marmarou A, Anderson RL, Ward JD, Choi SC, Young HF, Eisenberg HM, Foulkes MA, Marshall LF, Jane JA. Impact of ICP instability and hypotension on outcome in patients with severe head trauma. J Neurosurg. 1991;75:S59–66.
6. Schreiber MA, Aoki N, Scott BG, Beck JR. Determinants of mortality in patients with severe blunt head injury. Arch Surg. 2002;137:285–90.
7. Carney N, Totten AM, O'Reilly C, et al. Guidelines for the management of severe traumatic brain injury, fourth edition. Neurosurgery. 2016;81:1.
8. Meyfroidt G, Citerio G. Letter: guidelines for the management of severe traumatic brain injury, fourth edition. Neurosurgery. 2017;81:E1.
9. Picetti E, Iaccarino C, Servadei F. Letter: guidelines for the management of severe traumatic brain injury fourth edition. Neurosurgery. 2017;81:E2.
10. van Gijn J, Hijdra A, Wijdicks EF, Vermeulen M, van Crevel H. Acute hydrocephalus after aneurysmal subarachnoid hemorrhage. J Neurosurg. 1985;63:355–62.
11. Graff-Radford NR, Torner J, Adams HP, Kassell NF. Factors associated with hydrocephalus after subarachnoid hemorrhage. A report of the Cooperative Aneurysm Study. Arch Neurol. 1989;46:744–52.
12. Lowe GJ, Ferguson ND. Lung-protective ventilation in neurosurgical patients. Curr Opin Crit Care. 2006;12:3–7.
13. Frost EAM. Effects of positive end-expiratory pressure on intracranial pressure and compliance in brain-injured patients. J Neurosurg. 1977;47:195–200.
14. Burchiel KJ, Steege TD, Wyler AR. Intracranial pressure changes in brain-injured patients requiring positive end-expiratory pressure ventilation. Neurosurgery. 1981;8:443–9.
15. Cooper KR, Boswell PA, Choi SC. Safe use of PEEP in patients with severe head injury. J Neurosurg. 1985;63:552–5.
16. Boone MD, Jinadasa SP, Mueller A, Shaefi S, Kasper EM, Hanafy KA, O'Gara BP, Talmor DS. The effect of positive end-expiratory pressure on intracranial pressure and cerebral hemodynamics. Neurocrit Care. 2017;26:174–81.
17. Bein T, Kuhr LP, Bele S, Ploner F, Keyl C, Taeger K. Lung recruitment maneuver in patients with cerebral injury: effects on intracranial pressure and cerebral metabolism. Intensive Care Med. 2002;28:554–8.
18. Nemer SN, Caldeira JB, Azeredo LM, et al. Alveolar recruitment maneuver in patients with subarachnoid hemorrhage and acute respiratory distress syndrome: a comparison of 2 approaches. J Crit Care. 2011;26:22–7.
19. Parkinson D. Extradural neural axis compartment. J Neurosurg. 2000;92:585–8.
20. Tobinick E, Vega CP. The cerebrospinal venous system: anatomy, physiology, and clinical implications. MedGcnMed. 2006;8:53.
21. Epstein HM, Linde HW, Crampton AR, Ciric IS, Eckenhoff JE. The vertebral venous plexus as a major cerebral venous outflow tract. Anesthesiology. 1970;32:332–7.
22. Depauw PRAM, Groen RJM, Van Loon J, Peul WC, Malbrain MLNG, De Waele JJ. The significance of intra-abdominal pressure in neurosurgery and neurological diseases: a narrative review and a conceptual proposal. Acta Neurochir. 2019;161:855. https://doi.org/10.1007/s00701-019-03868-7.
23. De Laet I, Citerio G, Malbrain MLNG. The influence of intra-abdominal hypertension on the central nervous system: current insights and clinical recommendations, is it all in the head? Acta Clin Belg. 2007;62(Suppl 1):89–97.
24. Citerio G, Vascotto E, Villa F, Celotti S, Pesenti A. Induced abdominal compartment syndrome increases intracranial pressure in neurotrauma patients: a prospective study. Crit Care Med. 2001;29:1466–71.
25. Scalea TM, Bochicchio GV, Habashi N, McCunn M, Shih D, McQuillan K, Aarabi B. Increased intra-abdominal, intrathoracic, and intracranial pressure after severe brain injury: multiple compartment syndrome. J Trauma. 2007;62:647–56; discussion 656.
26. Qureshi AI, Suarez JI. Use of hypertonic saline solutions in treatment of cerebral edema and intracranial hypertension. Crit Care Med. 2000;28:3301–13.

27. Rossi S, Picetti E, Zoerle T, Carbonara M, Zanier ER, Stocchetti N. Fluid management in acute brain injury. Curr Neurol Neurosci Rep. 2018;18:74.
28. Hladky SB, Barrand MA. Mechanisms of fluid movement into, through and out of the brain: evaluation of the evidence. Fluids Barriers CNS. 2014;11:26.
29. Hladky SB, Barrand MA. Fluid and ion transfer across the blood-brain and blood-cerebrospinal fluid barriers; a comparative account of mechanisms and roles. Fluids Barriers CNS. 2016;13:19.

Diagnosis and Treatment of the Intracranial Compartment Syndrome

3

Etrusca Brogi, Federico Coccolini, Emanuele Russo, and Francesco Forfori

3.1 Introduction

The intracranial compartment syndrome is a condition that occurs when intracranial hypertension (IH) overcome the compensatory cerebral mechanisms. Excessive pressure within the rigid intracranial compartment leads to an insufficient blood supply to tissue within the skull and secondary irreversible brain injury. Several intracranial or extracranial disease can be responsible for IH [1]. Mass-occupying space disease (i.e. spontaneous intracerebral haemorrhage, aneurysmal subarachnoid haemorrhage, epidural–subdural haematoma, swelling, tumour), vasogenic/cytotoxic oedema, cerebral venous thrombosis or cerebrospinal fluid (CSF) disorders (i.e. hydrocephalus) represent intracranial causes of IH [2]. Instead, the extracranial causes of IH are due to the intrinsic interplay between intracranial pressure (ICP) and intrathoracic pressure (e.g. venous outflow obstruction, mechanical ventilation, lung recruitment manoeuvres or during coughing) and intrabdominal pressure (through the vertebral venous system) [3]. Consequently, therapeutic strategies

E. Brogi (✉)
Department of Anaesthesia and Intensive Care, University of Pisa, Pisa, Italy

Department of Anaesthesia and Intensive Care, Bufalini Hospital, Cesena, Italy

Department of Anaesthesia and Intensive Care, Azienda Ospedaliero Universitaria Pisana (AOUP), University of Pisa, Pisa, Italy

F. Coccolini
General, Emergency and Trauma Surgery Department, Pisa University Hospital, Pisa, Italy

E. Russo
Department of Anaesthesia and Intensive Care, Bufalini Hospital, Cesena, Italy

F. Forfori
Department of Anaesthesia and Intensive Care, University of Pisa, Pisa, Italy

© Springer Nature Switzerland AG 2021
F. Coccolini et al. (eds.), *Compartment Syndrome*, Hot Topics in Acute Care Surgery and Trauma, https://doi.org/10.1007/978-3-030-55378-4_3

that have effects on ITC and/or IAP (i.e. decompressive laparotomy) could present beneficial or a detrimental effect on ICP [4]. Furthermore, other conditions (e.g. fever, seizure) has to be promptly diagnosed and treated because are responsible for increased cerebral metabolic demand and oxygen consumption and, consequently, they may worsen a pre-existing brain disease [5, 6].

The diagnosis and the specific treatment of the cause responsible for elevated ICP (e.g. evacuation of mass-occupying space) has to be prompt in order to prevent and avoid an irreversible secondary cerebral insult and iatrogenic injuries. The therapeutic option should be tailored to each specific clinical case rather than on protocols. The reason is that any ICP-lowering therapies have potential side effects (e.g. hyperventilation/cerebral ischaemia) [7]. In this scenario, a multimodal monitoring approach is fundamental for patient assessment in order to make a specific diagnosis (i.e. spontaneous intracerebral haemorrhage, epidural–subdural haematoma, swelling, cerebral, meningitis) and guide the clinician in the right therapeutic choice [8]. This approach consists of clinical evaluation, neuroimaging and invasive/noninvasive tests. This multimodality monitoring approach, gathering data simultaneously from multiple sources, might combine the strengths of several techniques, providing a complete picture of a dynamic cerebral state. Unfortunately, the increasing amount and availability of data increase the complexity of interpretation of the information gathered. Consequently, the integration of different data obtained from various techniques through computer-assisted methods would represent a future challenge [9].

3.2 Diagnosis of the Intracranial Compartment Syndrome

Neurological examinations, neuroimaging, electrophysiologic tests (EEG) and invasive/noninvasive monitoring represent valuable tools for the diagnosis of intracranial compartment syndrome and to establish a precise aetiology. The fundamental importance of a multimodal approach is the early identification and treatment of a neurological decline for the prevention of an irreversible secondary cerebral insult. This approach helps the clinician in guiding patient management and monitoring the response to treatment.

3.2.1 Neurological Evaluation

The first approach to a patient with possible intracranial compartment syndrome is neurologic evaluation. Level of consciousness, eye examination, verbal and motor response and breathing pattern represent the first step of the patient clinical evaluation. Altered mental status can be due to primary brain disorders (e.g. traumatic brain injury, ischaemic stroke, spontaneous intracerebral haemorrhage, meningitis, tumours) or systemic disorders (e.g. overdose, sepsis, hepatic failure, hypothermia, hypoglycaemia, hypothyroidism, uraemia). However, it is vital to identify conditions that can mimic coma (i.e. catatonia, critical illness neuropathy, akinetic mutism, botulism, Guillain-Barré syndrome). The level of consciousness and the presence or absence of focal signs can orientate the clinician to a possible localization of a cerebral lesion. Eye examination consists of the evaluation of size, shape and reactivity to the light of the pupils. It is essential to evaluate the presence of anisocoria or to bilaterally fixed and dilated pupils and their response to medical treatment. Nevertheless, it is vital to recognize possible drugs that affect pupillary responses (e.g. opiate, atropine, cocaine, LSD). Even more, it is important to evaluate resting eye position, eye movement and the corneal reflex. Lateral and downwards deviation as well as nystagmus and saccade ocular movement have to be evaluated carefully because they can represent the clinical signs of a lesion of a cerebral hemisphere or non-convulsive seizure state, respectively. The motor response, during the neurological examination, represents another important moment of patient evaluation. The presence of focal signs and abnormal reflexes can help to localize the lesion or orientate the diagnosis. Finally, different breathing patterns can be observed in a comatose patient depending on the type and the location of the disease. Above all, we can find the following: apnoeic respiration, sustained hyperventilation, Kussmaul respiration, Cheyne-strokes respiration and agonal gasps.

Quantitative coma scales (Glasgow Coma scale, FOUR score) are used to estimate initial coma severity, to assess the progressive clinical decline/recovery and to predict mortality and neurological outcome. The Glasgow Coma Scale (GCS) is a widely adopted neurological scale used to assess the neurological status of a patient. The GCS scale correlates with survival and neurological outcome. The score is calculated by giving a numeric point to three categories: eye opening, verbal and motor response (as shown in Table 3.1). The score ranges from 3 to 15. Important limitations of GCS scale are represented by the inability to assess the verbal score in intubated patients and to evaluate brainstem reflexes. Then, the GCS-Pupils score was introduced in 2018 to combine assessment of patient responsiveness and brain stream function (i.e. pupil reaction) [10]. In addition to the general GCS score, GCS-P is calculated by subtraction Pupil Reactivity Score (PRS) from GCS score (as shown in Table 3.1). On the other hand, Glasgow Outcome Scale (GOS) and the Glasgow Outcome Scale Extended (GOSE—extended version of the GOS) are used to describe outcome in head injury patients (as shown in Table 3.1) [11, 12]. The Innsbruck Coma Score is an eight-items scale; however, it is rarely used in clinical practice [13]. In 2005, the Full Outline of Unresponsiveness (FOUR) score was developed to overcome the limitations of the GCS (assess intubated or aphasic patients and to evaluate brainstem reflexes) [14, 15]. In fact, the FOUR score included the evaluation of visual tracking, breathing pattern and respiratory drive. FOUR score scale evaluates four categories (i.e. eye, motor, brainstem and respiration). To each category is given a numeric point from 0 to 4 (as shown in Table 3.2); the total score ranges from 0 to 16. In comparison to GCS, FOUR score evaluates essential brain stem reflexes and provides information about brainstem injury. FOUR score allows the recognition of locked-in syndrome and persistent vegetative state. In addition to the aforementioned scale, specific scores were developed to assess ischaemic stroke, subarachnoid haemorrhage and intraparenchymal

Table 3.1 Glasgow Coma Score Pupils Score (GCS-P)

GCS-Pupils Score (GCS-P)							
Motor response		Verbal response		Eye opening		Pupils Unreactive to Light (PRS)	
Obeying commands	6	Orientated response	5	Spontaneous	4	Both pupils	2
Localized to pain	5	Confused conversation	4	In response to speech	3	One pupil	1
Flexion/withdraws to pain	4	Inappropriate words	3	To pain	2	Neither pupil	0
Abnormal muscle flexing to pain stimuli	3	Incomprehensible sounds	2	None	1	//	//
Extension to pain stimuli	2	None	1	//	//		
None	1	//	//				
GCS-P = GCS − PRS							
GOS							
Dead						1	
Vegetative state						2	
Severe disability						3	
Moderate disability						4	
Low disability						5	
GOS-E							
Dead						1	
Vegetative state						2	
Lower severe disability						3	
Upper severe disability						4	
Lower moderate disability						5	
Upper moderate disability						6	
Lower good recovery						7	
Upper good recovery						8	

The GCS-P is calculated by subtracting the Pupil Reactivity Score (PRS) from the Glasgow Coma Scale (GCS) total score. The Glasgow Outcome Scale Score (GOS) and the Glasgow Outcome Scale Score Extended (GOS-E) allow the objective assessment of patient's recovery after a brain injury

haemorrhage (ICH). The National Institutes of Health Stroke Scale (NIHSS) assesses the severity and the possible location of the stroke [16]. The NIHSS is a 15-item test, and it ranges from 0 to 42, and it is strongly associated with outcome. Even more, NIHSS represents a valid aid to identify those patients who are likely to benefit from reperfusion therapies and those who are at higher risk of developing complications. The Hunt and Hess Scale is used to grade the severity of a subarachnoid haemorrhage based on the patient's clinical condition. The scale correlates with patient's prognosis and outcome [17]. The World Federation of Neurosurgical Societies classification was developed as an alternative to Hunt and Hess scale. This score combines consciousness and motor deficit [18]. The ICH score was developed to provide a clinical grading scale for ICH and provide 30-day mortality [19]. The variables included in the ICH score are GCS, age, infratentorial origin (yes/no), ICH volume greater than 30 mL (yes/no) and intraventricular haemorrhage (yes/no). A score greater than 5 correlates with a bad outcome.

Table 3.2 The Full Outline of UnResponsiveness (FOUR) score is a 17-point, assessing eye responses, motor responses, brainstream reflexes and breathing pattern

FOUR score	
Eye opening	
Open eyes spontaneously, tracks, blink to command	4
Eyelids open but not tracking	3
Eyelids closed but open to loud voice	2
Eyelids closed but open to pain	1
Eyelids remain closed with pain	0
Motor response	
Thumbs-up, fist or peace sign	4
Localizing to pain	3
Flexion response to pain	2
Extension response to pain	1
No response to pain or generalized myoclonus status	0
Brainstem reflexes	
Pupil and corneal reflexes present	4
One pupil wide and fixed	3
Pupil or corneal reflexes absent	2
Pupil and corneal reflexes absent	1
Absent pupil, corneal and cough reflex	0
Respiration	
Not intubated, regular breathing pattern	4
Not intubated, Cheyne–Stokes breathing pattern	3
Not intubated, irregular breathing	2
Breathes above ventilator rate	1
Breathes at ventilator rate or apnoea	0

3.2.2   ICP Monitoring

Intracranial pressure (ICP) monitoring is vital to orientate clinical management and to detect life-threating complications [20]. This invasive monitoring is indicated when there is a high risk of elevated ICP based on clinical and imaging findings. Elevated ICP can result from any mechanism that increases the volume of the three intracranial components (i.e. brain tissue, blood, cerebrospinal fluid-CSF). When the compensatory system responsible for maintaining a stable ICP is depleted, the consequence of elevated ICP could be represented by cerebral ischaemia and/or cerebral herniation [2]. Consequently, the early identification and treatment of these complications are essential to prevent an irreversible secondary cerebral insult. However, ICP monitoring has to be evaluated in a context of a multimodal monitoring that involves neurological assessment, radiological imaging and other invasive and noninvasive monitoring. In fact, any therapeutic intervention that aims to lower ICP has potential side effects (e.g. hyperventilation/cerebral ischaemia, barbiturates/infection), consequently, it is fundamental to identify the precise aetiology of ICP increase and tailor to each patient the therapeutic option [7, 21]. Even more, to highlight the importance of a multimodal monitoring, brain metabolism may be altered (e.g. evaluated with jugular bulb catheters or $PbtO_2$) with a normal ICP and cerebral perfusion pressure (CPP) [22]. At the same time, the presence of mass lesions, midline shift or effacement of the basilar cisterns on a computed tomography (CT) scans may suggest an elevated ICP; however, patients without these finding on the basal CT scan may develop an altered ICP. In fact, brain injury is a dynamic state, and patients may develop CT scan abnormalities within the first hours or days after trauma or the insult; consequently, it is vital to monitor ICP to maintain strict surveillance. These evidences stress the importance of a multimodal approach, of the continuing ICP monitoring and the role of follow-up evaluation.

Intracranial hypertension is defined as an ICP > 20 mmHg [23]. However, the threshold that defines intracranial hypertension has been debated and moved from ages [22, 24, 25]. However, it is well recognized that not only an absolute value but also the trend over time and waveform analysis of ICP are important aspects that have to be analysed and are associated with outcome [26, 27]. Information that can be derived by ICP waveform analysis includes CPP, regulation of cerebral blood flow, cerebral compliance and brain compensatory reserve [28]. Only a single value of ICP cannot be considered a realist ICP. In fact, ICP is not a static value, and it is influenced by cardiac contraction, respiration and intracranial compliance. Consequently, mean ICP is derived by the average of at least 30 min of ICP waveform analysis [29].

The ICP waveform consists of three components that can be analysed in their different frequency domain:

- Respiratory waveform (influenced by the respiratory cycle);
- Pulse pressure waveform (heart rate);
- Vasogenic waveforms (Plateau waves or pathological A waves, B waves).

The compensatory reserve and regulation can be obtained by the analysis of these waveforms. The pulse pressure waveform can be subdivided into three components (i.e. P1, P2, P3) [30]. P1 is generated by systolic pulse wave. P2 reflects cerebral compliance. P3 reflects the closure of the aortic valve. The increase in the P2 component of the pulse pressure waveform is associated with elevated ICP and reduction in intracranial compliance. Furthermore, data processing systems allow the calculation of ICP-derived index, allowing a deeper understanding of ICP regulatory process. Cerebrovascular compensatory reserve (RAP) is an ICP-derived index and represent the correlation between pulse amplitude (AMP) and mean ICP [31]. Pulse amplitude (AMP) is evaluated with spectral analysis of arterial cycle; high AMP is associated with low compliance. Generally, 40 samples of AMP and ICP are obtained over a period of 6–10s. A RAP equal to 0 represents a good compensatory reserve, whereas a RAP equal to 1 indicates a low compensatory reserve. When ICP continues to increase, RAP becomes negative, showing an exhausted cerebral compensatory reserve. Furthermore, pressure reactivity index (PRx) is another ICP-derived index that allows the assessment of cerebral autoregulation

[32]. PRx is the time-averaged correlation coefficient between mean ICP and mean arterial pressure (MAP). A positive PRx reflects impaired autoregulation, while a negative PRx indicates a normal autoregulation capacity. Moreover, PRx plotted with CPP, in a 6-h time window, can allow the evaluation of optimal CPP value. This estimation allows an CPP oriented therapy to avoid too low CPP (with consequent cerebral ischaemia) or too high CPP (with consequent of hyperaemia and ICP increase) [33]. ICP, RAP and PRx indices are independent well-recognized predictors factor of outcome [34].

Several devices are available for the measurement of ICP, associated with specific advantages and disadvantages. Regardless of the specific device, ICP monitoring is associated with a risk of central nervous system (CNS) infection (risk increases the longer a device is in place), intracranial haemorrhage, displacement and accidental removal [29]. The gold standard for ICP monitoring is considered the external ventricular drain (EVD) [35]. The ventricular catheter is connected to a fluid-coupled external strain gauge. The intraventricular pressure equilibrates with the pressure into the catheter. In addition to ICP monitoring, EVD allows CSF drainage, consequently, it can be used as therapeutic option (e.g. hydrocephalus). Intraventricular monitoring has the advantage of accuracy; however, this device carries the specific risk of haemorrhage during placement. In addition, blockage of the drainage system may occur with an obstacle in CSF drainage and possible worsening of hydrocephalus. ICP can also be measured using microtransducers, pneumatic sensors and fibre-optic sensors. These sensors can be placed in intraventricular, intraparenchymal, subarachnoid, and epidural compartment. Intraparenchymal devices carry a lower risk of infection and haemorrhage than with intraventricular device; however, with this device, it is not possible to drain CSF for diagnostic or therapeutic purposes [36].

3.2.3 Noninvasive Systems

As already stated, the gold standard for ICP monitoring is represented by the placement of an intraventricular catheter connected to an external pressure transducer; unfortunately, this invasive method is associated with potential risks (e.g. infection, haemorrhage, obstruction, difficulty in placement, malposition). In the last years, several noninvasive ICP monitoring systems have been studied [37]. None of these techniques can replace ICP monitors for ICP evaluation; however, they can be used to screen patients for elevated ICP. Even more, noninvasive methods can be used to monitor the clinical course of a patient with brain injury and to help the clinician in the decision to use an invasive measurement device or as follow-up investigation. These diagnostic modalities provide non-continuous information, and they can be performed rapidly at the bedside without the use of ionizing radiation or the need of surgical installation. The high safe profile (no risk of infection/bleeding or the use of ionizing radiation) and the increasing availability make these methods appealing; however, they cannot completely replace invasive methods. In fact, one single method does not provide complete information on brain injury disease but has great potential when integrated into a multimodality monitoring approach [38].

There are several noninvasive neuromonitoring techniques:

- Transcranial Doppler (TCD) and transcranial colour-coded duplex (TCCD): TCD is based on Doppler effect. TCD blindly identifies cerebral arteries through Doppler signal obtained and consequent spectral display [39]. Spectral analysis can then be performed to monitor the velocity of proximal cerebral circulation. The parameter obtained from TCD are peak systolic velocity, end-diastolic velocity, pulsatility index and time-averaged mean maximum velocity. The TCD evaluation of internal carotid artery allows the evaluation of Lindegaard ratio (i.e. mean velocity in the MCA/mean velocity in ipsilateral extracranial internal carotid artery), and it is used to discriminate between hyperaemia and vasospasm. TCD is most commonly applied in the setting of subarachnoid haemorrhage (SAH) to predict vasospasm (as shown in Fig. 3.1). However, TCD is also a reliable method to confirm brain death. Even more, blood flow responses to changes in blood pressure and in end-tidal CO_2 can allow the evaluation of cerebral autoregulation and cerebral vasoreactivity, respectively [40]. On the other hand, TCCD allows the direct visualization of parenchymal structures and of the vessels, improving the angle corrected blood velocities [41]. TCCD combines pulsed wave Doppler with two-dimensional B-mode imaging. A 2.5 MHz probe is placed on transtemporal acoustic window to detect cerebral structures and circle of Willis. Other possible acoustic windows are represented by occipital, submandibular and transorbital window. TCCD-derived indices such as Gosling's Pulsatility index and estimated CPP formula may provide bedside information in neurocritical ill patients. Even more TCCD can allow the direct detection of midline shift, intracranial masses and cerebral haematoma. TCCD can be also used for detect vasospasm, evaluate autoregulation and for noninvasive ICP and CPP estimation [42, 43]. Both TCD and TCCD are subjected to operator variability and failure to insonate temporal window (10% of cases).
- Ocular sonography: The optic nerve sheath is surrounded by the dura sheat and by the subarachnoid space containing CSF. Therefore, an increase in ICP can be transmitted through the subarachnoid space with a consequent dilatation of optic nerve sheath. Ultrasound evaluation of optic nerve sheath diameter (ONSD) can provide a noninvasive measure of optic nerve sheath diameter (Fig. 3.2), which has been found to correlate with ICP with a sensitivity of 0.9 and a specificity of 0.85 [44]. A diameter >5–6 mm can be used to detect elevated ICP [45]. Interestingly, a combination of optic nerve sheat diameter and venous transcranial Doppler are proposed for noninvasive ICP measurement [46].

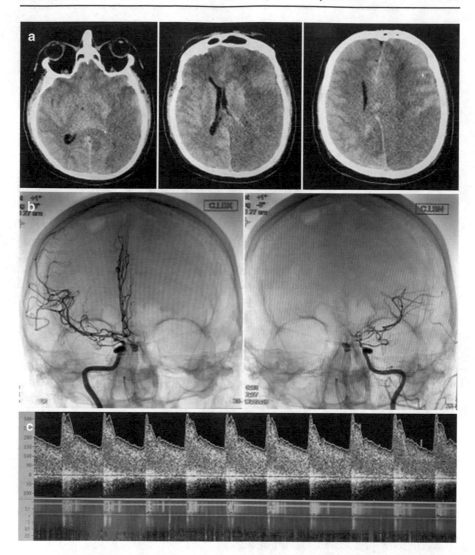

Fig. 3.1 Forty-two year-old patient with subarachnoid haemorrhage caused by ruptured aneurysm. During the intensive care stay, he developed severe vasospasm. (**a**) CT scan showing cortico-subcortical ischaemia with haemorrhagic cortical infarction, midline shifts to the right of the brain, transtentorial and subfalcine herniation; (**b**) Angiographic vasospasm of left anterior (A1-2) and middle (M1-2) cerebral arteries; (**c**) TCD waveform analysis shows a severe vasospasm of the left middle cerebral artery (mean velocity > 200 cm/s)

Several other noninvasive ICP monitoring techniques have been studied (i.e. tympanic membrane displacement, tissue resonance analysis, anterior fontanelle pressure monitoring, tonometry); however, they are not widely implemented into clinical practice [35].

Fig. 3.2 Ultrasound image
of the optic nerve

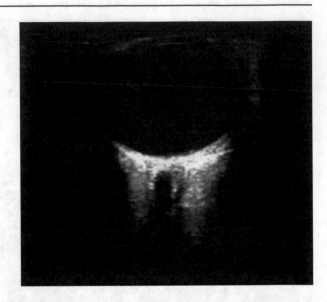

3.2.4 Advanced Monitoring

Multimodality brain monitoring includes also the evaluation of brain oxygenation and cerebral metabolism. The evaluation of tissue oxygenation allows the understanding of intracranial oxygen supply and demand. The goal of the evaluation of metabolic data, oxygen delivery and cerebral blood flow (CBF) is to identify and manage possible secondary brain injury. Brain oxygenation and metabolism measurements are recommended in patients at risk of ischaemia and/or hypoxia [20]. One important limitation to take into account is that these techniques represent focal metabolism measurement; consequently, the location of the probe and interpretation of the subsequent measurement have to be done based on probe location on post-insertion CT and the location of brain lesions. From this perspective, these techniques have to be integrated with other monitoring modalities.

Such techniques include the following:

- Jugular venous oximetry ($SjVO_2$):
  SjO_2 is obtained by performing a retrograde cannulation of the internal jugular vein. This parameter provides information on the balance between cerebral blood flow (CBF) and metabolic demand. Normal SjO_2 is considered between 55 and 75% [47]. SjO_2 below 55% advises that the cerebral demand exceeds the supply, and this value is considered a threshold for ischaemia. On the other hand, $SjO_2 > 75\%$ suggests hyperaemia. However, SjO_2 can be influenced by several factors (e.g. anaesthetics drug, blood pressure, hyperventilation, anaemia), and it fails to detect regional changes. SjO_2 represents a global evaluation of oxygen demand and supply; consequently, normal values of SjO_2 do not warrant the exclusion of regional ischaemia [48].

- Brain tissue oxygen ($PbtO_2$) monitoring:
  Brain tissue oxygen monitoring is the partial pressure of oxygen in the interstitial space. Normal $PbtO_2$ is 25–35 mmHg. $P_{bt}O_2$ measurements are strongly influenced by the distance from the site of focal injury. Tissue oxygen reactivity and oxygen reactivity index can be derived by $PbtO_2$ monitoring. Tissue oxygen reactivity can be calculated by the following formula: $([\Delta P_{btO2}/\Delta P_{aO2}]/P_{btO2}$ baseline) [49]. This parameter represents the relationship between $PbtO_2$ and PO_2. $PbtO_2$ varies in response to PaO_2 changes in patients without cerebral injuries. Oxygen reactivity index represents the ability to maintain $PbtO_2$ despite CPP variation, and it is used to assess the status of cerebral autoregulation [50]. A multimodal approach using $P_{bt}O_2$ and ICP monitoring led to a more favourable outcome [51].
- Cerebral microdialysis:
  Microdialysis allows in vivo sampling of cerebral metabolites and provides continuous information on metabolic cerebral status [52]. This technique allows the measurement of extracellular glucose, lactate, pyruvate and glutamate. However, microdialysis consents the evaluation of regional metabolism. In particular, the evaluation of the site where the probe is placed. Consequently, the catheter should be placed in 'at-risk' tissue.

In this section, we have briefly described few techniques for advanced multimodal neuromonitoring. A comprehensive exposition about the advantages/disadvantages, clinical application/data interpretation and how to avoid pitfall of the aforementioned techniques and of other interesting methods (e.g. Thermal diffusion flowmetry, Near Infrared Spectroscopy—NIRS) is outside the scope of this chapter.

3.3   Treatment of the Intracranial Compartment Syndrome

The first approach to a patient with brain injury is to prevent any possible factor that may aggravate or precipitate HI. As already explained, several intracranial or extracranial disease can be responsible for IH [1, 2]. Obstruction of venous return (head position, agitation), respiratory problems (airway obstruction, hypoxia, hypercapnia), fever, IAP, severe hypertension, hyponatremia, anaemia and seizure is possible reversible cause affecting ICP. Consequently, the first approach is to prevent and treat any trigger that can increase ICP [4–6, 53]. Then, medical management of increased ICP should include several lines of treatment (e.g. sedation, drainage of CSF and osmotherapy, barbiturate) that have to be chosen following a stepwise approach to therapy. This approach consists of escalating and deescalating treatment intensity on the base of the gravity of the medical condition and the response to therapy [54]. However, it is to keep in mind that in case of HI, the best therapeutic option is represented by the specific resolution of the cause of HI (e.g. evacuation of mass-occupying lesion, tumour resection, drainage of CSF in case of hydrocephalus).

HI is a medical emergency requiring a prompt diagnosis, treatment and close monitoring in Neurointensive care unit (NICU) [55]. As already stated, invasive ICP monitoring is indicated when there are high suspicions of intracranial hypertension, based on clinical and imaging findings [20]. Furthermore, it is crucial to monitor patient vital signs (e.g. ECG, invasive blood pressure, body temperature, haemogasanalysis, haemoglobin, blood glucose, diuresis). Unilateral or bilaterally fixed and dilated pupils, decorticate/decerebrate posturing, bradycardia, hypertension and respiratory depression are all signs suggesting elevated ICP during clinical evaluation and requiring urgent intervention. Then, consider further neuromonitoring tests (e.g. repeat CT scan) to address specific aetiology.

ICP-directed therapies include the following:

- Head position: head-up elevate to 30° and neutrally positioned to optimize venous outflow and improve CSF flow;
- Haemodynamic stability: maintain a CPP 50–70 mmHg (depending on the autoregulatory status of the patient). Systemic hypertension may have a detrimental effect on ICP and may worsen cerebral oedema and increase the risk of intracranial haemorrhage. However, the decision to treat systemic hypertension has to be tailored for each patient. In fact, in traumatic brain injury, an increase in systemic hypertension leads to an increase in ICP due to the loss of autoregulation. On the other hand, in patients with chronic hypertension, autoregulatory curve is right shifted, consequently, higher value of systemic pressure can be tolerated [56]. In case of the decision to treat systemic hypertension, short half-life drugs (i.e. clonidine) are to be preferred. Above all, large shifts in blood pressure should be minimized.
- Sedation and analgesia may prevent coughing and agitation. Even more, sedation and analgesia allow a better synchronism between the patient and the ventilator and enable seizure and systemic hypertension control. Furthermore, sedation has neuro-specific indications (i.e. reduction of cerebral metabolic rate of oxygen—$CMRO_2$). Up to now, there is no evidence on the superiority of one sedative agent in comparison to another [57]. Short-acting agents with minimal hypotensive effects should be preferred. In fact, these agents allow brief interruption of sedation to evaluate neurological status with minimum impact on systemic haemodynamic.
- Mechanical ventilation (MV): MV can present a double effect on ICP. Positive mechanical ventilation increases ITP and can reduce venous return, increase cerebral venous pressure and ICP. Furthermore, positive MV may present a detrimental effect on systemic haemodynamic, decreasing intrathoracic venous blood return and consequently, reducing systemic blood pressure [58]. Then, altered ventilation can lead to hypoxia and hypercapnia which present a negative effect on ICP. A balance between improving oxygenation without impact on cerebral haemodynamic is a crucial goal in neurocritical patients. Particular attention needs to be focused during recruitment manoeuvre. Furthermore, during intubation manoeuvre, care should be taken to minimize further elevation of ICP.
- Normothermia: Fever increases metabolic rate, and it is a potent vasodilator [59]. Fever can increase CBF and increase ICP, worsening brain injury. Fever should be treated with antipyretics and fluids.

- Seizures can increase metabolic rate and ICP and should be rapidly diagnosed and treated [60, 61]. Prophylactic treatment should be reserved for patients with specific risk factors (e.g. severe traumatic brain injury, brain contusion, subdural haematoma, depressed skull fracture, penetrating head wound, frontal and temporal contusion). Seizures may be subclinical and can be detected only with continuous EEG [62].
- Crystalloids are considered the preferred maintenance fluids in neurocritical ill patients, and they have to be used as the first-line resuscitation fluids in patients with low blood pressure [63]. Patients should be maintained euvolemic with strict electrolytes and plasma osmolarity control avoiding the use of colloids, hypotonic solution and albumin.

In case of refractory IH:

- Osmotic therapy: A recent consensus suggested that osmotherapy should be started in case of clinical decline and ICP above 25 mmHg (weak recommendation) [63]. Mannitol (0.5–1 g/Kg) and hypertonic saline (3% solution, 2.5–5 mL/Kg) can both be used empirically for ICP control [64]. They reduce intracranial volume thorough their osmotic properties. Important disadvantages to keep in mind is the hypotensive effects of mannitol. Even more, serum sodium, osmolarity and renal function have to be monitored. On the other hand, hypertonic saline presents hypertensive, hypervolemic and haemodilution effects. Serum sodium needs to be monitored (possible risk of osmotic demyelination). A 2019 meta-analysis concluded that hypertonic saline seems to be preferred as osmotherapy ICP lower therapy in TBI patients [65].
- Hyperventilation should be chosen only as a temporary measure, due to the risk of cerebral ischaemia, and only in case of refractory ICP. The target is mild hyperventilation (paCO$_2$ 30–32 mmHg); a more aggressive approach has to be avoided [66]. The effect of hypocapnia is rapid due to cerebral vasoconstriction and consequent reduction in cerebral blood flow; however, it lasts only 4–6 h [21]. In case of hyperventilation, advanced monitoring (i.e. SjO$_2$ and P$_{tb}$O$_2$) should be used for the evaluation of brain oxygenation and cerebral metabolism [67, 68].
- Barbiturates: Barbiturates suppress cerebral metabolism and reduce cerebral oxygen consumption [69]. These effects lead to a decrease in CBF, cerebral blood volume and ICP. However, barbiturates are associated with several adverse effects (e.g. cardiovascular instability, immune suppression, respiratory depression and paralytic ileus). Barbiturate should be considered only in patients with refractory HI [70].
- Decompressive craniotomy (DC) should be reserved when maximal medical management fails. In refractory intracranial hypertension, DC seems to improve outcome with a lower rate of severe disability [71, 72]. DC consists of the surgical removal of part of the skull allowing for herniation of brain through the bone with consequent pressure lowering. Possible complications are represented by infection, hydrocephalus, haemorrhage, subdural hygroma, herniation through the skull defect, seizure and CDSF fistulae [73].

3.4   Conclusions

The intracranial compartment syndrome is a medical emergency that requires a rapid diagnosis and treatment. The main goal is to preserve cerebral blood flow and to prevent a secondary brain injury. Medical management should include several lines of treatment following a stepwise approach. Escalating therapy should be reserved to refractory elevated ICP that do not respond to first-line treatment. However, the gold standard is to identify specific aetiology of intracranial hypertension and, then, tailor the medical strategy. Neuromonitoring has a central role in the rapid detection of intracranial compartment syndrome. In the last year, several monitoring techniques have gained importance. Future challenges would be represented by the integration of data gathered by different sources through computer-assisted methods. This multimodality monitoring would provide the clinician with real-time information on a dynamic cerebral state.

References

1. Kinoshita K. Traumatic brain injury: pathophysiology for neurocritical care. J Intensive Care. 2016;4:29.
2. Iencean SM, Ciurea AV. Intracranial hypertension: classification and patterns of evolution. J Med Life. 2008;1(2):101–7.
3. Rangel-Castillo L, Gopinath S, Robertson CS. Management of intracranial hypertension. Neurol Clin. 2008;26(2):521–41.
4. Scalea TM, Bochicchio GV, Habashi N, McCunn M, Shih D, McQuillan K, et al. Increased intra-abdominal, intrathoracic, and intracranial pressure after severe brain injury: multiple compartment syndrome. J Trauma. 2007;62(3):647–56; discussion 56.
5. Geeraerts T, Vigue B. [Cellular metabolism, temperature and brain injury]. Ann Fr Anesth Reanim. 2009;28:339–44. France.
6. Duncan R. Epilepsy, cerebral blood flow, and cerebral metabolic rate. Cerebrovasc Brain Metab Rev. 1992;4(2):105–21.
7. Godoy DA, Seifi A, Garza D, Lubillo-Montenegro S, Murillo-Cabezas F. Hyperventilation therapy for control of posttraumatic intracranial hypertension. Front Neurol. 2017;8:250.
8. Kirkman MA, Smith M. Multimodality neuromonitoring. Anesthesiol Clin. 2016;34:511–23. United States: 2016 Elsevier Inc.
9. John G, Peter JV, Chacko B, Pichamuthu K, Rao A, Subbalakshmi K, et al. A computer-assisted recording, diagnosis and management of the medically ill system for use in the intensive care unit: a preliminary report. Indian J Crit Care Med. 2009;13:136–42.
10. Brennan PM, Murray GD, Teasdale GM. Simplifying the use of prognostic information in traumatic brain injury. Part 1: the GCS-Pupils score: an extended index of clinical severity. J Neurosurg. 2018;128(6):1612–20.
11. Miller KJ, Schwab KA, Warden DL. Predictive value of an early Glasgow Outcome Scale score: 15-month score changes. J Neurosurg. 2005;103(2):239–45.
12. Wilson JT, Pettigrew LE, Teasdale GM. Structured interviews for the glasgow outcome scale and the extended glasgow outcome scale: guidelines for their use. J Neurotrauma. 1998;15(8):573–85.
13. Benzer A, Mitterschiffthaler G, Marosi M, Luef G, Puhringer F, De La Renotiere K, et al. Prediction of non-survival after trauma: Innsbruck Coma Scale. Lancet (London, England). 1991;338(8773):977–8.
14. Wijdicks EF, Bamlet WR, Maramattom BV, Manno EM, McClelland RL. Validation of a new coma scale: the FOUR score. Ann Neurol. 2005;58(4):585–93.

15. Iyer VN, Mandrekar JN, Danielson RD, Zubkov AY, Elmer JL, Wijdicks EF. Validity of the FOUR score coma scale in the medical intensive care unit. Mayo Clin Proc. 2009;84(8):694–701.
16. Kerr DM, Fulton RL, Lees KR. Seven-day NIHSS is a sensitive outcome measure for exploratory clinical trials in acute stroke: evidence from the Virtual International Stroke Trials Archive. Stroke. 2012;43(5):1401–3.
17. Oshiro EM, Walter KA, Piantadosi S, Witham TF, Tamargo RJ. A new subarachnoid hemorrhage grading system based on the Glasgow Coma Scale: a comparison with the Hunt and Hess and World Federation of Neurological Surgeons Scales in a clinical series. Neurosurgery. 1997;41(1):140–7; discussion 7–8.
18. Teasdale GM, Drake CG, Hunt W, Kassell N, Sano K, Pertuiset B, et al. A universal subarachnoid hemorrhage scale: report of a committee of the World Federation of Neurosurgical Societies. J Neurol Neurosurg Psychiatry. 1988;51(11):1457.
19. Hemphill JC 3rd, Bonovich DC, Besmertis L, Manley GT, Johnston SC. The ICH score: a simple, reliable grading scale for intracerebral hemorrhage. Stroke. 2001;32(4):891–7.
20. Le Roux P, Menon DK, Citerio G, Vespa P, Bader MK, Brophy GM, et al. Consensus summary statement of the International Multidisciplinary Consensus Conference on Multimodality Monitoring in Neurocritical Care: a statement for healthcare professionals from the Neurocritical Care Society and the European Society of Intensive Care Medicine. Neurocrit Care. 2014;21(Suppl 2):S1–26.
21. Muizelaar JP, Marmarou A, Ward JD, Kontos HA, Choi SC, Becker DP, et al. Adverse effects of prolonged hyperventilation in patients with severe head injury: a randomized clinical trial. J Neurosurg. 1991;75(5):731–9.
22. Stiefel MF, Udoetuk JD, Spiotta AM, Gracias VH, Goldberg A, Maloney-Wilensky E, et al. Conventional neurocritical care and cerebral oxygenation after traumatic brain injury. J Neurosurg. 2006;105(4):568–75.
23. Lundberg N. Continuous recording and control of ventricular fluid pressure in neurosurgical practice. Acta Psychiatr Scand Suppl. 1960;36(149):1–193.
24. Carney N, Totten AM, O'Reilly C, Ullman JS, Hawryluk GW, Bell MJ, et al. Guidelines for the management of severe traumatic brain injury, fourth edition. Neurosurgery. 2017;80(1):6–15.
25. Schreiber MA, Aoki N, Scott BG, Beck JR. Determinants of mortality in patients with severe blunt head injury. Arch Surg. 2002;137:285–90. United States.
26. Guiza F, Depreitere B, Piper I, Citerio G, Chambers I, Jones PA, et al. Visualizing the pressure and time burden of intracranial hypertension in adult and paediatric traumatic brain injury. Intensive Care Med. 2015;41(6):1067–76.
27. Vik A, Nag T, Fredriksli OA, Skandsen T, Moen KG, Schirmer-Mikalsen K, et al. Relationship of "dose" of intracranial hypertension to outcome in severe traumatic brain injury. J Neurosurg. 2008;109(4):678–84.
28. Czosnyka M, Pickard JD. Monitoring and interpretation of intracranial pressure. J Neurol Neurosurg Psychiatry. 2004;75(6):813–21.
29. Harary M, Dolmans RGF, Gormley WB. Intracranial pressure monitoring-review and avenues for development. Sensors (Basel). 2018;18(2):465.
30. Adolph RJ, Fukusumi H, Fowler NO. Origin of cerebrospinal fluid pulsations. Am J Physiol. 1967;212(4):840–6.
31. Zeiler FA, Donnelly J, Menon DK, Smielewski P, Hutchinson PJA, Czosnyka M. A description of a new continuous physiological index in traumatic brain injury using the correlation between pulse amplitude of intracranial pressure and cerebral perfusion pressure. J Neurotrauma. 2018;35(7):963–74.
32. Zweifel C, Lavinio A, Steiner LA, Radolovich D, Smielewski P, Timofeev I, et al. Continuous monitoring of cerebrovascular pressure reactivity in patients with head injury. Neurosurg Focus. 2008;25(4):E2.
33. Steiner LA, Czosnyka M, Piechnik SK, Smielewski P, Chatfield D, Menon DK, et al. Continuous monitoring of cerebrovascular pressure reactivity allows determination of optimal cerebral perfusion pressure in patients with traumatic brain injury. Crit Care Med. 2002;30(4):733–8.

34. Balestreri M, Czosnyka M, Steiner LA, Hiler M, Schmidt EA, Matta B, et al. Association between outcome, cerebral pressure reactivity and slow ICP waves following head injury. Acta Neurochir Suppl. 2005;95:25–8.

35. Nag DS, Sahu S, Swain A, Kant S. Intracranial pressure monitoring: gold standard and recent innovations. World J Clin Cases. 2019;7(13):1535–53.

36. Gupta DK, Bisht A, Batra P, Mathur P, Mahapatra AK. A cost effectiveness based safety and efficacy study of resterilized intra-parenchymal catheter based intracranial pressure monitoring in developing world. Asian J Neurosurg. 2016;11(4):416–20.

37. Narayan V, Mohammed N, Savardekar AR, Patra DP, Notarianni C, Nanda A. Noninvasive intracranial pressure monitoring for severe traumatic brain injury in children: a concise update on current methods. World Neurosurg. 2018;114:293–300. United States: 2018 Elsevier Inc.

38. Vinciguerra L, Bosel J. Noninvasive neuromonitoring: current utility in subarachnoid hemorrhage, traumatic brain injury, and stroke. Neurocrit Care. 2017;27:122–40. United States.

39. Bathala L, Mehndiratta MM, Sharma VK. Transcranial Doppler: technique and common findings (part 1). Ann Indian Acad Neurol. 2013;16(2):174–9.

40. Purkayastha S, Sorond F. Transcranial Doppler ultrasound: technique and application. Semin Neurol. 2012;32(4):411–20.

41. Krejza J, Mariak Z, Melhem ER, Bert RJ. A guide to the identification of major cerebral arteries with transcranial color Doppler sonography. AJR Am J Roentgenol. 2000;174(5):1297–303.

42. Khan MN, Shallwani H, Khan MU, Shamim MS. Noninvasive monitoring intracranial pressure—a review of available modalities. Surg Neurol Int. 2017;8:51.

43. Rasulo FA, Bertuetti R, Robba C, Lusenti F, Cantoni A, Bernini M, et al. The accuracy of transcranial Doppler in excluding intracranial hypertension following acute brain injury: a multicenter prospective pilot study. Crit Care. 2017;21(1):44.

44. Dubourg J, Javouhey E, Geeraerts T, Messerer M, Kassai B. Ultrasonography of optic nerve sheath diameter for detection of raised intracranial pressure: a systematic review and meta-analysis. Intensive Care Med. 2011;37(7):1059–68.

45. Rajajee V, Vanaman M, Fletcher JJ, Jacobs TL. Optic nerve ultrasound for the detection of raised intracranial pressure. Neurocrit Care. 2011;15(3):506–15.

46. Robba C, Cardim D, Tajsic T, Pietersen J, Bulman M, Donnelly J, et al. Ultrasound non-invasive measurement of intracranial pressure in neurointensive care: a prospective observational study. PLoS Med. 2017;14(7):e1002356.

47. Nakamura S. [Monitoring of jugular venous oxygen saturation]. Nihon Rinsho. 2011;69(4):704–7.

48. Muizelaar JP, Schroder ML. Overview of monitoring of cerebral blood flow and metabolism after severe head injury. Can J Neurol Sci. 1994;21(2):S6–11.

49. Ngwenya LB, Burke JF, Manley GT. Brain tissue oxygen monitoring and the intersection of brain and lung: a comprehensive review. Respir Care. 2016;61:1232–44. United States: 2016 by Daedalus Enterprises.

50. Dengler J, Frenzel C, Vajkoczy P, Horn P, Wolf S. The oxygen reactivity index and its relation to sensor technology in patients with severe brain lesions. Neurocrit Care. 2013;19(1):74–8.

51. Okonkwo DO, Shutter LA, Moore C, Temkin NR, Puccio AM, Madden CJ, et al. Brain tissue oxygen monitoring and management in severe traumatic brain injury (BOOST-II): a phase II randomized trial. Crit Care Med. 2017;45(11):1907–14.

52. Johnston AJ, Gupta AK. Advanced monitoring in the neurology intensive care unit: microdialysis. Curr Opin Crit Care. 2002;8(2):121–7.

53. Godoy DA, Lubillo S, Rabinstein AA. Pathophysiology and management of intracranial hypertension and tissular brain hypoxia after severe traumatic brain injury: an integrative approach. Neurosurg Clin N Am. 2018;29:195–212. United States: 2018 Elsevier Inc.

54. Tripathy S, Ahmad SR. Raised intracranial pressure syndrome: a stepwise approach. Indian J Crit Care Med. 2019;23(Suppl 2):S129–S35.

55. Ramesh Kumar R, Singhi SC, Singhi P. Raised intracranial pressure (ICP): management in emergency department. Indian J Pediatr. 2012;79(4):518–24.

56. Shekhar S, Liu R, Travis OK, Roman RJ, Fan F. Cerebral autoregulation in hypertension and ischemic stroke: a mini review. J Pharm Sci Exp Pharmacol. 2017;2017(1):21–7.
57. Oddo M, Crippa IA, Mehta S, Menon D, Payen JF, Taccone FS, et al. Optimizing sedation in patients with acute brain injury. Crit Care. 2016;20:128.
58. Asehnoune K, Roquilly A, Cinotti R. Respiratory management in patients with severe brain injury. Crit Care. 2018;22:76.
59. Rossi S, Zanier ER, Mauri I, Columbo A, Stocchetti N. Brain temperature, body core temperature, and intracranial pressure in acute cerebral damage. J Neurol Neurosurg Psychiatry. 2001;71(4):448–54.
60. Gabor AJ, Brooks AG, Scobey RP, Parsons GH. Intracranial pressure during epileptic seizures. Electroencephalogr Clin Neurophysiol. 1984;57:497–506. Ireland.
61. Shah AK, Fuerst D, Sood S, Asano E, Ahn-Ewing J, Pawlak C, et al. Seizures lead to elevation of intracranial pressure in children undergoing invasive EEG monitoring. Epilepsia. 2007;48:1097–103. United States.
62. Friedman D, Claassen J, Hirsch LJ. Continuous electroencephalogram monitoring in the intensive care unit. Anesth Analg. 2009;109:506–23. United States.
63. Oddo M, Poole D, Helbok R, Meyfroidt G, Stocchetti N, Bouzat P, et al. Fluid therapy in neurointensive care patients: ESICM consensus and clinical practice recommendations. Intensive Care Med. 2018;44:449–63. United States.
64. Farrokh S, Cho SM, Suarez JI. Fluids and hyperosmolar agents in neurocritical care: an update. Curr Opin Crit Care. 2019;25(2):105–9.
65. Gu J, Huang H, Huang Y, Sun H, Xu H. Hypertonic saline or mannitol for treating elevated intracranial pressure in traumatic brain injury: a meta-analysis of randomized controlled trials. Neurosurg Rev. 2019;42:499–509. Germany.
66. Stevens RD, Shoykhet M, Cadena R. Emergency neurological life support: intracranial hypertension and herniation. Neurocrit Care. 2015;23(Suppl 2):S76–82.
67. Stocchetti N, Maas AI, Chieregato A, van der Plas AA. Hyperventilation in head injury: a review. Chest. 2005;127:1812–27. United States.
68. Marion DW, Puccio A, Wisniewski SR, Kochanek P, Dixon CE, Bullian L, et al. Effect of hyperventilation on extracellular concentrations of glutamate, lactate, pyruvate, and local cerebral blood flow in patients with severe traumatic brain injury. Crit Care Med. 2002;30(12):2619–25.
69. Roberts I, Sydenham E. Barbiturates for acute traumatic brain injury. Cochrane Database Syst Rev. 2012;12:CD000033.
70. Stocchetti N, Zanaboni C, Colombo A, Citerio G, Beretta L, Ghisoni L, et al. Refractory intracranial hypertension and "second-tier" therapies in traumatic brain injury. Intensive Care Med. 2008;34(3):461–7.
71. Hutchinson PJ, Kolias AG, Timofeev IS, Corteen EA, Czosnyka M, Timothy J, et al. Trial of decompressive craniectomy for traumatic intracranial hypertension. N Engl J Med. 2016;375(12):1119–30.
72. Smith M. Refractory intracranial hypertension: the role of decompressive craniectomy. Anesth Analg. 2017;125(6):1999–2008.
73. Gopalakrishnan MS, Shanbhag NC, Shukla DP, Konar SK, Bhat DI, Devi BI. Complications of decompressive craniectomy. Front Neurol. 2018;9:977.

Definition, Pathomechanism of the Thoracic Compartment Syndrome

4

Eric M. Shurtleff and Joseph M. Galante

4.1 Introduction

Compartment syndrome can occur in any anatomical compartment when intra-compartmental pressure exceeds the perfusion pressure of the tissue or organ within that compartment [1]. The more common abdominal compartment syndrome is extensively described, and various principles of management are well established. Abdominal compartment syndrome manifests clinically with increased peak airway pressures, hypotension due to decreased venous return to the heart via a compressed inferior vena cava, increased bladder pressure, and renal impairment. Thoracic compartment syndrome (TCS) is simply this same pathophysiology in the mediastinum, pericardium, or pleural space(s). TCS can result from massive resuscitation or secondary to injuries such as tension pneumothorax or pericardial tamponade.

Tension pneumothorax clearly illustrates the basic pathophysiology underlying TCS: increased intrathoracic pressure compromises venous inflow into the right heart, subsequently decreasing blood flow through the pulmonary vasculature into the left heart, resulting in cardiopulmonary collapse.

TCS due to sternotomy or thoracotomy closure is among the most elusive of the TCSs, but when present has profound effects on clinical course and patient survival. While similar in terms of venous inflow compromise to abdominal compartment syndrome, TCS due to chest closure is a rare clinical entity, and its management is not well defined. This type of TCS is most prevalent in cardiothoracic and pediatric surgery, however still relatively rare, with approximately 200 cases reported in the

E. M. Shurtleff
Maine Medical Partners Acute Care Surgery, Portland, ME, USA
e-mail: emshurtleff@ucdavis.edu

J. M. Galante (✉)
University of California, Davis, UC Davis Medical Center, Sacramento, CA, USA
e-mail: jmgalante@ucdavis.edu

© Springer Nature Switzerland AG 2021
F. Coccolini et al. (eds.), *Compartment Syndrome*, Hot Topics in Acute Care
Surgery and Trauma, https://doi.org/10.1007/978-3-030-55378-4_4

adult cardiothoracic literature. The overall incidence of delayed sternal or thoracotomy closure, a primary risk factor for thoracic compartment syndrome, is estimated at 1.5–2.8% in the adult cardiothoracic surgery population [2].

In cardiothoracic surgery, TCS typically presents with increasing airway pressures and tamponade physiology on attempted chest closure. This phenomenon is not unique to non-traumatic cardiothoracic surgery and may develop in attempted chest closure for traumatic injury as well, particularly in cases where myocardial and pulmonary edema are present. Additionally, TCS may not develop at the time of operation, but can present hours to days postoperatively [2].

4.2   Definition of Thoracic Compartment Syndrome

Thoracic compartment syndrome (TCS) is defined as any process by which increased pressure in the mediastinum, pericardium, or pleural space(s) compromises tissue and organ perfusion within that space. Multiple spaces within the thorax may be affected simultaneously. It is similar to abdominal compartment syndrome (ACS) in that increased compartmental pressure compromises blood flow through a large venous conduit, i.e., the inferior vena cava is compressed in ACS, and both the inferior and superior vena cavae are compressed in TCS, leading in both cases to severely decreased blood flow.

In general, traumatic TCS is precipitated by tension pneumothorax, pericardial tamponade, or myocardial edema, illustrated in Fig. 4.1; the hemodynamic effects of these processes are quite similar. In fact, the hemodynamic changes seen in pericardial tamponade and in myocardial edema are essentially the same, but differ in etiology and the thoracic compartments involved: in pericardial tamponade the pericardial compartment is primarily involved, while in myocardial edema there is typically more generalized elevation of the mediastinal, pericardial, and hemi-thoracic compartments. There are a few significant differences that delineate tension pneumothorax from pericardial tamponade and myocardial edema. One significant difference is that the pulmonary artery pressure is elevated in tension pneumothorax, while in

Hemodynamic parameter (normal values)	Heart rate (80 BPM)	Cardiac output (4–6 L/min)	Cardiac index (2.5–4 L/min)	Central venous and right atrial pressure (5–7 mmHg)	Systemic vascular resistance (800–1100)	Pulmonary artery (15 mmHg)	Left atrial wedge (7–10 mmHg)
Tension pneumothorax	↑	↓	↓	↑↑	↑	↑↑	↑↓
Pericardial tamponade	↑	↓	↓	↑↑	↑	↓	↑
Myocardial edema	↑	↓	↓	↑↑	↑	↑↑	↑

Fig. 4.1 Pathophysiologic alterations in thoracic compartment syndrome

pericardial tamponade and myocardial edema it is decreased. This occurs because in tamponade and myocardial edema the entire heart is externally compressed and the right ventricular ejection fraction is low, whereas in tension pneumothorax, compression of the lung induces marked pulmonary hypertension and compromises compliance of the pulmonary vasculature. A second difference is that in pericardial tamponade and myocardial edema, the left atrial wedge pressure is elevated, while in tension pneumothorax it can be elevated or decreased. This is due again to direct external compression of the heart seen in pericardial tamponade and myocardial edema, whereas in tension pneumothorax there is poor left heart filling due to decreased pulmonary vascular flow in addition to external compression.

4.3   Pathophysiology of TCS

In its simplest form, TCS is compressive compromise of venous return. The pathophysiology of tension pneumothorax arises primarily from this loss of venous inflow into the chest. In tension pneumothorax, increased hemi-thoracic pressure shifts the heart and mediastinum to the contralateral side, which compresses the inferior and superior vena cavae, compromising right atrial and ventricular filling and therefore end diastolic volumes. Collapse of the ipsilateral lung and compression of the contralateral lung increase pulmonary vascular resistance, impeding right ventricular outflow. This combination of pressure effects—inferior and superior vena cavae compression, increased pulmonary vascular resistance, and decreased right atrial and ventricular volumes—results in profoundly decreased right ventricular output. Compromised right cardiac output results in impaired pulmonary vascular filling and flow, which manifests in the left heart as markedly decreased left atrial filling volume. The increased intrathoracic pressure also adversely affects left atrial volume (Fig. 4.2) [3].

In pericardial tamponade (and in myocardial edema), venous return is also compromised by compression of the superior and inferior vena cavae, but in addition there is twofold compression of both ventricles and subsequent impaired myocardial perfusion. Vena cava compression significantly decreases right heart output by restricting blood volume flow into the right atrium. External compression of the right ventricle further limits the volume of blood that can be delivered into the pulmonary vasculature, which in turn decreases left atrial filling volumes and therefore left ventricular output, with concomitant external compression of both chambers by pericardial fluid. The resultant decreased cardiac output leads to decreased blood pressure, coronary perfusion, and myocardial ischemia [3].

Myocardial edema due to acute ventricular dilatation, often coupled with traumatic pulmonary edema, can cause elevated compartmental pressures in the pericardium, mediastinum, and involved hemithorax [4]. In this setting, attempts to close the chest can induce tamponade physiology. Pulmonary edema increases mediastinal pressure, and, coupled with increased cardiac size due to edematous ventricular dilatation causes what is essentially pericardial and mediastinal loss of domain. This was first described in 1975 by Rahi et al. as "tight mediastinum" following prolonged cardiothoracic surgeries [5]. Attempts to return the heart to the pericardium

Fig. 4.2 Right-sided
tension pneumothorax: The
image demonstrates
marked mediastinal shift
away from the affected
right hemithorax, including
the superior vena cava
(SVC), an inferior vena
cava (IVC), total collapse
of the ipsilateral lung, and
compression of the
contralateral lung

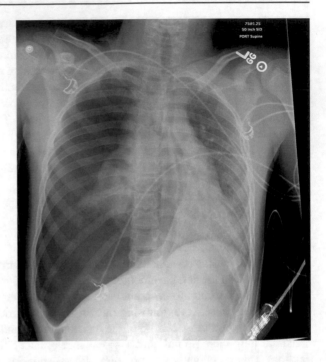

and to reduce the mediastinum cause decreased venous inflow from the superior and inferior vena cavae, which reduces diastolic volumes, compromising cardiac output, and precipitating hemodynamic collapse [4, 6].

The primary causes of prolonged open thoracotomy or sternotomy in cardiothoracic surgery are coagulopathy and uncontrolled bleeding, followed by cardiomegaly, decreased pulmonary compliance, and edema [4]. These processes are certainly present in chest injury, and case reports of traumatic TCS are consistent with the major causes of TCS described in the cardiothoracic literature [4, 6]. An additional factor seen in trauma that contributes to TCS and failure to close the chest is the massive resuscitation typically required in severe chest injury. The relative paucity of traumatic TCS case reports attests to the injury severity sustained by these patients, with their high mortality likely precluding even an attempt at delayed thoracic closure [4].

While management of traumatic TCS is evolving, several principles of abdominal compartment syndrome management do generalize to TCS. Stabilization and improvement of cardiac output, normalizing cardiac filling pressures and improving lung function prior to an attempt at thoracic closure are critical, as well as stabilizing other failing organ systems. Once this has been achieved, minimizing edema and volume overload in the massively resuscitated patient with aggressive diuresis or renal replacement therapy is critical [2]. Detailed descriptions of the technical aspects of thoracic closure in the face of TCS are beyond the scope of this chapter, but commonly used methods are skin flap closure over the sternotomy without fixation and synthetic prosthesis interposition if TCS prevents re-approximation of the sternum or thoracotomy [2].

4.4 Conclusion

TCS in trauma is a life-threatening process with a spectrum of etiologies, including tension pneumothorax, pericardial tamponade, myocardial, and pulmonary edema. Compression of venous return is the essential pathophysiology underlying all of the TCS causes listed above. TCS in trauma is associated with high injury severity and overall mortality. Current management involves emergent tube thoracostomy for tension pneumothorax, pericardial decompression via pericardiotomy, and thoracic skin closure without fixation of the sternum with or without prosthetic for tamponade on attempted chest closure, induced by myocardial and pulmonary edema. Ultimately, as with all compartment syndromes, TCS will persist until the underlying pathophysiology is treated.

References

1. Hurst JM, Fowl RJ. Vascular surgery and trauma. In: Civetta JM, Taylor RW, Kirby RR, editors. Critical care. 2nd ed. Philadelphia: J. B. Lippincott; 1992. p. 707–24.
2. Rizzo AG, Sample GA. Thoracic compartment syndrome secondary to a thoracic procedure. Chest. 2003;124:1164–8.
3. Blaisdell WF, Trunkey DD. Cardiovascular pathophysiology. In: Blaisdell WF, Trunkey DD, editors. Cervicothoracic trauma. 2nd ed. New York: Thieme Medical Publishers; 1994. p. 19–25.
4. Kaplan LJ, Trooskin SZ, Santora TA. Thoracic compartment syndrome. J Trauma Injury Infect Crit Care. 1996;40(2):29.
5. Rahi M, Tomatis LA, Schlosser RJ, et al. Cardiac compression due to closure of median sternotomy in open-heart surgery. Chest. 1975;67:113–4.
6. Wandling MW, An GC. A case report of thoracic compartment syndrome in the setting of penetrating chest trauma and review of the literature. World J Emerg Surg. 2010;5(22):1–5.

Thoracic Compartment Syndrome and Damage Control Surgery in Thoracic Trauma

5

Navjit Dharampal and Colin Schieman

5.1   Thoracic Compartment Syndrome

Compartment syndrome is a well-described phenomenon originally reported in the osteofascial space in orthopedic injuries [1]. It represents a process wherein tissue pressure exceeds capillary perfusion pressure within a confined anatomic space with resultant ischemia, necrosis, and organ dysfunction [2]. This process can occur in any body cavity constrained by fascia, including the abdomen, thorax, and extremities [2, 3]. The occurrence of this syndrome in the thoracic cavity was originally described in 1975 as a "tight mediastinum" following prolonged cardiac surgery [4]. It was later described in the trauma population secondary to a gunshot wound through the thorax [5].

By definition, thoracic compartment syndrome (TCS) implies an increase in intrathoracic pressure beyond tissue capillary perfusion pressure to the intrathoracic structures, such as the lungs, heart, and esophagus, with resultant organ ischemia and dysfunction. The syndrome may be manifested by increased peak, plateau, and mean airway pressures and decreased chest wall compliance [2, 6]. There are two main etiologies. Firstly, prolonged cardiac surgery may cause myocardial edema, mediastinal hematoma, pulmonary edema, or acute ventricular dilation, which results in cardiac tamponade physiology. Secondly, TCS may be precipitated by an accumulation of air or fluid within the thoracic cavity either by trauma, iatrogenic causes, or spontaneously.

The first description of TSC was originally published by Riahi et al. in 1975 [4]. They described the development of cardiac tamponade following closure of the sternum at the conclusion of prolonged open-heart surgery, most commonly in patients undergoing valvular procedures in the setting of cardiomegaly. Closure precipitated a decrease in arterial blood pressure and an increase in central venous pressure,

N. Dharampal · C. Schieman (✉)
University of Calgary, Calgary, AB, Canada
e-mail: Colin.schieman@albertahealthservices.ca

© Springer Nature Switzerland AG 2021
F. Coccolini et al. (eds.), *Compartment Syndrome*, Hot Topics in Acute Care
Surgery and Trauma, https://doi.org/10.1007/978-3-030-55378-4_5

which reversed by reopening of the sternum. They further describe resolution of hemodynamic instability with reopening of the sternum and delayed closure. Since this early description, TCS has been reported in adults and children undergoing cardiac surgery [3]. The mainstay of management of these patients has been an open chest with delayed closure. Initial concerns regarding mediastinal infections and sternal complication have been abated by low incidence rates [7–9].

TCS was first described in the non-cardiac surgery population in 1996 [5]. A case report by Kaplan et al. presented a 15-year-old male who sustained a single gunshot wound (GSW) to the left back and required a resuscitative left anterolateral thoracotomy, which was extended to a clamshell incision. The patients underwent evacuation of left hemothorax, evacuation of tense hemopericardium, and repair of two cardiac wounds in the emergency department, all while receiving open cardiac massage, massive transfusion of blood products, and vasopressor support. Eventually the patient was transferred to the operating room for definitive repair of an ascending aortic arch injury. At the cessation of the procedure, it was noted the patient's tissues were very edematous, secondary to local trauma, cardiac massage, cardiac defibrillation, and massive volume resuscitation. At time of closure of the left thoracotomy, the patient's arterial saturation dropped to 52%, mean and peak airway pressure increased dramatically leading to hypotension and asystole. The chest was emergently reopened and sinus rhythm was achieved. However, a second attempt at closure led to recurrence of hemodynamic collapse. Due to an inability to safely close the chest, the patient was taken to the ICU with packing in place for further resuscitation and correction of metabolic abnormalities. The patient underwent delayed closure of the chest once his core temperature, blood lactate level, and coagulation profile had returned to normal.

Although additional reports of noncardiac surgery-related TCS have been published, thoracic compartment syndrome still remains a rare entity in trauma patients [10–12]. This is likely due to high mortality rates associated with severe thoracic injuries [6]. The mainstay of management of the rare entity TCS in the trauma patient involves immediate decompression of the thoracic cavity and delayed closure.

5.2   Damage Control Surgery in Thoracic Trauma

5.2.1   Damage Control Surgery

The lethal triad of acidosis, coagulopathy, and hypothermia has long been recognized to increase the risk of mortality in severely injured trauma patients [13]. Traditionally patients would undergo prolonged procedures to identify and repair all injuries at a single operation. Many of these patients, however, would die in the operating room or in the intensive care unit (ICU) secondary to physiological derangements. In an attempt to avoid lengthy operations in hemodynamically unstable patients who have sustained significant blood loss, surgical management of these patients has evolved from a single extended, definitive operation to a staged approach allowing for appropriate resuscitation known as damage control surgery

(DCS) [14–16]. A common definition of DCS is a "multistep operative intervention, which included a brief initial surgical procedure that aimed to control mechanical bleeding, a massive air leak, and/or gross contamination" [17].

The core principle of DCS is to identify and address only life-threatening injuries in an abbreviated manner at the time of index operation and delay treatment of non-life-threatening injuries in severely injured patients until a later operation while they undergo correction of blood loss, coagulopathy, hypothermia, and acidosis [18]. Application of DCS has most commonly been for patients with major abdominal trauma and has resulted in marked improvement in mortality rates [15, 19, 20]. The specific stages for DCS and their objectives have been well outlined in literature [21–24]. Stage 1 (DC1) involves immediate laparotomy for control of exsanguination and contamination. In stage 2 (DC2), patients are transferred to the ICU to address hemodynamics and physiologic derangements. In stage 3 (DC3), patients undergo single or multiple reoperations for definitive management of abdominal injuries, management of non-life-threatening injuries, and closure of the abdomen.

5.2.2 History of Damage Control Surgery in Thoracic Trauma

The concepts established in abdominal DCS can also be applied in the thoracic cavity; however, the principles and objectives of thoracic damage control surgery (TDCS) have not been as clearly defined. The principles of rapid control of exsanguination, control of contamination, and temporary closure are similar in the two cavities. In the abdomen, DCS focusses on temporizing injuries with delayed definitive management, such rapid division and excision of bowel with re-anastomosis at a later operation. In the chest, however, the emphasis is on performing quick and simple definitive procedures that immediately threaten the patient's life in lieu of more complex anatomic resections. Rapid management of thoracic injuries was first described 1994 [14, 25]. Maneuvers to quickly address thoracic injuries in hemodynamically and physiologically stressed patients included packing of the pleural cavity and nonanatomic pulmonary parenchymal resections [26, 27]. Over the next few years, additional reports described pulmonary tractotomy and hilar twist procedures. Currently, there are a variety of damage control techniques that can be applied to thoracic injuries in polytrauma patients; these are outlined in Table 5.1.

Table 5.1 Interventions in damage control surgery for thoracic trauma	Pneumonorrhaphy
	Pulmonary tractotomy
	Pulmonary wedge resection
	Rapid, simultaneously staple pneumonectomy
	Drainage of esophagus and pleural space
	Mediastinal packing
	Pleural packing
	Temporary thoracic closure

5.2.3 Objectives of Damage Control Surgery in Thoracic Trauma

The purpose of damage control in the thoracic cavity is similar to DCS in the abdominal cavity: management of life-threatening injuries in an abbreviated fashion to facilitate adequate resuscitation and normalization of metabolic status in the ICU. The objectives fall into three main categories:

1. Cessation of hemorrhage
2. Control of hollow viscus injuries
3. Intrathoracic packing and temporary closure

5.2.4 Methods of Damage Control Surgery in Thoracic Trauma

5.2.4.1 Incisions and Gaining Access to the Chest

For a multitude of reasons, deciding upon the most suitable incision and approach for major thoracic injuries can at first seem challenging. Patients are often in extremis, there are often competing injuries, patients are positioned supine, there may be hemoptysis, lung isolation is not present, surgeon comfort with thoracotomies, intrathoracic anatomy and the associated instruments is often lacking. As a general rule, we advocate making a large anterior thoracotomy in approximately the fourth or fifth interspace in the inframammary crease, with liberal use of a transverse sternotomy with a saw or knife extended into a clamshell if required. This is typically done on the left and then extended to the right, but clearly it should be placed on the side suspected of harboring greatest injury [28]. The clamshell incision allows for a generous exposure to most intrathoracic structures. The median sternotomy should be reserved for cases wherein the surgeon has a high degree of confidence of a mediastinal or cardiac injury as it is limited by poor exposure to the remaining thorax. A posterior thoracotomy, although superb for elective intrathoracic exposure, is generally not appropriate for the critically ill and undifferentiated major thoracic trauma patient. It adds a layer of complexity and risk that is rarely appropriate.

5.2.4.2 Lung Parenchymal Injuries

Patients with serious parenchymal injuries may present with a hemothorax and varying degrees of hemodynamic instability. Patients necessitating an operative intervention will likely have a massive hemothorax apparent on chest X-ray or profuse bleeding from a thoracostomy tube. Upon entry into the chest, the initial objective should be rapid evacuation of blood followed by identification of bleeding.

A variety of surgical techniques are available to tackle lung parenchymal injuries. In a polytrauma patient, the objective should be to expediently address the injury with minimal disruption to normal lung tissue. Possible maneuvers include pneumonorrhaphy, pulmonary tractotomy, pulmonary wedge resection, packing, and rapid, simultaneously stapled pneumonectomy [29].

Pneumonorrhaphy describes the process of ligating injured vessels or small bronchi within the lung parenchyma [30]. Firstly, the lung must be stabilized in some fashion, such as with atraumatic lung clamps, such as Duval lung clamps. Secondly, gentle retraction and suction within the injury may expose bleeding vessels and leaking bronchi. These can be subsequently ligated using absorbable suture. Finally, edges of the parenchymal wound are approximated with a running suture. Often the injured surface bleeds diffusely, and simple en masse ligation with a running monofilament absorbable suture is most effective.

Pulmonary tractotomy is a surgical technique to manage through-and-through penetrating injuries of the lung parenchyma [30–33]. The first step in performing a tractotomy is to identify the entry and exit wounds of the penetrating injury. Atraumatic Duval lung clamps are placed parallel to the injury tract. The intraparenchymal component of the injury is then exposed by placing and firing a cutting linear stapler through the opening of the tract. The exposed parenchyma should subsequently be inspected for bleeding and air leaks, which should be ligated individually. Once the bleeding vessels and air leaks are controlled, the previously divided lung can be left splayed open or reapproximated with a running suture. This is one of the most commonly performed DCS maneuver in major trauma centers [26, 27].

Pulmonary wedge resection represents nonanatomic sublobar resections [29, 34, 35]. This procedure can be accomplished quickly with a cutting linear stapler. The injured parenchyma is identified by localizing bleeding or air leak. The involved lung is quickly transected and resected with adequate control of bleeding and air leak. This procedure is most appropriate for superficial parenchymal injuries; however, some deeper injuries may also be managed with a wedge resection. For injuries requiring a large sublobar resection, it is imperative to inspect the staple line for hemostasis and pneumostasis. In extreme cases, where the injury extends into the center of an anatomic lobe, a rapidly stapled deep wedge resection/lobectomy can be utilized. Unfortunately, the lung parenchyma in these situations are often congested, fragile, and under positive pressure ventilation, limiting the compressibility for the stapler cartridge to be safely applied.

A rapid, simultaneously stapled pneumonectomy is also often called a "trauma pneumonectomy" [36]. This is in contrast to an anatomic pneumonectomy performed in an elective setting, whereby all arterial, venous, and bronchial structure are identified, isolated, and individually ligated. In a trauma pneumonectomy, the mainstem bronchus, the mainstem pulmonary artery, and the superior and inferior pulmonary veins are controlled en bloc with a single right-angle stapler cartridge. This dramatic procedure should be reserved for patients in extremis who have failed lung sparing surgical techniques as the mortality rates may be prohibitively high [37]. The high mortality from a trauma pneumonectomy is likely multifactorial in etiology. Patients may have decompensated significantly while the surgeons attempt lung sparing techniques of managing parenchymal injuries. Also, ligation of the pulmonary artery may lead to dramatic right heart failure and cardiovascular collapse [38].

5.2.4.3 Hilar Injuries

Hilar injuries are associated with high mortality rates. Patients who present to the emergency department will often be in extremis due to massive blood loss into the ipsilateral pleural space or pericardial tamponade depending on the proximity of the injury [39]. Initial operative management involves evacuation of blood. In the case of intrapericardial bleeding, an immediate pericardiotomy is required. Manual compression of hilar bleeding is crucial. Once the bleeding is temporarily controlled, the surgeon must assess the injury to ascertain the extent of repair or resection required. If possible, a proximal cross clamp of the hilum to facilitate repair, or an emergency stapled pneumonectomy should be carried out without delay.

5.2.4.4 Cardiac

The severity of cardiac trauma can range widely [40, 41]. Blunt cardiac injuries are often mild and managed conservatively. Patients with penetrating cardiac trauma, however, are usually dead at the scene or present in extremis. The clinical presentation depends on whether the patient has cardiac tamponade due to bleeding into the pericardial sac or shock secondary to blood loss into the pleural space. These patients often require emergent operative intervention, usually via a resuscitative left anterolateral thoracotomy which may be extended into a clamshell incision.

Upon entry into the chest, a pericardiotomy should be performed taking care to avoid the phrenic nerve [40]. Once tamponade has been relieved, the heart should be inspected for injuries. Manual control of bleeding can be immediately accomplished by placing a finger over the injury site. A mechanism of temporary hemorrhage control includes placement of a Foley catheter into the wound with inflation and gentle traction of the balloon to occlude the wound. When placed into the atria, the Foley catheter may also be used for quick infusion of fluids and blood products. A skin stapler can also be used to rapidly approximate myocardial tissue. Once the patient is stabilized, cardiac wounds should be repaired with pledgeted, nonabsorbable sutures taking care to avoid coronary vessels. In the case of ventricular septal defects, repair should not be attempted at the index operation as the repair may be complex, and a majority of these may close spontaneously [40, 42].

Injuries to coronary arteries are particularly difficult to treat. Patients may present with cardiac tamponade or myocardial infarction. Bleeding from a laceration of distal coronary vessel should be managed with ligation of the vessel in a damage control setting [43]. Injury to a proximal artery, especially in the setting of myocardial infarction, is a challenging problem and will require expertise of a cardiac surgeon [44]. Repair of these injuries is ideally via coronary artery bypass. An additional layer of complexity in decision-making is introduced if the patient's hemodynamic instability is due to myocardial infarction, in which case the patient should be placed on cardiopulmonary bypass to facilitate definitive repair. This requires systemic anticoagulation and may not be feasible in a massively injured patient. Coronary injuries and repair can be associated with mortality rates up to 40% [45].

5.2.4.5 Chest Wall

Damage control surgery for the chest wall can be divided into two categories: management of chest wall bleeding and temporary closure of the chest wall [39].

Chest wall bleeding can occur from several sources. When patients are in profound shock, the source of bleeding from the chest wall may not be clearly visible.

For example, injured intercostal or internal mammary vessels may only bleed once the patient has been resuscitated. Regardless, initial attempts should be made identify and ligate the culprit vessel on the chest wall. In instances where the vessel has retracted, a "U"-stitch can be placed around the rib to occlude the vessel at multiple points. In the cases of tissue loss, a Foley or Fogarty catheter can be placed and inflated to tamponade the bleeding vessel. When localized measures fail and the patient in decompensating from a metabolic stand point, thoracic packing may be appropriate [46]. This may be particularly helpful in difficult areas of the thoracic cavity such as the apex and the paravertebral space [47]. Placement of thoracic packing requires temporary closure of the chest and a relook thoracotomy [27].

Several techniques have been described to temporarily close the chest wall. Options include packing the chest with gauze pads and leave an open wound, closing the chest with a Silastic sheet, with or without intrathoracic packing, or closing the skin incision alone with or without packing. The clinical indications for performing any of these maneuvers can include the surgeon's discretion for the requirement of a second-look thoracotomy, the development of thoracic compartment syndrome upon attempted closure of the thoracic cavity, or the patient exhibiting evidence of metabolic exhaustion. The mortality and morbidity of these patients can be quite high. In a case series of 11 patients undergoing abbreviated thoracotomy with temporary closure of the chest wall, 4 patients died in the ICU within 24 h and 7 survived [46]. Complications occurred in 100% of patients and included pneumonia, empyema, wound infection, and one occurrence of mediastinitis. The authors note the patient with mediastinitis had a dehiscence of an esophageal repair and was likely not related to the temporary chest wall closure. All seven who survived the initial 24 h were discharged from the hospital.

5.2.4.6 Esophagus

Traumatic thoracic esophageal injuries are quite rare, occurring almost exclusively in the setting of penetrating thoracic trauma [48]. In ideal circumstances, an esophageal injury is identified and repaired primarily. However, in the setting of a hemodynamically and metabolically challenged patient, this may not be the best option if simple sutures are inadequate. The DCS strategy of managing a traumatic esophageal injuries includes wide drainage of the pleural space and placement of a nasoesophageal tube for decompression [24]. Definitive repair can be completed during phase 3 of DCS. At the time of ultimate closure, thoughtful consideration must be given to the placement of a feeding jejunostomy tube to allow time for healing.

5.2.4.7 Diaphragm

Diaphragm injuries are unlikely to be the cause of hemodynamic instability. Instead, they may occur concurrently with other life-threatening injuries in a damage control setting. As such, surgeons should primarily address injuries that may lead to exsanguination or contamination initially. Once the patient has been stabilized, the diaphragm can be repaired in a non-emergent fashion.

Table 5.2 Indications for damage control surgery maneuvers in thoracic trauma[a]

Rapid lung sparing surgery
- This should always be the initial goal for parenchymal lung injuries, if possible
- Whenever emergent thoracotomy is indicated for thoracic trauma

Pulmonary tractotomy
- Penetrating through-and-through parenchymal injury not involving hilar structures AND hemodynamic instability in the OR

Rapid, simultaneous stapled pneumonectomy
- Irreparable central hilar vascular injury, main bronchial injury, AND hemodynamic instability in the OR

Therapeutic mediastinal/pleural space packing
- Coagulopathy in the OR
- Hypothermia AND coagulopathy in the OR
- Hypothermia, acidosis, AND coagulopathy in the OR
- Inability to control bleeding with conventional methods

Temporary thoracic closure
- Signs of thoracic compartment syndrome[b] during attempted closure
- Need to reassess intrathoracic organs in delayed fashion such as temporary packing
- Hypothermia, acidosis, AND coagulopathy in the OR

[a]Adapted from Roberts DJ, Bobrovitz N, Zygun DA, et al. Indications for use of thoracic, abdominal, pelvic, and vascular damage control interventions in trauma patients: A content analysis and expert appropriateness rating study. *The journal of trauma and acute care surgery.* 2015;79(4):568–579
[b]Sudden cardiopulmonary failure, hemodynamic instability, or increased airway pressure resulting in difficulty with ventilation

5.2.5 Indications for Damage Control Surgery in Thoracic Trauma

Once the benefits of DCS in abdominal trauma were well established, it was touted as the gold standard of management of patients with severe and multiple injuries [15]. It underwent widespread recommendation by trauma surgical societies and textbooks leading to a consequent extensive adoption by the early 2000s [14]. Recent studies, however, have examined its universally applicability, particularly in the setting improved resuscitation practices, and have reported over-utilization of DCS techniques [49]. These reports highlight the need for patient selection to appropriately manage patients with damage control principles in order to minimize complications related to DCS. Currently there are no clear guidelines regarding the indications for DCS in thoracic trauma. Expert opinion, however, suggests the indications included in Table 5.2 as appropriate for thoracic DCS [29].

References

1. Haljamäe H, Enger E. Human skeletal muscle energy metabolism during and after complete tourniquet ischemia. Ann Surg. 1975;182(1):9–14.
2. Saber A. Compartment syndromes. J Acute Dis. 2014;3(3):169–77.
3. Balogh ZJ, Butcher NE. Compartment syndromes from head to toe. Crit Care Med. 2010;38(9 Suppl):S445–51.

4. Riahi M, Tomatis LA, Schlosser RJ, Bertolozzi E, Johnston DW. Cardiac compression due to closure of the median sternotomy in open heart surgery. Chest. 1975;67(1):113–4.
5. Kaplan LJ, Trooskin SZ, Santora TA. Thoracic compartment syndrome. J Trauma. 1996;40(2):291–3.
6. Malbrain MLNG, Roberts DJ, Sugrue M, De Keulenaer BL, Ivatury R, Pelosi P, et al. The polycompartment syndrome: a concise state-of-the-art review. Anestezjol Intens Ter. 2014;46(5):433–50.
7. Boeken U, Assmann A, Mehdiani A, Akhyari P, Lichtenberg A. Open chest management after cardiac operations: outcome and timing of delayed sternal closure. Eur J Cardiothorac Surg. 2011;40(5):1146–50.
8. Hashemzadeh K, Hashemzadeh S. In-hospital outcomes of delayed sternal closure after open cardiac surgery. J Card Surg. 2009;24(1):30–3.
9. Mestres CA, Pomar JL, Acosta M, Ninot S, Barriuso C, Abad C, et al. Delayed sternal closure for life-threatening complications in cardiac operations: an update. Ann Thorac Surg. 1991;51(5):773–6.
10. Rizzo AG, Sample GA. Thoracic compartment syndrome secondary to a thoracic procedure: a case report. Chest. 2003;124(3):1164–8.
11. Wandling MW, An GC. A case report of thoracic compartment syndrome in the setting of penetrating chest trauma and review of the literature. World J Emerg Surg. 2010;5(1):22.
12. Parra MW, Rodas EB, Bartnik JP, Puente I. Surviving a delayed trans-diaphragmatic hepatic rupture complicated by an acute superior vena cava and thoracic compartment syndromes. J Emerg Trauma Shock. 2011;4(3):425–6.
13. Mikhail J. The trauma triad of death: hypothermia, acidosis, and coagulopathy. AACN Clin Issues. 1999;10(1):85–94.
14. Roberts DJ, Ball CG, Feliciano DV, Moore EE, Ivatury RR, Lucas CE, et al. History of the innovation of damage control for management of trauma patients. Ann Surg. 2017;265(5):1034–44.
15. Rotondo MF, Schwab CW, McGonigal MD, Phillips GR 3rd, Fruchterman TM, Kauder DR, et al. 'Damage control': an approach for improved survival in exsanguinating penetrating abdominal injury. J Trauma. 1993;35(3):375–82; discussion 82–3.
16. Moore EE, Burch JM, Franciose RJ, Offner PJ, Biffl WL. Staged physiologic restoration and damage control surgery. World J Surg. 1998;22(12):1184–91.
17. Roberts DJ, Bobrovitz N, Zygun DA, Ball CG, Kirkpatrick AW, Faris PD, et al. Indications for use of damage control surgery and damage control interventions in civilian trauma patients: a scoping review. J Trauma Acute Care Surg. 2015;78(6):1187–96.
18. Shapiro MB, Jenkins DH, Schwab CW, Rotondo MF. Damage control: collective review. J Trauma. 2000;49(5):969–78.
19. Kauvar DS, Lefering R, Wade CE. Impact of hemorrhage on trauma outcome: an overview of epidemiology, clinical presentations, and therapeutic considerations. J Trauma. 2006;60(6 Suppl):S3–11.
20. Johnson JW, Gracias VH, Schwab CW, Reilly PM, Kauder DR, Shapiro MB, et al. Evolution in damage control for exsanguinating penetrating abdominal injury. J Trauma. 2001;51(2):261–9; discussion 9–71.
21. Sugrue M, D'Amours SK, Joshipura M. Damage control surgery and the abdomen. Injury. 2004;35(7):642–8.
22. Hoey BA, Schwab CW. Damage control surgery. Scand J Surg. 2002;91(1):92–103.
23. Bashir MM, Abu-Zidan FM. Damage control surgery for abdominal trauma. Eur J Surg Suppl: Acta Chir Suppl. 2003;(588):8–13.
24. Chovanes J, Cannon JW, Nunez TC. The evolution of damage control surgery. Surg Clin North Am. 2012;92(4):859–75.
25. Hirshberg A, Wall MJ Jr, Mattox KL. Planned reoperation for trauma: a two year experience with 124 consecutive patients. J Trauma. 1994;37(3):365–9.
26. Garcia A, Martinez J, Rodriguez J, Millan M, Valderrama G, Ordoñez C, et al. Damage-control techniques in the management of severe lung trauma. J Trauma Acute Care Surg. 2015;78(1):45–51.

27. O'Connor JV, DuBose JJ, Scalea TM. Damage-control thoracic surgery: management and outcomes. J Trauma Acute Care Surg. 2014;77(5):660–5.
28. Hunt PA, Greaves I, Owens WA. Emergency thoracotomy in thoracic trauma—a review. Injury. 2006;37(1):1–19.
29. Roberts DJ, Bobrovitz N, Zygun DA, Ball CG, Kirkpatrick AW, Faris PD, et al. Indications for use of thoracic, abdominal, pelvic, and vascular damage control interventions in trauma patients: a content analysis and expert appropriateness rating study. J Trauma Acute Care Surg. 2015;79(4):568–79.
30. Petrone P, Asensio JA. Surgical management of penetrating pulmonary injuries. Scand J Trauma Resusc Emerg Med. 2009;17(1):8.
31. Wall MJ, Granchi T, Liscum K, Mattox KL. Penetrating thoracic vascular injuries. Surg Clin North Am. 1996;76(4):749–61.
32. Wall MJ Jr, Hirshberg A, Mattox KL. Pulmonary tractotomy with selective vascular ligation for penetrating injuries to the lung. Am J Surg. 1994;168(6):665–9.
33. Asensio JA, Demetriades D, Berne JD, Velmahos G, Cornwell EE, Murray J, et al. Stapled pulmonary tractotomy: a rapid way to control hemorrhage in penetrating pulmonary injuries. J Am Coll Surg. 1997;185(5):486–7.
34. Velmahos GC. Lung-sparing surgery after penetrating trauma using tractotomy, partial lobectomy, and pneumonorrhaphy. Arch Surg. 1999;134(2):186.
35. Wall MJ Jr, Soltero E. Damage control for thoracic injuries. Surg Clin North Am. 1997;77(4):863–78.
36. Wagner JW, Obeid FN, Karmy-Jones RC, Casey GD, Sorensen VJ, Horst HM. Trauma pneumonectomy revisited: the role of simultaneously stapled pneumonectomy. J Trauma. 1996;40(4):590–4.
37. Phillips B, Turco L, Mirzaie M, Fernandez C. Trauma pneumonectomy: a narrative review. Int J Surg. 2017;46:71–4.
38. Matsushima K, Aiolfi A, Park C, Rosen D, Strumwasser A, Benjamin E, et al. Surgical outcomes after trauma pneumonectomy: revisited. J Trauma Acute Care Surg. 2017;82(5):927–32.
39. Gonçalves R, Saad R Jr. Thoracic damage control surgery. Rev Col Bras Cir. 2016;43(5):374–81.
40. Embrey R. Cardiac trauma. Thorac Surg Clin. 2007;17(1):87–93.
41. Tyburski JG, Astra L, Wilson RF, Dente C, Steffes C. Factors affecting prognosis with penetrating wounds of the heart. J Trauma. 2000;48(4):587–90; discussion 90–1.
42. Rosenthal A, Parisi LF, Nadas AS. Isolated interventricular septal defect due to nonpenetrating trauma. N Engl J Med. 1970;283(7):338–41.
43. Espada R, Whisennand HH, Mattox KL, Beall AC Jr. Surgical management of penetrating injuries to the coronary arteries. Surgery. 1975;78(6):755–60.
44. Karin E, Greenberg R, Avital S, Aladgem D, Kluger Y. The management of stab wounds to the heart with laceration of the left anterior descending coronary artery. Eur J Emerg Med. 2001;8(4):321–3.
45. Rea WJ, Sugg WL, Wilson LC, Webb WR, Ecker RR. Coronary artery lacerations; an analysis of 22 patients. Ann Thorac Surg. 1969;7(6):518–28.
46. Vargo DJ. Abbreviated thoracotomy and temporary chest closure. Arch Surg. 2001;136(1):21.
47. Moriwaki Y, Toyoda H, Harunari N, Iwashita M, Kosuge T, Arata S, et al. Gauze packing as damage control for uncontrollable haemorrhage in severe thoracic trauma. Ann R Coll Surg Engl. 2013;95(1):20–5.
48. Rotondo MF, Bard MR. Damage control surgery for thoracic injuries. Injury. 2004;35(7):649–54.
49. Hatch QM, Osterhout LM, Podbielski J, Kozar RA, Wade CE, Holcomb JB, et al. Impact of closure at the first take back: complication burden and potential overutilization of damage control laparotomy. J Trauma. 2011;71(6):1503–11.

Definition, Pathophysiology, and Pathobiology of Intra-Abdominal Hypertension and the Abdominal Compartment Syndrome

6

Andrew W. Kirkpatrick, Federico Coccolini, Braedon McDonald, and Derek J. Roberts

6.1 Introduction

Knowing and understanding the effects of intra-abdominal pressure (IAP) are crucial to effectively manage critically ill and injured patients. Raised IAP, known as intra-abdominal hypertension (IAH), appears common in patients suffering from critical illness/injury. The pathophysiological consequences of IAH are complex: nearly every organ system may be affected through contiguous physical (polycompartment phenomenon) or biomediator (humoral and lymphatically-spread) effects. When IAH is sustained above 20 mmHg, and associated with new organ dysfunction, patients are diagnosed with abdominal compartment syndrome (ACS) [1, 2]. Although preventative, medical, and minimally invasive therapies are available, overt ACS is an emergency often warranting use of an open abdomen to decompress the abdominal cavity.

A. W. Kirkpatrick (✉)
Department of Surgery, University of Calgary and the Foothills Medical Centre, Calgary, AB, Canada

Critical Care Medicine, University of Calgary and the Foothills Medical Centre, Calgary, AB, Canada

Regional Trauma Program, University of Calgary and the Foothills Medical Centre, Calgary, AB, Canada
e-mail: Andrew.Kirkpatrick@albertahealthservices.ca

F. Coccolini
General, Emergency and Trauma Surgery Department, Pisa University Hospital, Pisa, Italy

B. McDonald
Department of Critical Care Medicine, Snyder Institute for Chronic Diseases, University of Calgary, Calgary, AB, Canada

D. J. Roberts
The Division of Vascular and Endovascular Surgery, Department of Surgery, University of Ottawa, Ottawa, ON, Canada

© Springer Nature Switzerland AG 2021
F. Coccolini et al. (eds.), *Compartment Syndrome*, Hot Topics in Acute Care Surgery and Trauma, https://doi.org/10.1007/978-3-030-55378-4_6

In 2006, standardized definitions of IAH and ACS were proposed by the WSACS—The Abdominal Compartment Society [3, 4]. Practical working definitions and later evidence-based management guidelines were felt critical to address the complex pathophysiologic challenges induced by these conditions [3, 4]. A notably missing topic from these highly referenced guidelines, however, is discussion of the relationship between IAH and the human microbiome, recognizing that humans are superorganisms, living in symbiosis with their gut microbiota. The symbiotic relationship between a healthy host human and a healthy microbiota within that host is critical for health. Given increasing basic science evidence that even modest IAH for short periods of time profoundly affect gut mucosa permeability, the presence of a dysbiome within a leaky gastrointestinal lining requires urgent study. Thus, the upcoming revisions of the Abdominal Compartment Society Consensus Guidelines will feature efforts to recognize the importance of new concepts regarding the human microbiome in critical illness, but remain grounded in established science.

6.2   Definitions

Internationally accepted definitions of the open abdomen (OA) and ACS are a relatively new phenomenon, for which the former World Society of the Abdominal Compartment Syndrome (WSACS), now the Abdominal Compartment Society (ACS former WSACS), is most responsible for [3, 4]. In 2006, the WSACS first promulgated consensus working definitions to describe standardized measurement techniques and reference standards to define what was considered abnormally high IAP. Further, raised IAP was termed IAH, recognizing that previously there was much controversy as to how to numerically define this, as the literature had variably defined measurements ranging from 12 to 25 mmHg [2].

The WSACS proposed that IAH constituted a gradient from mildly to severely abnormal, and suggested a grading scale ranging from grades I to IV (Table 6.1) [2]. The same year as the first WSACS definitions were published, authors from the Trauma Association of Canada reported that there was no standardization of terminology of the open abdomen, nor accepted guidelines for its use and attempted to survey their members to address these concepts [5, 6]. At this time, the concept known as the OA was previously referred to as laparostomy, temporary abdominal closure (TAC), "eteppenlavage", or simply the "open abdomen" [7–11]. Therefore, the WSACS addressed this issue in 2013, by defining an open abdomen as a case in which a temporary abdominal closure was required due to the skin and fascia not being closed after laparotomy [1].

The challenging mandate of the 2013 WSACS—The Abdominal Compartment Society guidelines was to update the previous highly cited definitions and

Table 6.1 Gradation of IAH as defined by the World Society of the Abdominal Compartment Syndrome	IAH is graded as follows:
	Grade I, IAP 12–15 mmHg
	Grade II, IAP 16–20 mmHg
	Grade III, IAP 21–25 mmHg
	Grade IV, IAP >25 mmHg

guidelines in response to advances in science and practice in order to retain the highest level of relevancy [12]. After an extensive systematic review, and online and face-to-face expert collaboration and debates, only modest changes to the existing definitions were required. In addition to formally defining the open abdomen, other important definitions were given to address important pathophysiological concepts, including lateralization of the abdominal musculature, polycompartment syndrome, abdominal compliance [13], and an improved system of open abdomen classification was given (in order to facilitate prognostication and comparison of cohorts of patients being treated with this technique between studies) [1, 14]. The most recent definitions are summarized in Table 6.2.

Table 6.2 Final 2013 consensus definitions of the World Society of the Abdominal Compartment Syndrome

No.	Definition
Retained definitions from the original 2006 consensus statements [2]	
1.	IAP is the steady-state pressure concealed within the abdominal cavity
2.	The reference standard for intermittent IAP measurements is via the bladder with a maximal instillation volume of 25 mL of sterile saline
3.	IAP should be expressed in mmHg and measured at end expiration in the supine position after ensuring that abdominal muscle contractions are absent and with the transducer zeroed at the level of the midaxillary line
4.	IAP is approximately 5–7 mmHg in critically ill adults
5.	IAH is defined by a sustained or repeated pathological elevation in IAP $\geq$12 mmHg
6.	ACS is defined as a sustained IAP >20 mmHg (with or without an APP <60 mmHg) that is associated with new organ dysfunction/failure

7.	IAH is graded as follows:
	  Grade I, IAP 12–15 mmHg
	  Grade II, IAP 16–20 mmHg
	  Grade III, IAP 21–25 mmHg
	  Grade IV, IAP >25 mmHg

8.	Primary IAH or ACS is a condition associated with injury or disease in the abdominopelvic region that frequently requires early surgical or interventional radiological intervention
9.	Secondary IAH or ACS refers to conditions that do not originate from the abdominopelvic region
10.	Recurrent IAH or ACS refers to the condition in which IAH or ACS redevelops following previous surgical or medical treatment of primary or secondary IAH or ACS
11.	APP = MAP − IAP
New definitions accepted by the 2013 consensus panel	
12.	A polycompartment syndrome is a condition where two or more anatomical compartments have elevated compartmental pressures
13.	Abdominal compliance is a measure of the ease of abdominal expansion, which is determined by the elasticity of the abdominal wall and diaphragm. It should be expressed as the change in intra-abdominal volume per change in IAP
14.	The open abdomen is one that requires a temporary abdominal closure due to the skin and fascia not being closed after laparotomy
15.	Lateralization of the abdominal wall is the phenomenon where the musculature and fascia of the abdominal wall, most exemplified by the rectus abdominis muscles and their enveloping fascia, move laterally away from the midline with time

ACS abdominal compartment syndrome, *APP* abdominal perfusion pressure, *IAH* intra-abdominal hypertension, *IAP* intra-abdominal pressure, *MAP* mean arterial pressure
Reproduced from Kirkpatrick et al. [1]

6.3 Definitions for the Next Decade

While the methodology to derive the optimal guidelines to best define and guide clinical practice regarding IAH/ACS and the open abdomen for the next decade are being formulated now, they will need to incorporate working definitions of patho-biological concepts regarding the microbiome. These include how to define and recognize the existence of a human pathobiome, and ideally how to quantify the degree and speed of transition between a healthy microbiome to a pathobiome, or at least how to begin to study these phenomena (Table 6.3). In health, the human "microbiota" refers to the communities of microbes (both commensal and patho-genic bacteria, viruses, and fungi) that inhabit the human gastrointestinal tract. The term "microbiome" refers to the related genes, gene products (proteins, metabo-lites), their community structure (distribution, diversity, evenness), and the environ-mental characteristics they reside in, and constitute the complete full microbial ecosystem of the body [15]. The microbiome is characterized by a state of symbiotic homeostasis between the host, microbial commensals, and potentially pathogenic bacteria [16]. The composition and ecological structure of the microbiome are con-tinuously evolving in response to environmental pressures (dietary intake, exposure to new microbes, antibiotics, etc.) as well as changes in host physiology [17]. A complex and diversified microbiome is advantageous, and it is important for regu-lating many aspects of host physiology, including immune function, gut mucosal barrier integrity, nutritional and metabolic functions, as well as colonization resis-tance against pathogens/infections [15, 18]. Dysbiosis defines a loss of microbial diversity and community structure that results in dysregulation of these physiologi-cal systems, and the outgrowth and overrepresentation of potentially pathogenic organisms within the gut. Consequently, gut microbiome dysbiosis has been linked to an extensive list of disease states, ranging from gastrointestinal disorders, auto-immunity, and infections, to cancer, metabolic syndrome, and neurological diseases [18, 19]. Severe Dysbiosis defines a state of catastrophic loss of microbial diversity during critical illness/injury [20]. While much remains to be learned about the impact of critical illness and extreme abnormalities of physiology on gut microbi-ome composition and the resulting pathological host–microbial interactions, it is believed that that this process serves as a central driver of critical illness.

Table 6.3 Definitions related to the human microbiome and the pathobiology of intra-abdominal hypertension

Microbiome	Aggregate of all microbiota that reside on or within human tissues and biofluids along with the corresponding anatomical sites in which they reside
Microbiota	Ecological communities of commensal, symbiotic, and pathogenic microorganisms found in and on all multicellular organisms from plants to animals. Microbiota includes bacteria, archaea, protists, fungi, and viruses
Dysbiosis	An imbalance between the types of organism present in a person's natural microflora, especially that of the gut, thought to contribute to a range of conditions of ill health
Severe dysbiosis	Catastrophic loss of microbial diversity during severe critical illness/injury
Holobiont	Assemblages of different species that form ecological units

6.4   Pathophysiology of IAH and ACS

IAH can somewhat simply be equated with a state of malperfusion. ACS therefore represents the extreme end of a pathophysiologic spectrum beginning with normal IAP and proceeding through worsening grades of IAH [1], and thus increasing malperfusion. We prefer the term "overt ACS" to describe a catastrophically ill/injured patient with severe IAH and new onset cardiorespiratory and/or renal failure. Although centered upon the abdominal cavity, the pathophysiology of IAH/ACS affects the entire body physically and biochemically. The effects of IAH/ACS are not limited to the intra-abdominal organs; they are enacted systemically through biomediator generation resulting in multiorgan dysfunction syndrome/multisystem organ failure and/or through polycompartmental pressure interactions [1, 3, 21].

The ACS has long been simplified as a physical phenomenon, being related to pathologically increased IAP which induces malperfusion and ischemia in addition to embarrassment of organ function. A classic description of overt ACS would report that the cardiac output is reduced owing to decreased preload and right heart volumes. Although increased systemic vascular resistance initially maintains apparent blood pressure, decreases in preload from the pooling of blood in splanchnic and lower extremity vascular beds eventually lead to reduced central venous return [22–26]. Cardiac underfilling also occurs despite apparently increased central hemodynamic measurements (central venous pressure and pulmonary artery occlusion pressure).

The respiratory system is profoundly affected. Abdominal distention with IAH physically compresses the lungs especially at the bases creating a restrictive lung disease. As respiratory compliance decreases, mechanical ventilation with increased ventilatory pressures and decreased volumes becomes difficult [23, 27, 28]. The partial pressures of oxygen will decrease, and carbon dioxide will increase [28, 29]. Even modest IAH appears to exacerbate acute lung injury and the acute respiratory distress syndrome (ARDS). When IAP levels greater than 20 mmHg are applied to critically ill animals, a dramatic exacerbation of ARDS-associated pulmonary edema is evident [28, 30]. Furthermore, elevated IAP results in a stiffer chest wall with much lower transpulmonary pressures, and therefore less susceptibility to ventilator-induced lung injury [31, 32].

Oliguria is a common manifestation of the ACS, and the degree of renal dysfunction has a dose-dependent relationship with IAH [33–35]. These effects are exaggerated by hypovolemia and positive end-expiratory pressure [29, 36], and renal failure is often multi-factorial in critical care settings. Blood flow to the kidney operates in series, with a high-pressure capillary bed in the glomerulus having a mean pressure of about 60 mmHg although mean capillary pressure of the peritubular capillary system operates at a mean pressure of approximately 13 mmHg [37]. Such pressure and flow relationships make the kidney very susceptible to IAH, and the renal recovery after decompression may be dramatic [38].

Beyond the heart, lungs, and kidneys, almost every other organ system is altered by IAH, even if the effects are not obvious clinically. IAH appears to contribute to increased intracerebral pressure (ICP) via transmitted intrathoracic pressure [39,

40] to the extent that laparotomy has been reported to reduce ICP in patients with secondary ACS [41, 42]. Patients in shock are at a particularly high risk for splanchnic malperfusion because even modest elevations in IAP greatly reduce hepatic and splanchnic perfusion [43]. This effect is exacerbated by prior hemorrhage [44] and is observed at much lower IAPs than required to induce other clinical features of ACS.

6.5   Pathobiology of IAH/ACS

From a pathophysiology perspective, "ground zero," or the epicenter of IAH, is the abdominal cavity, with the "fallout zone" being the entirety of the body. Evolutionary biology evolved a complex mammalian anatomy with the human holobiome being contained within the abdominal cavity within the gastrointestinal system (gut), which has a luxurious often redundant blood perfusion in health. Unfortunately, with critical illness and injury, a exponentially complex interplay of reduced gut perfusion due to shock, compartment induced vascular compression (related to the accumulation within the compartment of ascetic fluid, swollen viscera, and an edematous abdominal wall), and critical injury/illness-induced dysbiotic conditions may create the perfect storm of gut malperfusion-inducing dysbiotic conditions with a pathogenic microflora. This may induce translocation of pathogenic bacteria and their metabolic products to induce systemic inflammation.

As noted, owing to intra-compartment physiology, there is a marked reduction in perfusion to all the viscera inducing relative or actual organ ischemia related to intra-compartmental hypertension [45]. This ischemia initiates the inflammatory cascade of vasoactive biomediators common to sepsis. The effects of IAH on the gut are similar to those of prolonged hypoperfusion, and therefore these two issues are compounding. In the face of IAH, the damaged gut seems to act as a continued source of inflammation propagating the systemic inflammatory response syndrome and potentiating multiple organ dysfunction syndrome [46–48]. Even after resuscitation and normalization of hemodynamics, gut vasoconstriction persists and is further exacerbated by IAH. Even relatively mild IAH (e.g., an IAP of 15 mmHg) has been reported to decrease intestinal microcirculatory blood flow, increase bowel wall permeability, and induce irreversible gut histopathological changes, bacterial translocation, and multiorgan dysfunction syndrome [49–51]. Prolonged gut hypoperfusion can precipitate a severe inflammatory response due to mobilization of damage-associated molecular patterns (e.g., high mobility group box 1, heat shock proteins, s100 proteins, nucleic acids, and hyaluronan), pro-inflammatory cytokines, and other mediators [52].

This process itself may be exacerbated by a series of physiologic stresses associated with prior priming of the immune system elements, such that IAH/ACS will be potentiated due to sequential physiological "hits," which produce a self-perpetuating process termed the "acute intestinal distress syndrome" [53, 54]. In the first hit, resuscitation of patients in shock induces injury especially of the splanchnic circulation [49, 54, 55]. This "acute bowel injury" results in release of pro-inflammatory mediators into the peritoneum and systemic circulation, leading to neutrophil priming, increased intestinal wall permeability, extravasation of fluid into the bowel wall and mesentery, translocation of intestinal bacteria, and absorption of bacterial endotoxin [50, 56–59]. In any subsequent hit such as a severe infection or delayed bleeding requiring further resuscitation, the resultant abdominal visceral edema leads to further IAH, compressing intra-abdominal lymphatics and resulting in a progressive visceral malperfusion, mucosa-to-serosa intestinal necrosis, a further increase in bowel wall permeability, and heightened bacterial translocation/endotoxin absorption and release of pro-inflammatory mediators [50, 56]. Such a two-hit theory may explain why patients without a primary inciting cause of shock (e.g., during elective abdominal wall reconstruction) may sometimes tolerate IAH/ACS better than predicted [60, 61], if they do not suffer a secondary insult in the postoperative period.

6.6   Gut Dysfunction in the Shocked State

Hemodynamic shock is believed to be a prototypical precipitating factor that induces gut hypoperfusion and ultimately initiates a chain of events ultimately resulting in the occurrence of the multiple organ dysfunction syndrome. This series of events has long been suspected to implicate the gut as the "motor of multiple organ failure" [62, 63]. The initial insult to the gut lining is a result of splanchnic hypoperfusion and injury to the gut at the expense of other organ beds such as the heart and brain [1, 64]. Being metabolically very active, the gut mucosa is quite vulnerable. Despite even adequate resuscitation, the damage may be done in hours [49, 50], and the subsequent gut dysfunction promotes distant organ injury [1, 64]. This dysfunction likely results from mucosal ischemia, altered intestinal transit and luminal nutrient transportation, and disuse-associated villus atrophy, which results in an overall reduction in mucosal surface area with loss of barrier function and increased permeability [64]. This specific sensitivity of the gut to ischemic injury in shock also correlates with a secondary sensitivity of the lungs to gut-mediated lung injury, as by the gut-lymph hypothesis which suggests that translocating and dead bacteria, cytokines, and chemokines actually travel to injury the lungs through the mesenteric lymphatics to induce acute lung injury and propagate further distant organ dysfunction [64, 65].

While the gut has been considered integral to the propagation of MODS for over 50 years, when considering this gut motor theory for the next decade, a greater appreciation of the gut contents as a living holobiont interacting with the human host as an interactive unit will be required. It is not proven (but assumed) that the microbiome within is also profoundly and rapidly transformed into a pathobiome or dysbiome [66].

6.7   A Pressure-Cooked Motor of MODS?

We have previously speculated that IAH also potentiates multiple organ dysfunction syndrome, despite being a potentially treatable factor that is often ignored [3, 51, 67]. This can be conceptualized as placing the "motor" of multiple organ dysfunction syndrome within a "pressure cooker" (abdominal cavity), with the capability to squeeze out perfusing blood and thus inducing ischemia to supercharge the developing injury to the gut. In experimental animal modest, what might erroneously be considered "mild" grade I IAH (15 mmHg) had profound effects on mucosal blood flow, which was reduced by 50% after only 4 h. When IAH was even more severe (in the range commensurate with abdominal compartment syndrome) (defined as IAP >20 associated with new organ failure)) [1, 68], there was profound injury to the gut.

6.8 Conclusions

The consequences of excessive IAP within the closed abdominal container may be devastating to organ systems within that container as well as those distant to it due to both physical and biomediator-related consequences. The fact that the gut is one of the first and most severely compromised organ systems in IAH/ACS is also poorly understood and deserves urgent study. The authors therefore hope that this "Hot Topic" will evolve rapidly with new knowledge and understanding in the coming years. Although extensive evidence now exists to support that IAH/ACS results in a number of adverse physiologic effects in preclinical models, and that these conditions are associated with poor outcomes (including mortality) in critically ill/injured patients, future studies must determine whether strategies targeted at lowering IAP improve patient-important outcomes.

Acknowledgment This Chapter is an updated and revised version of the chapter "Intra-abdominal hypertension, Abdominal Compartment Syndrome, and the Open Abdomen: Looking Beyond the Obvious to New Understandings in Pathophysiology, Harm Reduction, and Systemic Therapies". Kirkpatrick AW, Roberts DJ, Coccolini F. In: E Picetti, Peireira BM, T Razek, M Narayan, JL Kashuk F (Eds). Intensive Care for Emergency Surgeons. Springer, Cham Switzerland, 2019 pps 237–262.

References

1. Kirkpatrick AW, Roberts DJ, De Waele J, Jaeschke R, Malbrain ML, De Keulenaer B, et al. Intra-abdominal hypertension and the abdominal compartment syndrome: updated consensus definitions and clinical practice guidelines from the World Society of the Abdominal Compartment Syndrome. Intensive Care Med. 2013;39(7):1190–206.
2. Malbrain ML, Cheatham ML, Kirkpatrick A, Sugrue M, Parr M, De Waele J, et al. Results from the International Conference of Experts on intra-abdominal hypertension and abdominal compartment syndrome. I. Definitions. Intensive Care Med. 2006;32(11):1722–32.
3. Kirkpatrick AW, Sugrue M, McKee JL, Pereira BM, Roberts DJ, De Waele JJ, et al. Update from the Abdominal Compartment Society (WSACS) on intra-abdominal hypertension and abdominal compartment syndrome: past, present, and future beyond Banff 2017. Anaesthesiol Intensive Ther. 2017;49(2):83–7.
4. Kirkpatrick AW, De Waele JJ, De Laet I, De Keulenaer BL, D'Amours S, Bjorck M, et al. WSACS—the Abdominal Compartment Society. A Society dedicated to the study of the physiology and pathophysiology of the abdominal compartment and its interactions with all organ systems. Anaesthesiol Intensive Ther. 2015;47(3):191–4.

5. Kirkpatrick AW, Laupland KB, Karmali S, Bergeron E, Stewart TC, Findlay C, et al. Spill your guts! Perceptions of Trauma Association of Canada member surgeons regarding the open abdomen and the abdominal compartment syndrome. J Trauma. 2006;60(2):279–86.
6. Karmali S, Evans D, Laupland KB, Findlay C, Ball CG, Bergeron E, et al. To close or not to close, that is one of the questions? Perceptions of Trauma Association of Canada surgical members on the management of the open abdomen. J Trauma. 2006;60(2):287–93.
7. Sugrue M, Jones F, Janjua KJ, Deane SA, Bristow P, Hillman K. Temporary abdominal closure: a prospective evaluation of its effects on renal and respiratory physiology. J Trauma. 1998;45:914–21.
8. Wittman DH, Apprahamian C, Bergstein JM. Etappenlavage: advanced diffuse peritonitis managed by planned multiple laparotomies utilizing zippers, slide fastener, and Velcro analogue for temporary abdominal closure. World J Surg. 1990;14:218–26.
9. Aprahamian C, Wittman DH, Bergstein JM, Quebbeman EJ. Temporary abdominal closure (TAC) for planned relaparotomy (Etappenlavage) in trauma. J Trauma. 1990;30:719–23.
10. Barker DE, Kaufman HJ, Smith LA, Ciraulo DL, Richart CL. Vacuum pack technique of temporary abdominal closure: a 7-year experience with 112 patients. J Trauma. 2000;48:201–7.
11. Swan MC, Banwell PE. The open abdomen: aetiology, classification and current management strategies. J Wound Care. 2005;14:7–11.
12. Kirkpatrick AW, Roberts DJ, Jaeschke R, De Waele JJ, De Keulenaer BL, Duchesne J, et al. Methodological background and strategy for the 2012-2013 updated consensus definitions and clinical practice guidelines from the abdominal compartment society. Anaesthesiol Intensive Ther. 2015;47 Spec No:s63–77.
13. Blaser AR, Bjorck M, De Keulenaer B, Regli A. Abdominal compliance: a bench-to-bedside review. J Trauma Acute Care Surg. 2015;78(5):1044 53.
14. Bjorck M, Kirkpatrick AW, Cheatham M, Kaplan M, Leppaniemi A, De Waele JJ. Amended classification of the open abdomen. Scand J Surg. 2016;105(1):5–10.
15. Alverdy JC, Hyoju SK, Weigerinck M, Gilbert JA. The gut microbiome and the mechanism of surgical infection. Br J Surg. 2017;104(2):e14–23.
16. Saei AA, Barzegari A. The microbiome: the forgotten organ of the astronaut's body—probiotics beyond terrestrial limits. Future Microbiol. 2012;7(9):1037–46.
17. Levy M, Kolodziejczyk AA, Thaiss CA, Elinav E. Dysbiosis and the immune system. Nat Rev Immunol. 2017;17(4):219–32.
18. Lynch SV, Pedersen O. The human intestinal microbiome in health and disease. N Engl J Med. 2016;375(24):2369–79.
19. Relman DA. The human microbiome and the future practice of medicine. JAMA. 2015;314(11):1127–8.
20. McDonald D, Ackermann G, Khailova L, Baird C, Heyland D, Kozar R, et al. Extreme dysbiosis of the microbiome in critical illness. mSphere. 2016;1(4):e00199–16.
21. Malbrain ML, De Laet I, De Waele JJ, Sugrue M, Schachtrupp A, Duchesne J, et al. The role of abdominal compliance, the neglected parameter in critically ill patients—a consensus review of 16. Part 2: measurement techniques and management recommendations. Anaesthesiol Intensive Ther. 2014;46(5):406–32.
22. Cothren CC, Moore EE, Johnson JL, Moore JB. Outcomes in surgical versus medical patients with secondary abdominal compartment syndrome. Am J Surg. 2007;194:804–8.
23. Cullen DJ, Coyle JP, Teplick R, Long MC. Cardiovascular, pulmonary, and renal effects of massively increased intra-abdominal pressure in critically ill patients. Crit Care Med. 1989;17:118–21.
24. Barnes GE, Laine GA, Glam PY, Smith EE, Granger HJ. Cardiovascular responses to elevation of intra-abdominal hydrostatic pressure. Am J Physiol Regul Integr Comp Physiol. 1985;248:208–13.
25. Malbrain ML. Intra-abdominal pressure in the intensive care unit: clinical tool or toy? In: Vincent JL, editor. Yearbook of intensive care and emergency medicine. Berlin: Springer; 2002. p. 792–814.

26. Malbrain ML, de Laet I. Functional hemodynamics and increased intra-abdominal pressure: same thresholds for different conditions ...? Crit Care Med. 2009;37(2):781–3.
27. Meldrum DR, Moore FA, Moore EE, Haenel JB, Cosgriff N, Burch JM. Cardiopulmonary hazards of perihepatic packing for major liver injuries. Am J Surg. 1995;170:537–42.
28. Pelosi P, Quintel M, Malbrain ML. Effect of intra-abdominal pressure on respiratory mechanics. Acta Clin Belg Suppl. 2007;1:78–88.
29. Richardson JD, Trinkle JK. Hemodynamic and respiratory alterations with increased intra-abdominal pressure. J Surg Res. 1976;20:401–4.
30. Quintel M, Pelosi P, Caironi P, Meinhardt JP, Luecke T, Herrmann P, et al. An increase of abdominal pressure increases pulmonary edema in oleic acid-induced lung injury. Am J Respir Crit Care Med. 2004;169(4):534–41.
31. Kirkpatrick AW, Meade MO, Mustard RA, Stewart TE. Strategies of invasive ventilatory support in ARDS. Shock. 1996;6:S17–22.
32. Gattinoni L, Chiumello D, Carlesso E, Valenza F. Bench-to-bedside review: chest wall elastance in acute lung injury/acute respiratory distress syndrome patients. Crit Care. 2004;8:350–5.
33. Sugrue M, Jones F, Deane SA, Bishop G, Bauman A, Hillman K. Intra-abdominal hypertension is an independent cause of postoperative renal impairment. Arch Surg. 1999;134:1082–5.
34. De Waele JJ, De Laet I, Kirkpatrick AW, Hoste E. Intra-abdominal hypertension and abdominal compartment syndrome. Am J Kidney Dis. 2011;57(1):159–69.
35. Mohmand H, Goldfarb S. Renal dysfunction associated with intra-abdominal hypertension and the abdominal compartment syndrome. J Am Soc Nephrol. 2011;22(4):615–21.
36. Kashtan J, Green JF, Parsons EQ, Holcroft JW. Hemodynamic effects of increased abdominal pressure. J Surg Res. 1981;30:249–55.
37. Formation of urine by the kidney: I. Renal blood flow, glomerular filtration, and their control. In: AC Guyton, editor. Textbook of medical physiology. 8th ed. Philadelphia: WB Saunders; 1991. p. 286–307.
38. McBeth PB, Dunham M, Ball CG, Kirkpatrick AW. Correct the coagulopathy and scoop it out: complete reversal of anuric renal failure through the operative decompression of extraperitoneal hematoma-induced abdominal compartment syndrome. Case Rep Med. 2012;2012:946103.
39. Malbrain ML. Is it wise not to think about intraabdominal hypertension in the ICU? Curr Opin Crit Care. 2004;10:132–45.
40. Citerio G, Vascotto E, Villa F, Celotti S, Pesenti A. Induced abdominal compartment syndrome increases intracranial pressure in neurotrauma patients: a prospective study. Crit Care Med. 2001;29:1466–71.
41. Miglietta MA, Salzano LJ, Chiu WC, Scalea TM. Decompressive laparotomy: a novel approach in the management of severe intracranial hypertension. J Trauma. 2003;55:551–5.
42. Joseph DK, Dutton RP, Aarabi B, Scalea TM. Decompressive laparotomy to treat intractable intracranial hypertension after traumatic brain injury. J Trauma. 2004;57:687–95.
43. Caldwell CB, Ricotta JJ. Changes in visceral blood flow with elevated intra-abdominal pressure. J Surg Res. 1987;43:14–20.
44. Friedlander MH, Simon RJ, Ivatury R, DiRaimo R, Machiedo GW. Effect of hemorrhage on superior mesenteric artery flow during increased intra-abdominal pressures. J Trauma. 1998;45(3):433–89.
45. Roberts DJ, Ball CG, Kirkpatrick AW. Increased pressure within the abdominal compartment: intra-abdominal hypertension and the abdominal compartment syndrome. Curr Opin Crit Care. 2016;22(2):174–85.
46. Marshall JC. Inflammation, coagulopathy, and the pathogenesis of multiple organ dysfunction, syndrome. Crit Care Med. 2001;29:S99–S106.
47. Johnson D, Mayers I. Multiple organ dysfunction syndrome: a narrative review. Can J Surg. 2001;48:502–9.
48. Fink MP, Delude RL. Epithelial barrier dysfunction: a unifying theme to explain the pathogenesis of multiple organ dysfunction at the cellular level. Crit Care Clin. 2005;21:177–96.
49. Cheng J, Wei Z, Liu X, Li X, Yuan Z, Zheng J, et al. The role of intestinal mucosa injury induced by intra-abdominal hypertension in the development of abdominal compartment syndrome and multiple organ dysfunction syndrome. Crit Care. 2013;17(6):R283.

50. Leng Y, Zhang K, Fan J, Yi M, Ge Q, Chen L, et al. Effect of acute, slightly increased intra-abdominal pressure on intestinal permeability and oxidative stress in a rat model. PLoS One. 2014;9(10):e109350.
51. Kirkpatrick AW, Roberts DJ, De Waele J, Laupland K. Is intra-abdominal hypertension a missing factor that drives multiple organ dysfunction syndrome? Crit Care. 2014;18(2):124.
52. Timmermans K, Kox M, Scheffer GJ, Pickkers P. Danger in the intensive care unit: damps in critically ill patients. Shock (Augusta, GA). 2016;45(2):108–16.
53. Malbrain ML, De Laet I. AIDS is coming to your ICU: be prepared for acute bowel injury and acute intestinal distress syndrome. Intensive Care Med. 2008;34(9):1565–9.
54. Malbrain ML, Vidts W, Ravyts M, De Laet I, De Waele J. Acute intestinal distress syndrome: the importance of intra-abdominal pressure. Minerva Anestesiol. 2008;74(11):657–73.
55. Shah SK, Jimenez F, Letourneau PA, Walker PA, Moore-Olufemi SD, Stewart RH, et al. Strategies for modulating the inflammatory response after decompression from abdominal compartment syndrome. Scand J Trauma Resus Emerg Med. 2012;20:25.
56. Carr JA. Abdominal compartment syndrome: a decade of progress. J Am Coll Surg. 2013;216(1):135–46.
57. Diebel LN, Dulchavsky SA, Brown WJ. Splanchnic ischemia and bacterial translocation in the abdominal compartment syndrome. J Trauma. 1997;43:852–5.
58. Shah SK, Jimenez F, Walker PA, Aroom KR, Xue H, Feeley TD, et al. A novel mechanism for neutrophil priming in trauma: potential role of peritoneal fluid. Surgery. 2010;148(2):263–70.
59. Shah SK, Jimenez F, Walker PA, Xue H, Feeley TD, Uray KS, et al. Peritoneal fluid: a potential mechanism of systemic neutrophil priming in experimental intra-abdominal sepsis. Am J Surg. 2012;203(2):211–6.
60. Petro CC, Raigani S, Fayezizadeh M, Rowbottom JR, Klick JC, Prabhu AS, et al. Permissive intra-abdominal hypertension following complex abdominal wall reconstruction. Plast Reconstr Surg. 2015;136(4):868–81.
61. Kirkpatrick AW, Nickerson D, Roberts DJ, Rosen MJ, McBeth PB, Petro CC, et al. Intra-abdominal hypertension and abdominal compartment syndrome after abdominal wall reconstruction: quaternary syndromes? Scand J Surg. 2017;106(2):97–106.
62. Clark JA, Coopersmith CM. Intestinal crosstalk: a new paradigm for understanding the gut as the "motor" of critical illness. Shock. 2007;28(4):384–93.
63. Silvestri L, van Saene HK, Zandstra DF, Marshall JC, Gregori D, Gullo A. Impact of selective decontamination of the digestive tract on multiple organ dysfunction syndrome: systematic review of randomized controlled trials. Crit Care Med. 2010;38(5):1370–6.
64. Patel JJ, Rosenthal MD, Miller KR, Martindale RG. The gut in trauma. Curr Opin Crit Care. 2016;22(4):339–46.
65. Moore FA, Moore EE, Poggetti R, McAnena OJ, Peterson VM, Abernathy CM, et al. Gut bacterial translocation via the portal vein: a clinical perspective with major torso trauma. J Trauma. 1991;31(5):629–36; discussion 36–8.
66. Krezalek MA, DeFazio J, Zaborina O, Zaborin A, Alverdy JC. The shift of an intestinal "microbiome" to a "pathobiome" governs the course and outcome of sepsis following surgical injury. Shock. 2016;45(5):475–82.
67. Kirkpatrick AW, Roberts DJ, De Waele J. High versus low blood-pressure target in septic shock. N Engl J Med. 2014;371(3):282–3.
68. Cheatham ML, Malbrain ML, Kirkpatrick A, Sugrue M, Parr M, De Waele J, et al. Results from the international conference of experts on intra-abdominal hypertension and abdominal compartment syndrome. II. Recommendations. Intensive Care Med. 2007;33(6):951–62.

Diagnosis and Treatment of the Abdominal Compartment Syndrome

7

Giovanni Scognamiglio, Emiliano Gamberini, Vanni Agnoletti, and Federico Coccolini

7.1   Introduction

During the last three decades, we have witnessed dramatic improvements in diagnosing and treating abdominal compartment syndrome. Abdominal compartment syndrome (ACS) has evolved from a poorly understood phenomenon in patients after emergency abdominal surgery to an established syndrome that contributes to organ dysfunction in different kinds of critically ill patients [1, 2]. Intra-abdominal hypertension (IAH) is a more common phenomenon and can proceed into ACS. ACS is just the most severe end point of increased intraperitoneal pressure, and it is recognized as a catastrophic disturbance of a patient's physiology that requires urgent intervention and guided therapies [1, 3]. Despite recent advances in both medical and surgical care, ACS still remains a significant cause of mortality: the full-blown syndrome without surgical decompression can still be lethal [4].

The creation of the multidisciplinary World Society of the Abdominal Compartment Syndrome (WSACS www.wsacs.org) in 2004 was an important milestone in the landmark of this disease. This is a multidisciplinary group, composed mostly of surgeons and intensivists. WSASC foundation was followed by the publication of consensus definitions and daily clinical guidelines in 2007. Five years later in 2013, those guidelines were updated according to an evidence-based methodology. A dedicated Pediatric Guidelines Sub-Committee was also created so that the definitions and guidelines can also be adapted to children.

G. Scognamiglio (✉) · E. Gamberini · V. Agnoletti
Anesthesia and Intensive Care Department, Surgery and Severe Trauma Division, Major Trauma Center "Maurizio Bufalini" Hospital, Cesena, Italy

F. Coccolini
General, Emergency and Trauma Surgery Department, Pisa University Hospital, Pisa, Italy

© Springer Nature Switzerland AG 2021
F. Coccolini et al. (eds.), *Compartment Syndrome*, Hot Topics in Acute Care Surgery and Trauma, https://doi.org/10.1007/978-3-030-55378-4_7

7.2   Definitions

Intra-abdominal hypertension is defined as a persistent or repeated pathologic elevation of intra-abdominal pressure >12 mmHg *without* any organ derangement. The
words "persistent or repeated" are important as a single value, maybe recorded
when the patient is in pain or when ventilator asynchrony arises, is therefore not
enough to define abdominal hypertension. The key difference between IAH and
ACS is presence or absence of concomitant organ dysfunction/failure.

IAH is further graded as follows:

1. IAP > 12–15 mmHg
2. IAP > 16–20 mmHg
3. IAP > 21–25 mmHg
4. IAP > 25 mmHg

A solely IAP value is less important than the duration of IAH. Prolonged high
elevations in IAP result in organ dysfunction or failure that can have a significant
impact upon patient morbidity and mortality.

In 2007 and lately in 2013, WSACS defined ACS as a *sustained* elevation of
intra-abdominal pressure >20 mmHg (with or without Abdominal Perfusion
Pressure APP <60 mmHg) associated with a new organ dysfunction or failure.

Trigger factors located within the abdominal cavity define primary compartment syndrome, whereas trigger factors out of the abdomino-pelvis region define
secondary syndrome. Most frequent causes of primary ACS are abdominal trauma,
abdominal aneurysm rupture, and pancreatitis: 30–53% of patients develop IAH
after major surgery or trauma. Secondary ACS may often occur after major trauma
followed by massive fluid resuscitation, sepsis, and burns. A third rare entity
known as tertiary ACS is defined as a recurrent ACS following either primary or
secondary ACS. Being an all or none entity and in contrast with IAH, ACS is not
graded [1].

7.3   IAH and Abdominal Perfusion Pressure

7.3.1   How to Measure

There are different methods to measure intra-abdominal pressure: these methods
can either be direct or indirect. Direct measurement of intra-abdominal pressure can
be done using an intraperitoneal catheter with a pressure transducer. Indirect measurements follow Pascal's law of fluids. Pascal states that any change in pressure in
an enclosed fluid is transmitted equally to every part of the fluid. Therefore, with the
abdomen considered an enclosed fluid-filled container, any change in pressure will
be equally distributed throughout the abdomen: inferior vena cava, rectal, uterine,
femoral vein, bladder, and gastric pressure measurements have all been advocated
and suggested as IAP surrogates and indirect estimates. Nevertheless, over the

years, bladder pressure measurements have been regarded as the gold standard technique since it is simple, precise, and minimally invasive.

According to WSACS definition, intra-abdominal pressure is the steady-state pressure concealed within the abdominal cavity, measured via the bladder at end expiration, in supine position.

IAP should be measured via a Foley catheter in supine position, after instilling a minimum volume of 25 mL of sterile saline into the bladder. Over-distending the bladder with more saline is just useless as it may return a false result [5]. Measurement should be made at end expiration (or end expiratory pause, if mechanically ventilated) with transducer zeroed at midaxillary line. Furthermore, IAP should be measured 30–60 s after instillation to allow bladder detrusor muscle relaxation.

A nasogastric tube with an esophageal and a gastric balloon can be indicated whenever gastric drainage and enteral nutrition have to be combined with abdominal pressure measurements (peritonitis, obesity, polytraumatized patient) and/or pleural/trans-pulmonary pressure measurements (mechanically ventilated patients) [6, 7]. Moreover, it grants an incontinuous IAP measurement which can be very useful in the operating theater during surgical decompression.

The abdomen and pelvis collectively form one compartment, bounded by the diaphragm, abdominal wall, back, and the peritoneal reflection at the bony pelvis. The size and volume of the abdomen may be affected by the varying location of the diaphragm, the shifting position of the costal arch, the contractions of the abdominal wall, and the amount of contents (air, liquid, feces, fetus, or even blood) contained within the boundaries.

Normal IAP in a wealthy adult is about 2–5 mmHg and varies inversely with intrathoracic pressure during normal breathing [8]. Confounding factors such as BMI (body mass index) should always be considered when assessing basal IAP value; indeed, it can go up to 12 mmHg in an obese adult [9]. Given IAP dependency from the abdominal content, baseline IAP is also increased during pregnancy, in patients undergoing chronic ambulatory peritoneal dialysis, and after laparotomy [9].

ICU patients who have undergone massive fluid resuscitation after shock often have basal IAP values right above 7 mmHg.

After measuring IAP, abdominal perfusion pressure can be easily calculated by simply subtracting IAP from systemic MAP. A 60 mmHg APP is desirable since organ dysfunction may begin to occur just below this threshold. APP can be thought as analogous to cerebral perfusion pressure: as for Intra Cranic Pressure and Cerebral Perfusion Pressure, APP can be used as a better predictor of visceral perfusion than MAP and IAP alone. It represents an easily calculated parameter for guiding the resuscitation and management of the patient with IAH/ACS [10].

7.3.2   When to Measure

Early identification of patients at risk is the first step in diagnosing and preventing both IAH and ACS. According to WSACS, IAP should be measured when any known risk factor for IAH/ACS is present, and protocolized measurement series should be performed. Multiple studies have been conducted to identify the current state of awareness, knowledge, and use of evidence-based medicine regarding IAH and ACS [11].

IAH should be considered in any patient who presents with one or more of the following risk factors [12]:

- intra-abdominal infection or abscess
- liver dysfunction with ascitis
- obesity
- prolonged shock (acidosis, hypothermia, hemorrhage, coagulopathy),
- visceral ischemia or perforation and major abdominal surgery,
- major trauma and burns, damage control laparotomy,
- sepsis,
- polytransfusion and massive fluid resuscitation (>5 L crystalloids in 24 h),
- prone positioning (i.e. in severe respiratory failure),
- ruptured abdominal aneurysm,
- retroperitoneal hemorrhage,
- abdominal neoplasm,
- liver dysfunction/ascites,
- peritoneal dialysis,
- pancreatitis,
- ileus/gastroparesis.

The recommendation is to assess the IAP at baseline and then IAP should be measured every 4–6 h, i.e. at least once in a nurse shift.

7.4   Epidemiology

Epidemiological studies conducted in the last decades vastly differ in their report of incidence and prevalence. The previous lack of consensus definitions before WSACS came out, different IAP measurement techniques and the different case-mix of both medical and surgical patients add to the dearth of concurrence in data. Both IAH and ACS, however, still remain unrecognized or underdiagnosed even though they are much more common than expected [13]. There is an agreement however that the occurrence of IAH during the intensive care unit stay is an independent predictor of patients' outcome [14].

The reported incidence of IAH ranges between 21 and 58%, while for ACS it ranges between 1 and 12% among general ICU patients. A recent individual patient data meta-analysis of 1669 adult general ICU patients reported that 27.7% had IAH and 2.7% had ACS (as defined by the WSACS) at ICU admission [11]. In both medical and surgical critical care patients, the presence of IAH or ACS is associated with a significant increase in mortality [11]. When compared to mixed populations of adult ICU patients, trauma and emergency general surgery patients and those with ruptured AAAs, severe acute pancreatitis, and burns appear to have a substantially higher incidence and prevalence of IAH and ACS [15]. In a study by Vidal and colleagues, 53% of trauma and emergency surgery patients developed IAH, while more than 12% developed ACS during their ICU stay [14].

7.5 Physiopathology

Primary ACS may be a no-turning back point of pathologies concealed within the abdominal region and usually follows abdominal trauma, pancreatitis, rupture of abdominal aneurysm.

Secondary ACS is usually the presentation of the syndrome in patients who have had no abdominal injuries nor abdominal surgical intervention [16]. Typically, these patients suffer the sequence of events after a major traumatic event resulting in hemorrhagic shock and needing of exsanguino-transfusions (complete replacement of blood volume) [16–18]. Secondary ACS patients develop ACS from delayed definitive hemorrhage control and cyclic and substantial crystalloid loading [19].

Regardless of what the primary event is, whether it be trauma with hemorrhagic shock, sepsis, or burns, all lead to a capillary leak syndrome resulting in the extravasation of fluid into the interstitium and massive bowel edema [19]. Fluid-filled bowel will increase pressure within the abdominal cavity. Increased IAP leads to organ dysfunction of all abdominal organs due to arterial blood flow limitation, venous outflow obstruction, and impaired microcirculatory flow: this derangement of local tissue perfusion will necessitate more fluid loading, finally triggering a vicious cycle.

Trauma patients in hemorrhagic shock are often aggressively resuscitated with IV crystalloid fluid and blood products to maintain intravascular volume and restore normal perfusion. Unfortunately, measurements of blood pressure, heart rate, urine output, and central venous pressure commonly used as clinical end points of adequate resuscitation are inadequate indicators of tissue perfusion. Thus, conventional IV resuscitation from trauma and hemorrhagic shock sometimes culminates in multisystem organ failure, over resuscitation, and delayed primary abdominal closure in case of laparotomy.

The application of damage control principles, as well as the understanding of the advantage of whole blood resuscitation, and the development of massive transfusion protocols are important recent advances in the management of the bleeding patient [16, 20].

7.6 ACS: Systemic Effects and Organ Derangement

IAH reduces perfusion to all intra-abdominal organs, and it has been recognized to affect extra-abdominal organs as well. As the intra-abdominal pressure rises, multiple organs will progressively start to fail.

While IAH is a graded and often a gradual phenomenon, ACS is an all or none condition causing dysfunction of neurological, respiratory, cardiovascular, renal, and hepatic organ systems, leading, in most severe situations, to multi-organ failure.

7.6.1   Pulmonary

Increased IAP leads to elevation of the diaphragm and costal arch, reducing thoracic volume, functional residual capacity, and compliance while increasing intrapleural pressure. Compressive basal atelectasis increases physiological dead space. Chest wall compliance is decreased and elastic recoil (1/C) augmented, creating a restrictive syndrome resulting in respiratory failure. Diminished chest wall compliance will result in shifting the lower inflection point on the pressure–volume curve to the right, flattening the initial inspiratory part of the curve with an associated rise in airway resistance. Furthermore, the trans-pulmonary pressure will be decreased (Pleural pressure—alveolar pressure): higher Plateau pressures will be needed for alveolar opening and recruitment maneuvers [21]. Respiratory failure observed in ACS is also attributed to a more complex problem related to hypoxia: release of pro-inflammatory cytokines results in inflammatory edema and, in worst cases, ARDS (adult respiratory distress syndrome) [22]. Setting the right PEEP value can be very challenging since high PEEP might be needed: indeed attempts at matching IAP with PEEP could be detrimental because of uncontrolled pressure created in the chest which could have negative effects on both cardiac preload and output, without any improvement in oxygenation [23].

Esophageal pressure today is a key parameter for patient ventilation because it accurately estimates pleural pressure and allows for the determination of trans-pulmonary pressure [24, 25].

A nasogastric tube for esophageal and trans-pulmonary pressure measurements can help calculating the best PEEP value and diminishing respiratory driving pressure (Pplat − PEEP = the lower, the better! ≤15 cmH$_2$O). Tailored protective ventilation (i.e., 6–7 mL/kg Vt, right PEEP value, Pplat <30 cmH$_2$O) is mandatory to relieve ventilator-associated lung injury. Trans-pulmonary pressure is also useful for respiratory weaning, when lung injury abates.

Elevated intrathoracic pressure and hypoxia increase pulmonary vascular resistance and right ventricular strain with risk of right heart failure. A Swan-Ganz catheter (a pulmonary catheter) can be useful to assess heart–lung interactions.

7.6.2   Heart and Hemodynamics

IAP increase affects both preload and afterload: it leads to a decreased venous return by compressing inferior vena cava and a greatly increased afterload. Preload is further reduced by pooling of blood in the pelvis and lower limbs. These changes result in augmented stroke volume variation (SVV%) and reduced cardiac output, which may be exacerbated by concomitant hypovolemia. Relative hypovolemia is usually associated to IAH and ACS: after massive crystalloid resuscitation, resulting capillary leak syndrome will proceed in the extravasation of fluid into the interstitium. This is important to understand why increasing venous return by administration of crystalloids may initially help to restore a proper cardiac output [16, 19]. Beware that additional crystalloid infusion only creates a futile cycle of crystalloid filling. Indeed, additional crystalloids only worsen the gut edema, increases IAP, and propagates the cycle. Unfortunately, blood pressure, heart rate, urine output, and central venous pressure commonly used as clinical end points of adequate resuscitation are inadequate indicators of tissue perfusion. Because of the increased abdominal pressure compressing the vena cava and increasing the intrathoracic pressure as well, the central venous pressure may be misleading to evaluate patient's fluid status.

A bed-side fast ecocardiography is the first step to correctly evaluate patient's volemic state: it is noninvasive, replicable, and any intensivist should be able to perform it.

Invasive hemodynamic monitoring is mandatory (a Swan-Ganz Catheter as stated above or Pulse Wave Form Analysis methods if SWG catheter is not immediately available). Therefore, Cardiac Index (CI), Stroke Volume Variation (SVV%, strictly related to Δ-Ups & Δ-Downs in invasive blood pressure wave form), Right Ventricular End Diastolic Volume Index (RVEDI), and arterial lactate have proven themselves to be the most reliable variables in resuscitation of patients suffering from IAH/ACS.

7.6.3 Renal

Renal dysfunction is highly associated to ACS and often the first to occur. It presents as oliguria (≤0.5 mL/kg/h urine output) progressing to anuria, despite increases in fluid administration. As asserted earlier, crystalloid boluses, often suggestively addressed as Fluid Challenge Therapies, are not the key to obtain a physiological urine output, as it may only trigger IAH vicious cycle. IAH associated cardiac dysfunction (see above), and impaired renal perfusion may contribute to oliguria. Furthermore, the anatomical position of the kidneys in the retroperitoneal space makes them vulnerable to direct parenchymal compression. The underlying pathological process that induces renal failure from IAH is exacerbated by increased renal venous resistance and arteriolar resistance, which lead to reduction of glomerular filtration rate [3]. In addition, alterations in systemic and renal hemodynamics upregulate the renin–angiotensin–aldosterone system, which further increases renal vascular resistance to retain salt and water to compensate for low cardiac output and eventually worsens bowel edema.

7.6.4 Gastrointestinal and Liver

Along with the kidneys, all of the structures within the abdominal cavity are also compressed, and this will cause regional hypoperfusion. This effect may be most pronounced in the liver. Hepatic dysfunction can arise, even when not directly injured after trauma, with a low-grade IAH. Hepatic derangement manifests through impaired clearance of plasmatic lactate, resulting in metabolic acidosis that is not solely attributable to increased mismatch of O_2 demand/delivery. This flawed lactate clearance can confuse the clinical interpretation of lactate levels, making their interpretation more difficult in their common use as a resuscitation end point, if used alone. Several animal studies have demonstrated an association between raised IAP and bacterial translocation, supporting the hypothesis that gut barrier function is also compromised. Indeed, it is likely that the gut is the initial motor of Multi-Organ Disfunction Syndrome, also during extra-abdominal sepsis [20, 26, 27]. The loss of intestinal barrier function and the increase of permeability will result in intestinal edema, ascites formation, and exacerbated bacterial translocation.

7.6.5   Central Nervous System

Elevated IAP raises intrathoracic pressure and central venous pressure (CVP), eventually resulting in elevated intracranial pressure (ICP) due to a functional obstruction to cerebral venous outflow. Clinical observations in major trauma patients with concomitant brain and abdominal injuries have shown that decompressive laparotomy for ACS would also relieve intracranial hypertension [28].

7.7   Treatment

A deep knowledge of the physiopathologic implications of IAH is essential to understand the reasoning behind the therapeutic tactics hereby advocated. First of all, the awareness a patient is at risk of IAH is the key point in approaching and treating this polyhedral pathology. Many medical treatment options are already part of routine daily management in the ICU (analgo-sedation, nasogastric and rectal tube, prokinetics, enemas, body position) [29].

Current management of IAH and ACS is based upon the latest up-to-date, evidence-based recommendations provided by the World Society of the abdominal compartment syndrome (WSACS).

Appropriate management of IAH/ACS is based upon four general principles:

1. Basal measurement of IAP in patients at risk and then serial monitoring of IAP (every 4–6 h if any risk factor is present and IAH is established, i.e. at least once in a nurse shift);
2. Optimization of systemic and local perfusion;
3. Monitoring of end-organ function and institution of organ-specific therapies to reduce IAP;
4. Prompt surgical decompression for refractory IAH/ACS.

Treatment of ACS requires rapid normalization of IAP, thereby restoring normal abdominal visceral perfusion and resolving contemporary organ dysfunction. Definitive management of ACS from most causes other than tense ascites involves emergent surgical decompression of the abdomen to release the abdominal pressure and provide a temporary abdominal closure until the disease process is reversed and the swelling abates. Lower grade IAH may be temporized or relieved using nonsurgical measures. Nonoperative medical management plays a vital role in both the prevention and treatment of IAP-induced organ dysfunction and failure.

As stated above, IAP is determined by several factors, thus management of high IAP must therefore be taken into account:

1. abdominal wall compliance,
2. organ intraluminal contents,

3. presence of space-occupying substances,
4. abdominal organ volume,

As stated earlier, only one IAP high value is not sufficient to determine any organ dysfunction. Indeed, the amount of time during which IAP is elevated is much more critical to trigger organ and systemic derangements.

Medical management may play an increasingly important role in the prevention and management of intra-abdominal hypertension (IAH). Nonoperative management can be divided into the following steps: sedation and paralysis to relax the abdominal wall; evacuation of intraluminal contents; evacuation of large abdominal fluid collections; optimization of APP and correction a positive fluid balance. Surgical decompressive laparotomy is still the only viable option for refractory IAH/ACS (Figs. 7.1 and 7.2).

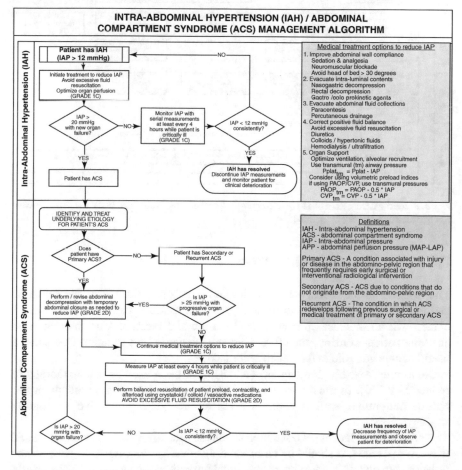

Fig. 7.1 IAH and ACS management algorithm, WSACS guidelines—Intensive Care Med. 2013 Jul; 39(7): 1190–1206

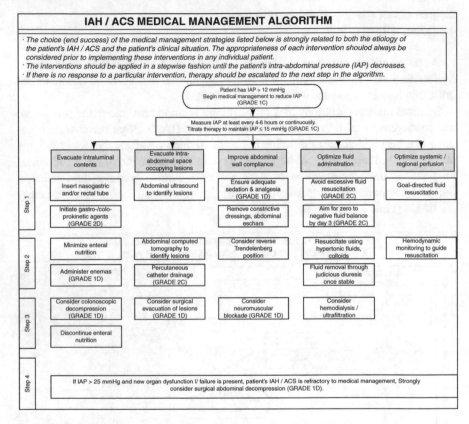

IAH / ACS MEDICAL MANAGEMENT ALGORITHM

· The choice (end success) of the medical management strategies listed below is strongly related to both the etiology of the patient's IAH / ACS and the patient's clinical situation. The appropriateness of each intervention should always be considered prior to implementing these interventions in any individual patient.
· The interventions should be applied in a stepwise fashion until the patient's intra-abdominal pressure (IAP) decreases.
· If there is no response to a particular intervention, therapy should be escalated to the next step in the algorithm.

Patient has IAP > 12 mmHg
Begin medical management to reduce IAP
(GRADE 1C)

Measure IAP at least every 4-6 hours or continuously.
Titrate therapy to maintain IAP ≤ 15 mmHg (GRADE 1C)

	Evacuate intraluminal contents	Evacuate intra-abdominal space occupying lesions	Improve abdominal wall compliance	Optimize fluid administration	Optimize systemic / regional perfusion
Step 1	Insert nasogastric and/or rectal tube	Abdominal ultrasound to identify lesions	Ensure adequate sedation & analgesia (GRADE 1D)	Avoid excessive fluid resuscitation (GRADE 2C)	Goal-directed fluid resuscitation
Step 1	Initiate gastro-/colo-prokinetic agents (GRADE 2D)		Remove constrictive dressings, abdominal eschars	Aim for zero to negative fluid balance by day 3 (GRADE 2C)	
Step 2	Minimize enteral nutrition	Abdominal computed tomography to identify lesions	Consider reverse Trendelenberg position	Resuscitate using hypertonic fluids, colloids	Hemodynamic monitoring to guide resuscitation
Step 2	Administer enemas (GRADE 1D)	Percutaneous catheter drainage (GRADE 2C)		Fluid removal through judicious diuresis once stable	
Step 3	Consider colonoscopic decompression (GRADE 1D)	Consider surgical evacuation of lesions (GRADE 1D)	Consider neuromuscular blockade (GRADE 1D)	Consider hemodialysis / ultrafiltration	
Step 3	Discontinue enteral nutrition				
Step 4	If IAP > 25 mmHg and new organ dysfunction I/ failure is present, patient's IAH / ACS is refractory to medical management, Strongly consider surgical abdominal decompression (GRADE 1D).				

Fig. 7.2 Medical treatment of IAH/ACS according to the latest guidelines by WSACS—Intensive Care Med. 2013 Jul; 39(7): 1190–1206

7.7.1 Analgesia (First!), Sedation, and Paralysis

The first step in the management of elevated IAP is to ensure adequate analgesia and, if necessary, sedation and muscle paralysis. Anxiety, pain, ventilation asynchrony will all increase abdominal wall tension and increase IAP. In addition to ensuring patient comfort, therefore adequate analgesia and sedation also serve a useful therapeutic role in the patient with IAH.

Neuromuscular blocking agents (NMB) have been used as rescue therapy to reduce IAP [30]. In most severe cases, muscle relaxation can be mandatory to reduce abdominal wall tension and set an adequate protective ventilation strategy.

According to Vincent [31], sedation should be secondary to proper analgesia and whenever possible, it should be based on drugs that can be titrated to prespecified sedation targets: this introduces the breakthrough concept of eCASH—**E**arly **C**omfort using **A**nalgesia with a minimum of **S**edatives and a maximum of **H**umanity.

While opioids are very effective at treating pain, they also have important side effect: addiction, ileus, respiratory depression among others. On the sedative side, nowadays, benzodiazepines have been pushed aside by new molecules such as dexmedetomidine, a selective α2-agonist, whose price is rapidly dropping. Dexmedetomidine has a rapid onset, distribution, and elimination that does not accumulate and therefore could be ideally suitable for reliable and fast neurological examination. Propofol is widely used as sedative of choice, but it has an important hemodynamic impact and can trigger the propofol infusion syndrome (↓ heart rate, ↓ pH, ↑ lactate, ↑ CPK, myocardial failure). Ketamine has been gaining some consensus for long-term sedation since it does not alter systemic hemodynamics or respiratory drive, and has an analgesic effect too. In the last few years, Ketamine has proven itself safe even in the traumatic brain injury patient [32].

Thanks to adequate control of the pain, the level of sedation can be reduced. The new paradigm is multimodal analgesia which can be considered as a more rational approach to pain management: by using different ways of administration and different drugs, it is possible to reduce the need for sedation, opioids, and side effects. The combined use of different analgesics (opioids, NSAIDs, local anesthetics) produces synergistic analgesia and enables clinicians to use lower total doses [33].

In the last years, ICU doctors have shifted from a renowned sedo-analgesia concept to a more modern analgo-sedation approach [34]. Analgo-sedation can be an "analgesia-based sedation" which refers to the use of a long action analgesic instead of a sedative to reach the sedative goal. On the other hand, analgo-sedation can also be interpreted as "analgesia-first sedation" which refers to the use of an analgesic before a sedative to reach the sedative goal. Moving from using sedative drugs like benzodiazepines to using much more analgesics with some sedatives has proven to be quite a good strategy. "Low dose, long action opioids" like Sufentanil and Fentanyl along with acetaminophen can grant a valid analgesia with a mild sedation. Morphine should be avoided whenever possible as there is a risk of overdosing in patients with acute renal failure, which is quite common in ICU setting and ACS patients. Multimodal means also different way of administration: epidural catheters in trauma patients with local anesthetic continuous infusion (for example, Ropivacaine 0.2–0.3%, along with adjuvants, clonidine, or morphine) can reduce patient's pain. Regional anesthesia can also help reducing rehabilitation time.

Cis-Atracurium or Rocuronium (IV bolus + IV continuous infusion) are commonly used for muscle paralysis.

7.7.2 Abdominal Decompression

Many critically ill patients will at some point develop gastrointestinal ileus. Gastric, small bowel, and colonic distension can all increase IAP substantially. Nasogastric and/or rectal drainage, enemas, and even endoscopic decompression are relatively noninvasive methods for reducing IAP and treating mild to moderate IAH [35]. Therefore, all patients with elevated IAP should have a nasogastric tube placed.

Administration of pro-kinetic motility agents such as:

- metoclopramide (IV bolus, 10 mg ×3/daily),
- neostigmine (IV continuous infusion, up to 5 mg/daily; or IV bolus 0.5 mg up to ×6/daily),
- levosulpiride (IV bolus, 25 mg ×3/daily),
- erythromycine (NGT 300 mg/daily),
- naloxone (NGT, 0.4 mg up to ×6/daily to prevent opioid-related ileus),

is also useful in promoting gastrointestinal dumping and decreasing visceral volume. If gastric stagnation is present, re-administering bile salt-rich secretion can stimulate gastric emptying and intestinal transit.

Patients with ascites can benefit from drainage [36].

Percutaneous drainage of the fluid in these situations has shown great success in burn and oncology patients, avoiding the need for a decompressive laparotomy. Albumin administration can be useful after paracentesis.

Unfortunately in trauma patients, ACS is much more commonly due to swollen bowel from massive fluid resuscitation rather than free fluid [19].

Appropriate patient positioning in bed can also help reducing significantly IAP. Semi-recumbent position is associated with a higher IAP: the higher the head of bed elevation, the higher the IAP [37, 38].

7.7.3 Optimization of APP and Fluid Balance

Hypovolemia aggravates the physiopathologic effects of elevated IAP, while hypervolemia (i.e., excessive crystalloid volume resuscitation) is an independent predictor for the development of ACS.

In critically ill patients, invasive hemodynamic monitoring technologies can be very useful in assessing intravascular volume status and optimizing patient resuscitation. A Swan-Ganz catheter with incontinuous CO (Cardiac Output) and SvO_2 monitoring is a good choice to assess volemic status of patients.

Any intensivist should be able to perform a rapid bed-side echo exam to assess fluid status, while the best way to ameliorate fluid balance is by weighing patients every day: ICU beds with weighing scales are commercially available.

Traditional pressure-based parameters such as central venous pressure may be misleading in the presence of elevated intra-abdominal and intrathoracic pressure and can lead to erroneous clinical decisions regarding fluid status.

Because the central venous pressure will likely be artificially elevated, the right ventricular end diastolic volume index (RVEDVI) and Right Ventricle Ejection Fraction (RVEF) are much more reliable to guide resuscitation. Random boluses or fluid challenges should be discouraged because a transient increase in blood pressure will do nothing to ameliorate the underlying problem, and excessive fluid infusion will worsen the gut edema.

Blood products can be preferred over crystalloids to ameliorate perfusion without worsening bowel edema even if Hb is >10 g/dL. Another option is to use hypertonic crystalloid resuscitation [39] (saline 3 or 7.4%) along with albumin, which is associated with a substantially decreased fluid requirement.

The following can be considered good resuscitation endpoints: $ScvO_2$ (every ICU patient should have an IV central line available), incontinuous SvO_2 and RVEF/RVEDI if a SWG catheter is available, arterial lactate, differential AV CO_2, and diuresis.

Inotropic amine infusion can be useful to counterbalance depressive effect of acidosis on myocardium, while vasopressors, such as high-dose norepinephrine, can worsen splanchnic vasoconstriction and visceral ischemia: amine support should be implemented only after ensuring adequate intravascular volume. In most severe cases, administration of hydrocortisone (IV 250 mg bolus + 250 mg continuous infusion/daily) can revert tissue unresponsiveness to amines.

Early continuous hemofiltration/ultrafiltration may be more appropriate than continuing to volume load the patient to obtain a proper urine output and increase the likelihood of secondary ACS. Continuous Renal Replacement Therapies help revert acidosis and can have a role in cytokine absorption and washout [40–42].

7.7.4   Nutritional Support

These patients are hyper-catabolic, that is why nutritional support has such an important role [43]. Enteral feeding should be started as soon as possible in all patients with intestinal continuity as it promotes gut-mediated immunity, maintains microbial diversity, and increases intestinal blood flow [44]. High-protein/high-calorie products can be a good choice as they can reduce enteral feeding volume. A post-pyloric NGT will be needed whenever gastric ileus inhibits reaching proper daily intake and can be mandatory in pancreatitis.

High-dose ascorbic acid (Vitamin C) has proposed to be a useful adjunct in minimizing the effects of free radical injury [45] since it attenuates post-burn lipid peroxidation: daily dose is 1–2 g by parenteral infusion. Micronutrient deficiency is often described, thus losses of vitamins and minerals should always be counterbalanced. In the last decades, Alanine and Glutamine have been addressed as the primary fuel of the intestinal mucosa, and they contribute to intestinal villous integrity.

Here is an easy scheme to understand how to address nutritional needings in ICU patients:

2 g–2.5 g/kg/daily protein and 30 kCal/kg/daily, plus micronutrients (minerals and vitamins), can be a good starting point.

Administering drugs to prevent stress gastric ulcer (proton pump inhibitors, H_2-antagonists) cannot be recommended as it has been demonstrated that raising gastric inner pH can expose to inhalation and pneumonia. Early enteral feeding is the best prophylaxis against stress ulcer [44, 46].

As stated above, pro-kinetic drugs can play an important role.

7.7.5 New Drugs

Theophylline: According to Bodnar et al. [47], theophylline can be useful to counteract the effects of serum interleukin 10 and adenosine. The authors experienced a dramatic reduction of both IAP values (19.2 mmHg vs and 9.5 mmHg) and mortality (0% vs 55%).

Octreotide [48]: It can reduce oxidative tissue damage and have a therapeutic role as a reperfusion injury-limiting agent among patients with IAH and ACS. Further studies are needed to confirm these findings.

7.7.6 Surgical Decompression

Surgical decompression is still the only viable treatment in case of refractory IAH/ACS, and it can be lifesaving. Multi-organ derangement, hemodynamics, and the need for high-level amine support should guide the physician to consider damage control and open abdomen techniques. Delayed abdominal decompression and disregard of high IAP levels are associated with significant increases in patient mortality. Prophylactic decompression and creation of a temporary abdominal closure in surgical patients at risk for elevated IAP significantly reduce the subsequent development of IAH/ACS and improve survival [17]. Recent experimental and clinical work has suggested that the open abdomen technique with temporary abdominal wall closure using negative pressure therapy methods (i.e., Bogota Bag, Ab Thera) is associated with superior outcomes. With decompression, there is an immediate decrease in IAP [4, 49]. However, the pressure may not decrease to normal levels while an immediate recovery for some organs can be noticed. After decompression, monitoring of IAP continues as, contrary to popular belief, IAH and ACS can recur, and visceral perfusion can still be inadequate despite an open abdomen.

7.8 Summary

Despite recent advances in both medical and surgical care, IAH and ACS still remains a significant cause of morbidity and mortality. The creation of the multidisciplinary World Society of the abdominal compartment syndrome (WSACS www. wsacs.org) in 2004 was an important event in the landmark of this entities.

Intra-abdominal hypertension is defined as a persistent or repeated pathologic elevation of intra-abdominal pressure >12 mmHg without any organ derangement. ACS is a sustained elevation of intra-abdominal pressure >20 mmHg (with or without APP <60 mmHg) associated with a new organ dysfunction or failure. While IAH is a graded and often gradual phenomenon, ACS is an all or none condition causing dysfunction of neurological, respiratory, cardiovascular, renal, and hepatic organ systems, leading, in most severe situations, to Multi-Organ Failure.

IAP should be measured when any know risk factor for IAH/ACS is present in clinically ill or injured patients. IAP should be measured via a Foley catheter in supine position, after instilling a minimum volume of 25 mL of sterile saline into the bladder. Measurement should be made at end expiration (or end expiratory pause if mechanically ventilated) with transducer zeroed at midaxillary line.

Appropriate management of IAH/ACS is based upon four general principles:

1. Serial monitoring of IAP (every 4–6 h if any risk factor is present and IAH is established, i.e. at least once in a nurse shift).
2. Optimization of systemic perfusion and end-organ function.
3. Institution of organ-specific therapies to reduce IAP and avoid the detrimental end-organ consequences of IAH/ACS.
4. Prompt surgical decompression for refractory IAH/ACS.

References

1. Malbrain ML, Cheatham ML, Kirkpatrick A, Sugrue M, Parr M, DeWaele J, Balogh Z, Leppaniemi A, Olvera C, Ivatury R, D'Amours S, Wendon J, Hillman K, Johansson K, Kolkman K, Wilmer A. Results from the international conference of experts on intra-abdominal hypertension and abdominal compartment syndrome. I. Definitions. Intensive Care Med. 2006;32(11):1722–32.
2. Ivatury RR, Sugerman HJ. Abdominal compartment syndrome: a century later, isn't it time to pay attention? Crit Care Med. 2000;28(6):2137–8.
3. Balogh Z, McKinley BA, Holcomb JB, Miller CC, Cocanour CS, Kozar RA, Valdivia A, Ware DN, Moore FA. Both primary and secondary abdominal compartment syndrome can be predicted early and are harbingers of multiple organ failure. J Trauma. 2003;54(5):848–59; discussion 859–61.
4. De Waele JJ, Hoste EA, Malbrain ML. Decompressive laparotomy for abdominal compartment syndrome: a critical analysis. Crit Care. 2006;10(2):R51.
5. Fusco MA, Martin RS, Chang MC. Estimation of intra-abdominal pressure by bladder pressure measurement: validity and methodology. J Trauma. 2001;50(2):297–302.
6. Pelosi P, Vargas M. Mechanical ventilation and intra-abdominal hypertension: 'Beyond Good and Evil'. Crit Care. 2012;16(6):187.
7. Yoshida T, Brochard L. Esophageal pressure monitoring: why, when and how? Curr Opin Crit Care. 2018;24(3):216–22.
8. Cobb WS, Burns JM, Kercher KW, Matthews BD, Norton HJ, Heniford BT. Normal intraabdominal pressure in healthy adults. J Surg Res. 2005;129(2):231–5.
9. Malbrain ML, De Keulenaer BL, Oda J, De Laet I, De Waele JJ, Roberts DJ, et al. Intra-abdominal hypertension and abdominal compartment syndrome in burns, obesity, pregnancy, and general medicine. Anaesthesiol Intensive Ther. 2015;47(3):228–40.
10. Cheatham ML, White MW, Sagraves SG, Johnson JL, Block EF. Abdominal perfusion pressure: a superior parameter in the assessment of intra-abdominal hypertension. J Trauma. 2000;49(4):621–6; discussion 626–7.
11. Malbrain ML, Chiumello D, Cesana BM, Reintam Blaser A, Starkopf J, Sugrue M, et al. A systematic review and individual patient data meta-analysis on intra-abdominal hypertension in critically ill patients: the wake-up project. World initiative on abdominal hypertension epidemiology, a unifying project (WAKE-Up!). Minerva Anestesiol. 2014;80(3):293–306.
12. Holodinsky JK, Roberts DJ, Ball CG, et al. Risk factors for intra-abdominal hypertension and abdominal compartment syndrome among adult intensive care unit patients: a systematic review and meta-analysis. Crit Care. 2013;17(5):R249.

13. Malbrain ML, Chiumello D, Pelosi P, Wilmer A, Brienza N, Malcangi V, et al. Prevalence of intra-abdominal hypertension in critically ill patients: a multicentre epidemiological study. Intensive Care Med. 2004;30(5):822–9.
14. Vidal MG, Ruiz Weisser J, Gonzalez F, Toro MA, Loudet C, Balasini C, et al. Incidence and clinical effects of intra-abdominal hypertension in critically ill patients. Crit Care Med. 2008;36(6):1823–31.
15. De Waele JJ, Ejike JC, Leppaniemi A, De Keulenaer BL, De Laet I, Kirkpatrick AW, et al. Intra-abdominal hypertension and abdominal compartment syndrome in pancreatitis, paediatrics, and trauma. Anaesthesiol Intensive Ther. 2015;47(3):219–27.
16. Balogh Z, McKinley BA, Cocanour CS, Kozar RA, Holcomb JB, Ware DN, Moore FA. Secondary abdominal compartment syndrome is an elusive early complication of traumatic shock resuscitation. Am J Surg. 2002;184(6):538–43; discussion 543–4.
17. Biffl WL, Moore EE, Burch JM, Offner PJ, Franciose RJ, Johnson JL. Secondary abdominal compartment syndrome is a highly lethal event. Am J Surg. 2001;182(6):645–8.
18. Maxwell RA, Fabian TC, Croce MA, Davis KA. Secondary abdominal compartment syndrome: an underappreciated manifestation of severe hemorrhagic shock. J Trauma. 1999;47(6):995–9.
19. Balogh Z, McKinley BA, Cocanour CS, Kozar RA, Valdivia A, Sailors RM, Moore FA. Supranormal trauma resuscitation causes more cases of abdominal compartment syndrome. Arch Surg. 2003;138(6):637–42; discussion 642–3.
20. Neal MD, Hoffman MK, Cuschieri J, et al. Crystalloid to packed red blood cell transfusion ratio in the massively transfused patient: when a little goes a long way. J Trauma Acute Care Surg. 2012;72(4):892–8.
21. Pelosi P, Quintel M, Malbrain ML. Effect of intra-abdominal pressure on respiratory mechanics. Acta Clin Belg. 2007;62(Suppl 1):78–88.
22. Gattinoni L, Pelosi P, Suter PM, et al. Acute respiratory distress syndrome caused by pulmonary and extrapulmonary disease. Different syndromes? Am J Respir Crit Care Med. 1998;158(1):3–11.
23. Sugrue M, D'Amours S. The problems with positive end expiratory pressure (PEEP) in association with abdominal compartment syndrome. J Trauma. 2001;51(2):419–20.
24. Yoshida T, Marcelo B, Amato P, Grieco DL, Chen L, Lima CAS, Roldan R, Morais CCA, Gomes S, Costa ELV, Cardoso PFG, Charbonney E, Richard J-CM, Brochard L, Kavanagh BP. Esophageal manometry and regional transpulmonary pressure in lung injury. Am J Respir Crit Care Med. 2018;197(8):1018–26.
25. Talmor D, Sarge T, O'Donnell CR, Ritz R, Malhotra A, Lisbon A, Loring SH. Esophageal and transpulmonary pressures in acute respiratory failure. Crit Care Med. 2006;34(5):1389–94.
26. Assimakopoulos SF, Triantos C, Thomopoulos K, Fligou F, Maroulis I, Marangos M, Gogos CA. Gut-origin sepsis in the critically ill patient: pathophysiology and treatment. Infection. 2018;46(6):751–60.
27. Deitch EA. Gut-origin sepsis: evolution of a concept. Surgeon. 2012;10(6):350–6.
28. De Laet I, Citerio G, Malbrain ML. The influence of intra-abdominal hypertension on the central nervous system: current insights and clinical recommendations, is it all in the head? Acta Clin Belg. 2007;62(Suppl 1):89–97.
29. Vachharajani V, Scott LK, Grier L, Conrad S. Medical management of severe intra-abdominal hypertension with aggressive diuresis and continuous ultra-filtration. Internet J Emerg Intensive Care Med. 2003:6.
30. De Waele J, Delaet I, Hoste E, Verholen E, Blot S. The effect of neuromuscular blockers on intraabdominal pressure. Crit Care Med. 2006;34(12):A70.
31. Vincent JL, Shehabi Y, Walsh TS, Pandharipande PP, Ball JA, et al. Comfort and patient-centred care without excessive sedation: the eCASH concept. Intensive Care Med. 2016;42(6):962–71.
32. Oddo M, Crippa IA, Mehta S, Menon D, Payen J-F, Taccone FS, Citerio G. Optimizing sedation in patients with acute brain injury. Crit Care. 2016;20:128.
33. Devlin JW, Skrobik Y, Gélinas C, Needham DM, Slooter AJC, Pandhari-pande PP, et al. Clinical practice guidelines for the prevention and management of pain, agitation/sedation,

delirium, immobility, and sleep disruption in adult patients in the ICU. Crit Care Med. 2018;46(9):e825–73.
34. Faust AC, Rajan P, Sheperd LA, Alvarez CA, McCorstin P, Doebele RL, et al. Impact of an analgesia-based sedation protocol on mechanically ventilated patients in a medical intensive care unit. Anesth Analg. 2016;123(4):903–9.
35. Peces R, Vega C, Peces C, Trebol J, Gonzalez JA. Massive gastric dilatation and anuria resolved with naso-gastric tube decompression. Int Urol Nephrol. 2010;42(3):831–4.
36. Etzion Y, Barski L, Almog Y. Malignant ascites presenting as abdominal compartment syndrome. Am J Emerg Med. 2004;22(5):430–1.
37. Cheatham ML, De Waele JJ, De Laet I, et al. The impact of body position on intra-abdominal pressure measurement: a multicenter analysis. Crit Care Med. 2009;37(7):2187–90.
38. Vasquez DG, Berg-Copas GM, Wetta-Hall R, Vasquez DG, Berg-Copas GM, Wetta-Hall R. Influence of semi-recumbent position on intra-abdominal pressure as measured by bladder pressure. J Surg Res. 2007;139(2):280–5.
39. Oda J, Ueyama M, Yamashita K, Inoue T, Noborio M, Ode Y, Aoki Y, Sugimoto H. Hypertonic lactated saline resuscitation reduces the risk of abdominal compartment syndrome in severely burned patients. J Trauma. 2006;60(1):64–71.
40. Hawchar F, László I, Öveges N, Trásy D, Ondrik Z, Molnar Z. Extracorporeal cytokine adsorption in septic shock: a proof of concept randomized, controlled pilot study. J Crit Care. 2019;49:172–8.
41. Kogelmann K, Jarczak D, Scheller M, Drüner M. Hemoadsorption by CytoSorb in septic patients: a case series. Crit Care. 2017;21(1):74.
42. Bonavia A, Groff A, Karamchandani K, Singbartl K. Clinical utility of extracorporeal cytokine hemoadsorption therapy: a literature review. Blood Purif. 2018;46(4).337–49.
43. Moore SM, Burlew CC. Nutrition support in the open abdomen. Nutr Clin Pract. 2016;31(1):9–13.
44. Byrnes MC, Reicks P, Irwin E. Early enteral nutrition can be successfully implemented in trauma patient with an "open abdomen". Am J Surg. 2010;199(3):359–62; discussion 363.
45. Kremer T, Harenberg P, Hernekamp F, et al. High-dose vitamin C treatment reduces capillary leakage after burn plasma transfer in rats. J Burn Care Res. 2010;31(3):470–9.
46. Krag M, Perner A, Møller MH. Stress ulcer prophylaxis in the intensive care unit. Curr Opin Crit Care. 2016;22(2):186–90.
47. Bodnar Z, Keresztes T, Kovacs I, Hajdu Z, Boissonneault GA, Sipka S. Increased serum adenosine and interleukin 10 levels as new laboratory markers of increased intra-abdominal pressure. Langenbecks Arch Surg. 2010;395(7):969–72.
48. Kacmaz A, Polat A, User Y, Tilki M, Ozkan S, Sener G. Octreotide: a new approach to the management of acute abdominal hypertension. Peptides. 2003;24(9):1381–6.
49. Hong JJ, Cohn SM, Perez JM, Dolich MO, Brown M, McKenney MG. Prospective study of the incidence and outcome of intra-abdominal hypertension and the abdominal compartment syndrome. Br J Surg. 2002;89(5):591–6.

Compartment Syndrome of the Extremities: Pitfalls in Diagnosis and Management

Luigi Branca Vergano and Philip F. Stahel

8.1 Historical Perspective

The sequelae of untreated compartment syndrome were first described by Volkmann in 1881; he described the clinical features of the syndrome as a paralytic contracture of a limb due to a tight bandage [1]. A better description of the syndrome was provided by Bywaters and BeallI based on a case series of British victims during World War II in 1941 [2]. The authors underlined the general consequences of the syndrome, described as a "crush" syndrome with impending gangrene of the limb, systemic shock, progressive renal failure, and ultimately death. A better understanding of the pathophysiology of the syndrome is attributed to Carter in 1949 [3]. Carter's description related to a muscle trauma leading to increased pressure within a muscular compartment, with consequent impairment of blood supply, ultimately leading to muscle necrosis.

The importance of time from the onset of the syndrome was well understood and described in the early literature. Most authors reported that tissue ischemia lasting for less than 1 h is associated with reversible neuropraxia, while prolonged ischemia over 4 h will induce irreversible axonotmesis. Irreversible muscle necrosis was described beyond 6–8 h of ischemia [4].

The historic basic principles related to the evolution of compartment syndrome and subsequent tissue injury remain valid until present [5].

Traumatic etiologies of acute compartment syndrome can be divided into three main groups: fracture related, soft tissue injury-related, and vascular injury-related [6].

Extremity fractures after high-energy trauma mechanisms represent the most frequent cause of acute compartment syndromes [7].

L. Branca Vergano (✉) · P. F. Stahel
Department of Orthopaedics and Traumatology, Ospedale M. Bufalini, Cesena, FC, Italy

Rocky Vista University, College of Osteopathic Medicine, Parker, CO, USA

© Springer Nature Switzerland AG 2021
F. Coccolini et al. (eds.), *Compartment Syndrome*, Hot Topics in Acute Care Surgery and Trauma, https://doi.org/10.1007/978-3-030-55378-4_8

Crush injuries are responsible for around 20% of acute compartment syndromes in absence of fractures.

Traumatic vascular injuries can induce acute compartment syndrome as a consequence of ischemia-reperfusion injury [8, 9].

Nontraumatic root causes include exertional compartment syndrome, thermal/burning injuries, constricting casts or wraps, bleeding disorders, soft tissue infections, and iatrogenic complications [5, 10, 11].

8.2 Definition

The definition of acute compartment syndrome of the extremities is an increase in pressure within a defined compartment of the limb, demarcated by a fascia. The increase in the intracompartmental pressure causes a decrease in perfusion pressure, leading to hypoxemia of the tissues. If this situation is prolonged, irreversible impairment of the muscles can occur, leading to tissue necrosis and devastating subsequent patient outcomes.

8.3 Pathophysiology

In the extremities, there are many anatomic compartments, containing muscle groups and neurovascular structures, separated and demarcated by fasciae. The fascia is composed by dense connective tissue; this fibrous tissue envelopes delimit anatomical space, with low compliance. This means that little increase in volume causes high-pressure elevation.

In case of traumatic event and in some nontraumatic accident (burns, ischemia and reperfusion), the injured tissue responds with precapillary vasodilation in the arteriole system of the muscles, along with collapsing venules and increased permeability of the capillary bed. This leads to increased capillary filtration and raise of interstitial fluid; the pressure of interstitial fluid (normally lower than 10 mmHg) raises in injured tissue, with the clinical aspect of edematous limb, and consequently the intracompartmental pressure raises [12–14].

In case of nontraumatic compartment syndrome (e.g., extravasation of drugs), there is a direct increase of extravascular fluid.

The increase in intracompartmental pressure has the direct consequence of external compression of the microvasculature. Efferent capillaries and venules, with their small diameter and lack of intramural musculature, are extremely sensitive to pressure changes, and collapse first. The compression of outflow system, along with venous congestion, diminishes the arterio-venous gradient. This reduction of the gradient leads to a decrease in local perfusion pressure and consequently to tissue ischemia [4, 12, 15, 16].

The congestion of the microcirculation causes an increase in the permeability of the vessel walls, worsening the fluid extravasation in the interstitial space. The increased fluid volume in third space produces tissue edema and increased interstitial pressure, generating a feedback loop, which increases external pressure on the intra-compartmental vasculature, with consequent worsening of tissue ischemia.

Lymphatics, which, in healthy tissues, assist with outflow and decompression, fail rapidly under the increased pressure [17].

Once perfusion pressure reaches a critically low level, severe tissue hypoxemia evolves.

When muscles are deprived of oxygen and metabolic supply, changes in cellular metabolism occur, resulting in the production of reactive oxidative species, which damage endothelial cells, further increasing vascular permeability.

The combination of hypoxia, increase in oxidant stress, and development of hypoglycemia in tissue causes cell edema, cellular swelling, and necrosis.

Furthermore, in reperfusion injury, after a prolonged period of ischemia, the production of oxygen radicals, lipid peroxidation, and calcium influx leads to disturbances of mitochondrial oxidative phosphorylation and, ultimately, cell-membrane destruction; this worsens the extravasation of the fluid in the interstitial space [4, 13, 14, 18].

Neutrophils and other inflammatory cells are drawn to the ischemic regions and release cytokines and chemical mediators, which exacerbate the vascular permeability.

This cycle is perpetuated till complete necrosis of the tissues occurs unless a surgical procedure (fasciotomy) interrupts the loop.

The time from the initial event to the onset of the compartment syndrome can vary from minutes to hours, and different tissues respond in different manners to reduction of aerobic metabolism consequent to ischemia [17].

Peripheral nerves are highly susceptible to ischemia: after 1 h, reversible neurapraxia occurs, and after 4 h irreversible axonotmesis [4].

Muscles are slightly more resistant to the anaerobic metabolism due to compartment syndrome, but when ischemia persists for more than 8 h, irreversible changes are likely to occur. The inflammatory response, if not treated, evolves in irreversible changes and finally to necrosis and fibrotic tissue.

Rhabdomyolysis after acute compartment syndrome has been reported as more than 40%; the massive release of myoglobin in the circulation can lead to acute kidney injury and kidney failure [19].

8.4   Diagnostic Pitfalls: The "5 P's" Revisited

Acute extremity compartment syndrome can be diagnosed on the basis of clinical symptoms, by measurement of intracompartmental pressure, or both.

The clinical symptoms designated by the mnemonic of "5 P's" (pallor, poikilothermia, pulselessness, paresthesia, and paralysis) were historically considered to be the typical signs for the diagnosis of compartment syndrome [16, 17]. However, these clinical signs are typically the signs of arterial ischemia and delayed presentation of a "missed" compartment syndrome [20]. Thus, the guiding principle is represented by pain out of proportion as the only cardinal symptom of acute compartment syndrome of the extremities. In the current age, the classic "5 P's" have been replaced by "Pain, pain, pain, pain, pain", and the burden is on the physician to either diagnose or rule out the presence of acute compartment syndrome, independent of the mechanism of injury [16, 17, 20].

Severe pain, not proportionated to the severity of the injury ("pain out of proportion"), that does not improve with i.v. painkillers and adequate analgesia should raise the suspicion of acute extremity compartment syndrome. Clinical symptoms appear in the early phases of the development of compartment syndrome in conscious and wakeful patients. Much attention has to be paid to overuse of painkillers, for the risk of hiding the subjective symptoms of the syndrome.

Another early sign is pain on passive stretching of the affected muscles, especially in case of compartment syndrome of the forearm (pain with extension of the fingers) and of the leg (pain with dorsi- or plantarflexion of the toes).

As mentioned before, nerves (especially sensory ones) are very susceptible to hypoxia. For this reason, neurological signs can appear in the onset of compartment syndrome: paresthesia in the affected extremity is common, while complete anesthesia or paresis appears late and not constantly. However, the absence of neurological signs must not rule out compartment syndrome; motor nerves have some resistance to ischemia, and waiting for complete motor deficits to make the diagnosis could be extremely risky [5, 6, 11].

Unless all these clinical signs have high sensitivity, they were shown to have low sensitivity and poor predictive value [16, 17].

All clinical symptoms lack completely in case of non-evaluable patients because of altered mental status: intubated, obtunded, or non-collaborative patients cannot communicate early symptoms of compartment syndrome. Even in awake patients sometimes the pain could be well tolerated, in presence of preexisting neurological disorders (neuropathy in diabetes or nephropathy) or, as mentioned before, due to pharmacological sedation (large use of painkillers, regional anesthesia, epidural pain catheters). Moreover, anxiety or other distracting injuries can contribute to misdiagnose an initial compartment syndrome [10, 12, 13].

On the basis of clinical examination, the limb involved appears swollen and distended and can be very hard at palpation (Fig. 8.1). The presence of distal pulses does not exclude acute compartment syndrome. In fact they can be completely normal for hours; blood flow through large arteries is preserved till the compartment

Fig. 8.1 Swollen leg after fracture of the distal third of tibia, with impending compartment syndrome

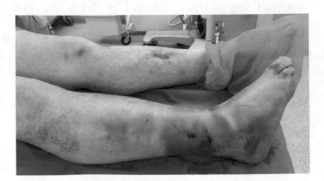

pressure rises above systolic blood pressure, which occurs in the late phase of compartment syndrome [17].

If the clinical diagnosis is equivocal, measurement of intracompartmental tissue pressure can be extremely useful for the diagnosis. The physiological compartment pressures in adults are around 8–10 mmHg. There are many portable devices for the measurement of intracompartmental pressure: the needle is inserted perpendicular to the skin into the muscle compartment under exam. Less than 1 mL of sterile saline is injected through the needle into the compartment. When equilibrium is reached, that it takes a few seconds, the compartmental pressure is then read on a digital screen. If these devices are not available, an arterial line transducer system with side-port needles can be effective as well. The needle should be inserted near the fracture site (not farther than 5 cm). Pressure measurements should be obtained in all compartments of the extremities involved, especially when analyzing forearm and leg. It is not infrequent to miss the development of acute extremity compartment syndrome in a neighboring compartment [16, 17, 21–24].

A measured pressure greater than 30 mmHg is thought to be an indication for emergency surgical decompression. The use of an absolute value, however, has been questioned because the perfusion pressure necessary for oxygenation is partly dependent on the patients' blood pressure. On one hand, this means that a relatively high pressure in a well-perfused compartment could suggest unnecessary fasciotomy. On the other hand, low compartment pressure in a poor perfused patient (shock) could be alarming and the muscle compartment should be considered hypoxygenated and at risk. Some researchers have suggested the use of differential pressure (Δp = diastolic blood pressure – intracompartmental pressure), with a proposed threshold of 30 mmHg. In a prospective study, McQueen et al. examined the use of a pressure differential ($\Delta p > 30$ mmHg) as diagnostic criteria for acute compartment syndrome. They showed no missed diagnoses of compartment syndrome with this value [14, 25–29].

Compartment syndrome is a dynamic process, and the limb can worsen its edema along minutes and hours. The compartment pressure, even if normal at the initial examination, can raise till high value. For this reason, it is imperative to repeat frequent examinations of the extremities of the patient, especially if consciousness. Continuous measurement of intracompartmental pressure can be made by attaching a catheter to an arterial transducer. This method is controversial, first of all because it measures only one compartment at a time, then because some studies have suggested that the use of continuous measurement can lead to unnecessary fasciotomy [30–32].

8.5   Management of Acute Compartment Syndrome: A Surgical Emergency

Once the diagnosis of compartment syndrome is sure, fasciotomy should be carried out emergently; it is proved that an extended time period between onset of compartment syndrome and surgical treatment worsens the outcome. Animal studies suggest that tissue necrosis occurs within 6–12 h of onset of hypoxemia. The optimum

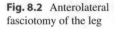

Fig. 8.2 Anterolateral
fasciotomy of the leg

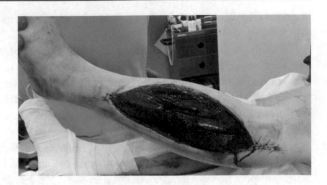

timing for fasciotomy is within 8 h from the development of acute extremity compartment syndrome, but the rationale is to perform fasciotomy as soon as possible [33–35] (Fig. 8.2).

In case of missed diagnosis of compartment syndrome for more than 24 h, it is questionable to perform fasciotomy. In fact, in such cases, muscle necrosis has already occurred and simple fasciotomy could pose the patients at high risk of bacterial colonization of necrotic tissues. If necrotic muscles become infected, repeated debridement is needed, and amputation might be necessary if the infection cannot be controlled. On the other hand, if acute extremity compartment syndrome has been missed for longer than 24–48 h without evidence of infection, nonsurgical management should be applied.

The fasciotomy must be complete in length, with decompression of all the muscle compartments affected. Multiple techniques exist that might be used for closing or dressing fasciotomy wounds. It is important to avoid any constrictive dressing: the muscles, especially in the first hours, can worsen their swelling, and they should be allowed to fully expand. The fascia, the subcutaneous tissue, and the skin should left be open. Loose tension-based suture, as shoelace technique with vessel loops, can be applied; this suture can be tightened the following days, when swelling decreases [35–38].

Wet gauzes dressing or vacuum-assisted medication can be alternatively used. Standard wet gauzes should be changed every 24 h. VAC therapy allows 2–4 days of permanence on the wound. The goal of fasciotomy dressing is to facilitate delayed primary closure of the wound. The literature does not show completely agreement on the superiority of VAC dressing over wet gauzes. However, many studies support the evidence that use of VAC is associated with significantly higher rates of primary closure than traditional dressings [37, 38] (Fig. 8.3).

The wound should be closed when feasible: the fascia could left be open in case of excessive tension of the suture. Early closure of fasciotomy wounds has been associated with recurrence of compartment syndrome. When direct suture is not possible, skin graft may be used. Even if primary closure without tension is the gold standard, some authors strongly recommend the use of skin graft for fasciotomy closure: Johnson et al. show less infection and significantly less pain in grafted patients compared to them with primary closure of the wound [39, 40].

Fig. 8.3 Shoelace technique for closure of an anterolateral fasciotomy of the leg

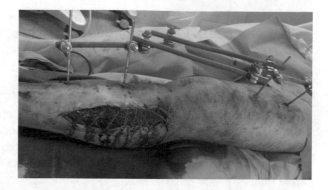

Complications to soft tissues and skin after fasciotomy are not rare. Nearly one-third of patients have postoperative complication: soft tissue necrosis, wound dehiscence, skin graft infection or necrosis, or need for tissue debridement. Even without occurrence of complications, patients treated with fasciotomy often complain of altered sensation and dry skin with pruritus, besides cosmetic issues [41, 42].

8.6   Specific Compartment Syndrome Locations

Acute compartment syndrome can occur in any location of the upper and lower extremities, from the shoulder to the hands and from the gluteal compartment to the foot. The lower leg represents the most frequent and vulnerable location for acute compartment syndrome, followed by the forearm, thigh, and upper arm [10].

8.6.1   Lower Extremity

8.6.1.1 Gluteal Region

Gluteal compartment syndrome is rare when compared to other anatomical regions. Only about 20% of the cases of gluteal compartment syndrome is secondary to pelvic trauma. More frequently the syndrome is the consequence of nontraumatic conditions, such as prolonged immobilization due to loss of consciousness in patients with history of drug or alcohol abuse, incorrect position during orthopedic or urological surgeries with long operative time, infections, intramuscular drug abuse [43–45].

There are three compartments in this region: tensor fascia lata laterally, gluteus medium and minimus deeper, gluteus maximus posteriorly. Sciatic nerve runs through these compartments, between gluteus maximus and pelvis external rotator complex. When these muscles are swollen, the nerve is at high risk of compression. The consequence might be a neuropathy, with paresthesia in the early stage, and complete palsy if the syndrome remains untreated.

In case of massive necrosis of the gluteus muscles, high quantity of myoglobin is released in the blood stream. The consequences of the rhabdomyolysis are well known, carrying finally to acute kidney failure.

The literature does not reveal precise indications for surgery. Nearly 30% of the patients were treated conservatively, with careful monitoring. The other 70% were treated with emergent decompression of the three compartments [45, 46].

8.6.1.2 Thigh

Acute compartment syndrome of the thigh is a potentially devastating condition. The causes of the syndrome can be traumatic (femur fractures with or without vascular injury, contusion with muscular hematoma) or nontraumatic (external compression in consciousness people caused by narcotic overdose, incorrect intraoperative positioning during orthopedic procedures in patients with epidural anesthesia) [47–49].

The thigh has three compartments: anterior, medial, and posterior.

Clinical presentation of acute compartment syndrome is characterized by excessive painful and tensely swollen thigh. Measurement of the thigh circumference may be helpful to monitoring the condition, determining progression of the swelling.

Some studies strongly recommend the treatment of acute compartment syndrome of the thigh with emergent fasciotomy. Often large inter or intramuscular hematoma is evacuated during surgery. Delayed fasciotomy was associated with increased complications. But has to be noticed that fasciotomy of the thigh results in large scars, with wound infection reported in up to 67% of the cases. On the other hand, thigh musculature can tolerate elevated compartment pressure for long period, if compared to other muscular regions [16, 48–50]. In fact, the compartment has large volume and its fasciae have a relatively elasticity.

For the reasons above, the course of the thigh compartment syndrome is variable. Some patients have high morbidity and mortality, others have an uncomplicated course with excellent outcomes. Consequently, there is not a strict recommendation for the treatment of acute thigh compartment syndrome (surgical versus conservative).

In the literature, the overall death rate in patients with acute thigh compartment syndrome was reported to be very high (till 47%). Other authors have instead reported mortality of 11%, caused by associated injuries rather than by direct consequences of the syndrome [47–49].

8.6.1.3 Lower Leg

The lower leg is the most common location of acute extremity compartment syndrome. In general, up to 70% of all cases of compartment syndrome are associated with fractures, and nearly 40% of all cases are secondary to diaphyseal fractures of the tibia [6].

The lower leg consists of four compartments: anterior (containing ankle extensor muscles), lateral (peronei muscles), superficial posterior (sural triceps), and deep posterior (ankle flexor muscles). The anterior and lateral compartments are the most frequently affected by compartment syndrome.

Fractures of the diaphysis of the tibia are most commonly associated with acute extremity compartment syndrome of the lower leg (from 2 to 9% reported in the literature). Even fractures of proximal and distal metaphysis of the tibia can provocate compartment syndrome, with different rate of occurrence described in the literature (1.4–17%). The predominance of compartment syndrome occurring in the middle third of the tibia can be attributed to the fact that diaphyseal portion of the tibia is surrounded by bulky muscle mass. Among tibial shaft fractures, displaced, comminuted, and segmental patterns are the most prone to develop compartment syndrome. Even then high-energy tibia fractures are associated with increased risk of developing compartment syndrome, a significant association between fracture type (A, B, or C sec. Ao classification) and compartment syndrome is yet debated. An open tibia fracture does not exclude the possibility of developing acute extremity compartment syndrome [6, 29, 34, 51–54].

Younger patients have higher risk to develop lower leg compartment syndrome, compared to old ones. This may be explained by the difference in muscle mass between young and old patients; younger have more muscle mass that can potentially swell against relatively noncompliant fascia in limited space. Even the property of the fascia can change during the years because of the different proportion and characteristics of collagen fibers between young and old people [51, 52, 55, 56].

The definitive treatment is emergency fasciotomy and decompression of the four compartments. This is usually achieved with two incisions, one centered over the intermuscular septum laterally (decompression of anterolateral and lateral compartments) and the other posterior to the subcutaneous posteromedial border of the tibia (decompression of superficial and deep posterior compartments). A four-compartment decompression by a single incision has been described [57]. The incision is lateral, and can be done with or without fibulectomy. The procedure is usually performed by general or epidural anesthesia, but even bedside fasciotomy under local anesthesia could be an option in very unstable patients.

8.6.1.4 Foot

Each foot has nine compartments: medial, lateral, four interossei, and three central. Measurement of intracompartmental pressure of all compartments is virtually impossible because of the difficulty to target every compartment with the misuration needle. Although emergency fasciotomy is indicated in practically all other acute extremity compartment syndromes, its recommendation in the foot lacks consensus and is still debated. To make multiple large incisions on swollen and injured foot posed the extremity at high risk of wound complications; some surgeons thus prefer to manage the sequelae of untreated compartment syndrome [58–62].

8.6.2   Upper Extremity

8.6.2.1 Shoulder

Deltoid compartment syndrome is extremely rare, with few cases described. The reported cause is usually nontraumatic: prolonged compression in obtunded patients, drug or anabolic abuse with intracompartmental injection of heroin or hormone, long operation time in lateral decubitus. The fasciotomy is mandatory, with decompression of the three deltoid compartments [63–65].

8.6.2.2 Upper Arm

Upper arm includes two compartments, anterior (flexor) and posterior (extensor). The brachial fascia surrounds the two compartments that are separated by medial and lateral intermuscular septa.

Upper arm compartment syndrome is very rare; the few reported causes are traumatic (fracture, tendon rupture) and nontraumatic (anticoagulants, prolonged use of tourniquet).

Decompression can be achieved by a lateral incision (in case of concomitant fracture fixation) or by a medial incision (in case of revision of vascular lesion). There is no consensus on whether a release of both the anterior and posterior compartments should be performed when only one compartment is affected [17, 66, 67].

8.6.2.3 Forearm

The forearm is the most common site of compartment syndrome in the upper extremity. In the forearm there are four compartments, divided by fascia layers: superficial and deep volar compartments, dorsal compartment, and the mobile wad (posterolateral compartment).

Deep volar compartment is the most susceptible to ischemic and compression injury. It lays between the interosseous membrane, virtually inextensible, and the superficial volar compartment. It contains flexor pollicis longus and flexor digitorum profundus.

Superficial volar compartment, divided by fascia from the deep volar one, includes pronator teres, palmaris longus, flexor digitorum superficialis, flexor carpi radialis, and flexor carpi ulnaris.

Within the volar compartments run the median nerve, the anterior interosseous nerve, and the ulnar nerve. The median nerve runs in the forearm between the flexor digitorum superficialis and the flexor digitorum profundus, and is the most commonly injured in forearm compartment syndrome. It can also be compressed under the transverse carpal ligament.

The dorsal compartment lays on the interosseous membrane and contains extensor of the thumb and extensor of the long fingers.

The mobile wad includes the brachioradialis, extensor carpi radialis longus, and extensor carpi radialis brevis.

Fractures of the forearm, both open and closed, are the most common causes of forearm compartment syndrome. There are also nontraumatic causes of forearm compartment syndrome, including reperfusion injury, angioplasty or angiography, intravenous line extravasations, injection of drugs, coagulopathies, or bleeding disorders [68, 69] (Fig. 8.4).

In awake patients, pain out of proportion and pain with passive stretching of the fingers in a swollen forearm are considered very sensitive signs of compartment syndrome. In the early phases, it is fundamental to remove any bandages or splints that may be causing external compression on the forearm. The fractures should be realigned. If the suspect of compartment syndrome persists, fasciotomy should be urgently executed.

Fig. 8.4 Compartment syndrome and fasciotomies of the upper extremity after an electrocution

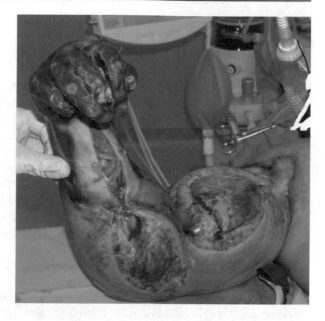

Even if the compartment could involve only one or two compartments, many authors suggest to decompress all the four compartments: this is accomplished with two incisions, one on the volar aspect and one on the dorsal aspect of the forearm. The volar incision begins proximal and medial to the antecubital fossa and extends distally in a curvilinear fashion till the midline, at the level of the carpal tunnel (that should be released). The dorsal compartment and mobile wad are decompressed with a single incision beginning at the level of the lateral epicondyle and extending to the distal radioulnar joint in line with Lister tubercle [68–70].

Delay to decompress the forearm is predictive of long-term complications. If patients underwent fasciotomy after 6 h of presentation, then they were significantly more likely to develop complications. The overall complication rate, as described in a recent systematic review, is about 40%, including neurologic deficits, contracture, delayed fracture union, muscle necrosis, complex regional pain syndrome, and tethering of skin graft to tendon limiting motion [71, 72].

8.6.2.4 Hand

The hand is composed of ten myotendinous compartments. Although anatomic studies suggest the presence of variability among individuals, the hand compartments are the thenar, hypothenar, adductor, and seven interosseous compartments. The carpal tunnel is mostly considered part of the forearm. Each of these compartments is bound by its own fascial envelope. The digits, despite the absence of muscle bellies, are considered by some authors to contain individual compartments, delimited by the boundaries of Grayson and Cleland ligaments [73].

Due to the low incidence of hand compartment syndrome, few large studies exist, with the literature describing small case series or case report. The underlying causes slightly differ from other compartment syndrome of the extremities: complications related to intravenous infiltrations, crush injuries, fractures, prolonged external compression, insect bites, snake envenomation, high-pressure injections, infection, and burns [74, 75].

In the event of suspected compartment syndrome, any dressing should be removed. If the suspicious persists, decompression must be carried out urgently. The release of the dorsal and volar interossei is obtained with separate longitudinal dorsal incisions over the second and fourth metacarpal. Dissection is carried down along the sides of each metacarpal, and the fascia is incised. Deeper dissection is continued along the radial aspect of the second metacarpal to release the adductor compartment. A similar technique is used along the radial and ulnar side of each metacarpal to decompress the volar interossei. To release the thenar and hypothenar compartments, volar incisions are needed. Digital decompression is performed using midaxial incisions, releasing the Cleland ligaments, taking caution to avoid the neurovascular bundles [74–76].

If not treated, acute compartment syndrome of the hand will evolve in intrinsic contracture. The muscle bellies, after ischemia and necrosis, become fibrotic and shortened. The hand will assume an intrinsic minus position, with the metacarpophalangeal joints in extension and the interphalangeal joints in flexion. The contracture of the first webspace, due to retraction of adductor muscles, can be associated to the other deformities. The prognosis for functional recovery is extremely low [74, 75].

8.7 Considerations in the Pediatric Population

Acute compartment syndrome in children is a rare but potentially devastating condition affecting orthopedic patients. The reported causes are the same of those of the adult population, with traumatic as the most common. In the upper extremity supracondylar humerus fractures and both bone forearm fractures are the most frequently involved in acute compartment syndrome; in the lower limb, tibia fractures are the main causes. Nontraumatic causes can be iatrogenic, due to casting complications, intravenous infiltrations, or intravenous medication administration [26, 77].

The diagnosis of acute extremity compartment syndrome in children is particularly difficult and is often delayed because the classic signs commonly described in adults are not constant. The three A's can be helpful when formulate a suspicious of compartment syndrome in children: anxiety, agitation, and increasing analgesic requirement. As described, the pressure threshold that mandates fasciotomy is debatable. In adults an absolute pressure of 30–45 mmHg has been suggested as an indication for decompression. Because normal compartment pressures are higher in children, and these values cannot be used as reliable standards in children. Furthermore, direct measurement of intracompartmental pressure using a needle and catheter is invasive and can be difficult in children. With this, compartment syndrome remains fundamentally a clinical diagnosis even in children [26, 77, 78].

When compartment syndrome is suspected, circumferential dressings should be split and casts should be bi-valved. If the clinical diagnosis of compartment syndrome is made, emergent fasciotomy and decompression is indicated. Despite a long period from injury to surgery in many cases reported in the literature, excellent results were achieved with fasciotomy in most patients. The reason is that children can tolerate increased intracompartmental pressure for longer periods of time than adults before tissue necrosis becomes irreversible [77, 79].

8.8 "Crush" Syndrome

Crush injury, literally, is a lesion resulting from direct physical crushing of the muscles due to something heavy. When the limbs are subject to prolonged pressure or are tightly restrained, rupture of muscle cells releases myoglobin. Myoglobin is filtered out of the glomerulus, but once the renal threshold is exceeded, it precipitates in the distal convoluted tubules causing obstruction. Furthermore, other substances such as potassium, magnesium, phosphate, acids, enzymes like creatine phosphokinase and lactate dehydrogenase are released into the blood stream. These are essential for cell function, but are toxic when released into circulation in large amounts. The consequent metabolic changes rapidly leads to the so-called crush syndrome [2, 18, 19, 80].

The muscles are grossly swollen, hard, cold, insensitive, and necrotic (Fig. 8.5). Kidneys also tend to be edematous and increase in volume. The released potassium in the circulation causes alteration in cardiac rhythm; respiratory gas exchange due to lung edema. Ultimately, shock develops, followed by ARDS, SIRS, sepsis, and finally death.

The majority of crush syndrome reported in literature are associated with disaster (earthquake, explosion, terroristic attack), with a large number of victims. In daily practice, crush syndrome can be occasionally seen in comatose patients, after prolonged rescue in traffic accident, in patients receiving surgery in tight position [80, 81].

Most of these patients are conscious at rescue; crush injuries, in fact, are not common after head and chest injuries because the prolonged pressure necessary to cause this syndrome often results in death for massive brain injury or for hypoxia.

After rescue and initial resuscitation, the key is to recognize the signs and symptoms of the syndrome: petechiae, blisters, muscle bruising, and superficial injuries

Fig. 8.5 Muscle necrosis after crush syndrome of the leg

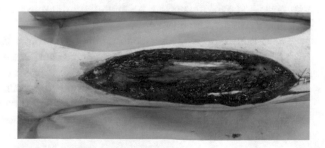

are common. Myalgia, muscle paralysis and sensory deficit, fever, cardiac arrhythmia, pneumonia, oliguria, and renal failure are the natural consequence of crush injuries. After rescue of these patients, reperfusion of the muscles can worsen the general status. Large amounts of potentially toxic substance are suddenly released into the blood stream, reaching rapidly brain, heart, lung, and kidneys. The keys of treatment are replacement of fluid, maintenance of effective kidney function, and decompression of the suffering muscular compartments [80, 81].

8.9   Acute Exertional Compartment Syndrome: A Rare Occurrence That Is Frequently Missed

Nontraumatic root causes of acute compartment syndrome of the extremities were described earlier in this chapter. One of the most concerning entities is related to acute exertional compartment syndrome which can occur after any extent of physical exercise in absence of a preceding trauma mechanism [16, 20]. A multiplicity of case reports have been published on the rare entity of acute exertional compartment syndrome of the leg, foot, and upper extremity [82–88]. All these reports unequivocally emphasize the notion that a missed diagnosis leading to delayed surgical treatment is associated with dismal patient outcomes, and most frequently related to the absence of a trauma mechanism which decreases the level of suspicion by the treating physician [82–88]. These findings corroborate the notion that the presence of pain out of proportion, reflected by the revised "5 P's" (Pain, pain, pain, pain, pain!), frequently represents the exclusive cardinal symptom suggestive of presence of acute compartment syndrome of the extremities, independent of the underlying etiology and absence of a preceding trauma mechanism [20, 89]. Thus, as a general rule of thumb, it is highly prudent for any physician, independent of the medical specialty, to consider presence of acute compartment syndrome in ANY patient with pain to the extremities, independent of the root cause, until proven otherwise [20, 89].

8.10   Outcomes of Compartment Syndrome and Sequelae

Acute compartment syndrome is related to high costs for the community: hospitalization increased threefold and overall costs are 2.3 times higher than for uncomplicated patients. Acute compartment syndrome can be a reason for legal dispute; late diagnosis and subsequent late treatment are the most important factors related to indemnity compensation [90–92].

The overall mortality after compartment syndrome has been reported to be as high as 15%, but the correlation is suggested to be more with the concomitant traumatic injury than with the extremity lesion itself. Among survived patients, loss of limb is obviously the worst complication after development of compartment syndrome. The reported amputation rate after compartment syndrome is 5.7–12.9%. Risk factors for amputation include male gender, associated vascular injury, and delayed fasciotomy [16, 20, 89].

Fig. 8.6 Typical deformity of ankle and foot after compartment syndrome of the lower leg

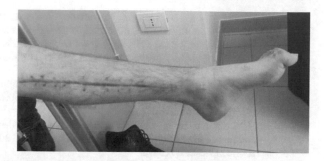

When fasciotomies are performed more than 8 h after injury, rate of complications, and consequently bad outcomes, progressively increases. Consequently, even in case of saving the limb, the patient can still develop tremendous disability. A delay in the diagnosis of acute compartment syndrome can have devastating consequences for the function of the extremity of the patient. Physicians and patients might believe that a delay in diagnosis is due to abnormal presentation and symptoms; on the other hand, inadequate training and poor culture of trauma could represent important risk factors for missed diagnosis [91, 92].

When acute extremity compartment syndrome of the lower leg is missed or treatment is delayed, late functional disabilities mostly consists in limited range of movement of the ankle, reduced functional strength of the foot extensors, contractures of the foot flexors, abnormal superficial sensibility, and chronic pain. The ischemic insult to the nerves might result in decreased proprioception and sensation. Lesser-toe deformities (claw toes) and cavus foot deformity are common sequelae as well. It has to be noted that the degree of subsequent functional disability is strongly influenced by the severity of the primary soft tissue trauma [38, 56, 59, 60] (Fig. 8.6).

In the upper limb, Volkmann contracture is the result of irreversible tissue ischemia, muscle necrosis with consequent fibrotic evolution and retraction. In the forearm, the typical posture that develops includes elbow flexion, forearm pronation, wrist flexion, and thumb adduction with the metacarpophalangeal joints in extension and the interphalangeal joints in flexion. The median nerve is often affected because it lays in the deeper zone of the forearm, that is more severely compromised by ischemia. The main goal in the management of Volkmann contracture is to restore function; however, normal function of the upper extremity should not be expected. Affected muscles are exposed, fibrotic tissue is removed, tenolysis and neurolysis of the median and ulnar nerves should be performed. Tendon transfer may be a solution to improve the long-term residual function [68, 69, 72, 74].

References

1. Konig F, Richter E, Volkmann R. Die ischaemischen Muskellahmungen und Kontrakturen. Centralblatt fur Chirurgie. 1881;51:801–3.
2. Bywaters EG, Beall D. Crush injuries with impairment of renal function. Br Med J. 1941;1:427–32.

3. Carter AB, Richards RL, Zachary RB. The anterior tibial syndrome. Lancet. 1949;2:928–34.
4. Hargens AR, Romine JS, Sipe JC, et al. Peripheral nerve-conduction block by high muscle-compartment pressure. J Bone Joint Surg Am. 1979;61:192–200.
5. Hope MJ, McQueen MM. Acute compartment syndrome in the absence of fracture. J Orthop Trauma. 2004;18:220–4.
6. Stella M, Santolini E, Sanguineti F, et al. Aetiology of trauma-related acute compartment syndrome of the leg: a systematic review. Injury. 2019;50(Suppl 2):S57–64. https://doi.org/10.1016/j.injury.2019.01.047.
7. Janzing HM. Epidemiology, etiology, pathophysiology and diagnosis of the acute compartment syndrome of the extremity. Eur J Trauma Emerg Surg. 2007;33(6):576–83. https://doi.org/10.1007/s00068-007-7151-0.
8. Meskey T, Hardcastle J, O'Toole RV. Are certain fractures at increased risk for compartment syndrome after civilian ballistic injury? J Trauma. 2011;71(5):1385–9. https://doi.org/10.1097/TA.0b013e31822fec25.
9. Steele HL, Singh A. Vascular injury after occult knee dislocation presenting as compartment syndrome. J Emerg Med. 2012;42(3):271–4. https://doi.org/10.1016/j.jemermed.2008.08.029. Epub 2009 Apr 2.
10. Ulmer T. The clinical diagnosis of compartment syndrome of the lower leg: are clinical findings predictive of the disorder? J Orthop Trauma. 2002;16:572–7.
11. Branco BC, Inaba K, Barmparas G, et al. Incidence and predictors for the need for fasciotomy after extremity trauma: a 10-year review in a mature level I trauma centre. Injury. 2011;42:1157–63.
12. Leversedge FJ, Moore TJ, Peterson BC, et al. Compartment syndrome of the upper extremity. J Hand Surg Am. 2011;36(3):544–59. https://doi.org/10.1016/j.jhsa.2010.12.008; quiz 560.
13. Kleshinski J, Bittar S, Wahlquist M, et al. Review of compartment syndrome due to group A streptococcal infection. Am J Med Sci. 2008;336:265–9.
14. Matsen FA 3rd. Compartmental syndromes. N Engl J Med. 1979;300:1210–1.
15. Odeh M. The role of reperfusion-induced injury in the pathogenesis of the crush syndrome. N Engl J Med. 1991;324:1417–22.
16. Von Keudell AG, Weaver MJ, Appleton PT. Diagnosis and treatment of acute extremity compartment syndrome. Lancet. 2015;386(10000):1299–310. https://doi.org/10.1016/S0140-6736(15)00277-9.
17. Schmidt AH. Acute compartment syndrome. Injury. 2017;48(Suppl 1):S22–5. https://doi.org/10.1016/j.injury.2017.04.024. Epub 2017 Apr 24.
18. Blaisdell FW. The pathophysiology of skeletal muscle ischemia and the reperfusion syndrome: a review. Cardiovasc Surg. 2002;10:620–30.
19. Chen CY, Lin YR, Zhao LL, et al. Clinical factors in predicting acute renal failure caused by rhabdomyolysis in the ED. Am J Emerg Med. 2013;31:1062–6.
20. Ipaktchi K, Stahel PF. Musculoskeletal trauma and hand injuries. In: Markovchick VJ, Pons PT, Bakes KM, Buchanan JA, editors. Emergency medicine secrets. 6th ed. St. Louis: Elsevier; 2016. p. 603–17.
21. Wong JC, Vosbikian MM, Dwyer JM, et al. Accuracy of measurement of hand compartment pressures: a cadaveric study. J Hand Surg Am. 2015;40:701–6.
22. Boody AR, Wongworawat MD. Accuracy in the measurement of compartment pressures: a comparison of three commonly used devices. J Bone Joint Surg Am. 2005;87:2415–22.
23. Matava MJ, Whitesides TE Jr, Seiler JG 3rd, et al. Determination of the compartment pressure threshold of muscle ischemia in a canine model. J Trauma. 1994;37:50–8.
24. Heckman MM, Whitesides TE Jr, Grewe SR, et al. Compartment pressure in association with closed tibial fractures. The relationship between tissue pressure, compartment, and the distance from the site of the fracture. J Bone Joint Surg Am. 1994;76:1285–92.
25. Mubarak SJ, Owen CA, Hargens AR, et al. Acute compartment syndromes: diagnosis and treatment with the aid of the wick catheter. J Bone Joint Surg Am. 1978;60:1091–5.
26. Matsen FA 3rd, Veith RG. Compartmental syndromes in children. J Pediatr Orthop. 1981;1:33–41.

27. Matsen FA 3rd, Winquist RA, Krugmire RB Jr. Diagnosis and management of compartmental syndromes. J Bone Joint Surg Am. 1980;62:286–91.
28. Whitesides TE, Haney TC, Morimoto K, et al. Tissue pressure measurements as a determinant for the need of fasciotomy. Clin Orthop Relat Res. 1975;(113):43–51.
29. McQueen MM, Court-Brown CM. Compartment monitoring in tibial fractures. The pressure threshold for decompression. J Bone Joint Surg Br. 1996;78:99–104.
30. Harris IA, Kadir A, Donald G. Continuous compartment pressure monitoring for tibia fractures: does it influence outcome? J Trauma. 2006;60:1330–5.
31. Janzing HM, Broos PL. Routine monitoring of compartment pressure in patients with tibial fractures: beware of overtreatment! Injury. 2001;32:415–21.
32. Al-Dadah OQ, Darrah C, Cooper A, et al. Continuous compartment pressure monitoring vs. clinical monitoring in tibial diaphyseal fractures. Injury. 2008;39:1204–9.
33. McQueen MM, Duckworth AD. The diagnosis of acute compartment syndrome: a review. Eur J Trauma Emerg Surg. 2014;40(5):521–8. https://doi.org/10.1007/s00068-014-0414-7.
34. McQueen MM, Christie J, Court-Brown CM. Acute compartment syndrome in tibial diaphyseal fractures. J Bone Joint Surg Br. 1996;78(1):95–8.
35. Rorabeck CH, Clarke KM. The pathophysiology of the anterior tibial compartment syndrome: an experimental investigation. J Trauma. 1978;18:299–304.
36. Ritenour AE, Dorlac WC, Fang R, et al. Complications after fasciotomy revision and delayed compartment release in combat patients. J Trauma. 2008;64(2 Suppl):S153–62.
37. Zannis J, Angobaldo J, Marks M, et al. Comparison of fasciotomy wound closures using traditional dressing changes and the vacuum-assisted closure device. Ann Plast Surg. 2009;62:407–9.
38. Kakagia D, Karadimas EJ, Drosos G, et al. Wound closure of leg fasciotomy: comparison of vacuum-assisted closure versus shoelace technique. A randomised study. Injury. 2014;45:890–3.
39. Giannoudis PV, Nicolopoulos C, Dinopoulos H, et al. The impact of lower leg compartment syndrome on health related quality of life. Injury. 2002;33(2):117–21.
40. Johnson SB, Weaver FA, Yellin AE, et al. Clinical results of decompressive dermotomy-fasciotomy. Am J Surg. 1992;164(3):286–90.
41. Kosir R, Moore FA, Selby JH, et al. Acute lower extremity compartment syndrome (ALECS) screening protocol in critically ill trauma patients. J Trauma. 2007;63:268–75.
42. Fitzgerald AM, Gaston P, Wilson Y, et al. Long-term sequelae of fasciotomy wounds. Br J Plast Surg. 2000;53(8):690–3.
43. Diaz Dilernia F, Zaidenberg EE, Gamsie S, et al. Gluteal compartment syndrome secondary to pelvic trauma. Case Rep Orthop. 2016;2016:2780295. https://doi.org/10.1155/2016/2780295.
44. Henson JT, Roberts CS, Giannoudis PV. Gluteal compartment syndrome. Acta Orthop Belg. 2009;75(2):147–52.
45. Hilland SL, Bianchi J. The gluteal compartment syndrome. Am Surg. 1997;63(9):823–6.
46. Schmalzried TP, Neal WC, Eckardt JJ. Gluteal compartment and crush syndromes: a report of three cases and review of the literature. Clin Orthop Relat Res. 1992;(277):161–5.
47. Mithöfer K, Lhowe DW, Vrahas MS, et al. Clinical spectrum of acute compartment syndrome of the thigh and its relation to associated injuries. Clin Orthop Relat Res. 2004;(425):223–9.
48. Schwartz JT Jr, Brumback RJ, Lakatos R, et al. Acute compartment syndrome of the thigh. A spectrum of injury. J Bone Joint Surg Am. 1989;71(3):392–400.
49. Robinson D, On E, Halperin N. Anterior compartment syndrome of the thigh in athletes—indications for conservative treatment. J Trauma. 1992;32(2):183–6.
50. Rööser B, Bengtson S, Hägglund G. Acute compartment syndrome from anterior thigh muscle contusion: a report of eight cases. J Orthop Trauma. 1991;5(1):57–9.
51. DeLee J, Stiehl JB. Open tibia fracture with compartment syndrome. Clin Orthop Relat Res. 1981;160:175–84.
52. Blick SS, Brumback RJ, Poka A, et al. Compartment syndrome in open tibial fractures. J Bone Joint Surg Am. 1986;68-A:1348–53.

53. McQueen MM, Gaston P, Court-Brown CM. Acute compartment syndrome: who is at risk? J Bone Joint Surg Br. 2000;82-B:200–3.
54. Halpern AA, Nagel DA. Anterior compartment pressures in patients with tibial fractures. J Trauma. 1980;20:786–90.
55. Barei DP, Nork SE, Mills WJ, et al. Complications associated with internal fixation of high-energy bicondylar tibial plateau fractures utilizing a two incision technique. J Orthop Trauma. 2004;18:649–57.
56. Egol KA, Tejwani NC, Capla EL, et al. Staged management of high energy proximal tibia fractures (OTA types 41): the results of a prospective, standardized protocol. J Orthop Trauma. 2005;19:448–55.
57. Ebraheim NA, Siddiqui S, Raberding C. A single-incision fasciotomy for compartment syndrome of the lower leg. J Orthop Trauma. 2016;30(7):e252–5. https://doi.org/10.1097/BOT.0000000000000542.
58. Brink F, Bachmann S, Lechler P, et al. Mechanism of injury and treatment of trauma-associated acute compartment syndrome of the foot. Eur J Trauma Emerg Surg. 2014;40(5):529–33. https://doi.org/10.1007/s00068-014-0420-9.
59. Santi MD, Botte MJ. Volkmann's ischemic contracture of the foot and ankle: evaluation and treatment of established deformity. Foot Ankle Int. 1995;16:368–77.
60. Mittlmeier T, Mächler G, Lob G, et al. Compartment syndrome of the foot after intraarticular calcaneal fracture. Clin Orthop Relat Res. 1991;(269):241–48.
61. Dodd A, Le I. Foot compartment syndrome: diagnosis and management. J Am Acad Orthop Surg. 2013;21:657–64.
62. Brey JM, Castro MD. Salvage of compartment syndrome of the leg and foot. Foot Ankle Clin. 2008;13:767–72.
63. Diminick M, Shapiro G, Cornell C. Acute compartment syndrome of the triceps and deltoid. J Orthop Trauma. 1999;13:225–7.
64. Rohde RS, Goitz RJ. Deltiod compartment syndrome: a result of operative positioning. J Shoulder Elb Surg. 2006;15:383–5.
65. Wijesuriya JD, Cowling PD, Izod C, et al. Deltoid compartment syndrome as a complication of lateral decubitus positioning for contralateral elbow surgery in an anabolic steroid abuser. Shoulder Elbow. 2014;6(3):200–3. https://doi.org/10.1177/1758573214530607.
66. Thomas N, Cone B. Acute compartment syndrome in the upper arm. Am J Emerg Med. 2017;35(3):525.e1–2. https://doi.org/10.1016/j.ajem.2016.10.029.
67. Maeckelbergh L, Colen S, Anné L. Upper arm compartment syndrome: a case report and review of the literature. Orthop Surg. 2013;5(3):229–32. https://doi.org/10.1111/os.12054.
68. Kistler JM, Ilyas AM, Thoder JJ. Forearm compartment syndrome: evaluation and management. Hand Clin. 2018;34:53–60. https://doi.org/10.1016/j.hcl.2017.09.006.
69. Prasarn ML, Ouellette EA. Acute compartment syndrome of the upper extremity. J Am Acad Orthop Surg. 2011;19(1):49–58. Erratum in: J Am Acad Orthop Surg. 2011;19(5):50A.
70. Friedrich JB, Shin AY. Management of forearm compartment syndrome. Crit Care Nurs Clin North Am. 2012;24(2):261–74. https://doi.org/10.1016/j.ccell.2012.03.003.
71. Alexander CM, Ramseyer M, Beatty JS. Missed extravasation injury from peripheral infusion of norepinephrine resulting in forearm compartment syndrome and amputation. Am Surg. 2016;82(7):e162–3.
72. Kalyani BS, Fisher BE, Roberts CS, et al. Compartment syndrome of the forearm: a systematic review. J Hand Surg Am. 2011;36(3):535–43. https://doi.org/10.1016/j.jhsa.2010.12.007.
73. Guyton GP, Shearman CM, Saltzman CL. Compartmental divisions of the hand revisited. Rethinking the validity of cadaver infusion experiments. J Bone Joint Surg Br. 2001;83(2):241–4.
74. Rubinstein AJ, Ahmed IH, Vosbikian MM. Hand compartment syndrome. Hand Clin. 2018;34(1):41–52. https://doi.org/10.1016/j.hcl.2017.09.005.
75. Oak NR, Abrams RA. Compartment syndrome of the hand. Orthop Clin North Am. 2016;47(3):609–16. https://doi.org/10.1016/j.ocl.2016.03.006.

76. Turkula SC, Fuller DA. Extensile fasciotomy for compartment syndrome of the forearm and hand. J Orthop Trauma. 2017;31(Suppl 3):S50–1. https://doi.org/10.1097/BOT.0000000000000903.
77. Kanj WW, Gunderson MA, Carrigan RB, et al. Acute compartment syndrome of the upper extremity in children: diagnosis, management, and outcomes. J Child Orthop. 2013;7(3):225–33. https://doi.org/10.1007/s11832-013-0492-9.
78. Bae DS, Kadiyala RK, Waters PM. Acute compartment syndrome in children: contemporary diagnosis, treatment, and outcome. J Pediatr Orthop. 2001;21(5):680–8.
79. Grottkau BE, Epps HR, Di Scala C. Compartment syndrome in children and adolescents. J Pediatr Surg. 2005;40(4):678–82.
80. Yokota J. Crush syndrome in disaster. JMAJ. 2005;48(7):341–52.
81. Rajagopalan S. Crush injuries and the crush syndrome. Med J Armed Forces India. 2010;66(4):317–20. https://doi.org/10.1016/S0377-1237(10)80007-3.
82. Lambert J, Ceulemans R. Acute exertional compartment syndrome in a young amateur soccer player: a case report. J Belg Soc Radiol. 2016;100:59.
83. Popovic N, Bottoni C, Cassidy C. Unrecognized acute exertional compartment syndrome of the leg and treatment. Acta Orthop Belg. 2011;77:265–9.
84. Anderson KD. Missed diagnosis of acute exertional compartment syndrome, occurring after a short run. Am J Emerg Med. 2005;23:215–6.
85. Stollsteimer GT, Shelton WR. Acute atraumatic compartment syndrome in an athlete: a case report. J Athl Train. 1997;32:248–50.
86. Jefferies JG, Carter T, White TO. A delayed presentation of bilateral leg compartment syndrome following non-stop dancing. BMJ Case Rep. 2015;2015:bcr2014208630. https://doi.org/10.1136/bcr-2014-208630.
87. Kelsey NR, Edmonds LD, Biko DM. Acute exertional medial compartment syndrome of the foot in a teenager. Radiol Case Rep. 2015;10:1092.
88. DeFilippis EM, Kleiman DA, Derman PB, DiFelice GS, Eachempati SR. Spinning-induced rhabdomyolysis and the risk of compartment syndrome and acute kidney injury: two cases and a review of the literature. Sports Health. 2014;6:333–5.
89. Forsh DA, Wolinsky PR. Compartment syndrome. In: Smith WR, Stahel PF, editors. Management of musculoskeletal injuries in the trauma patient. New York: Springer; 2014. p. 225–42.
90. Schmidt AH. The impact of compartment syndrome on hospital length of stay and charges among adult patients admitted with a fracture of the tibia. J Orthop Trauma. 2011;25(6):355–7. https://doi.org/10.1097/BOT.0b013e3181f18ad8.
91. Bhattacharyya T, Vrahas MS. The medical-legal aspects of compartment syndrome. J Bone Joint Surg Am. 2004;86-A(4):864–8.
92. Marchesi M, Marchesi A, Calori GM, et al. A sneaky surgical emergency: acute compartment syndrome. Retrospective analysis of 66 closed claims, medico-legal pitfalls and damages evaluation. Injury. 2014;45(Suppl 6):S16–20. https://doi.org/10.1016/j.injury.2014.10.017.

Polycompartment Syndrome

9

Andrea Minini, Moataz M. Emara,
and Manu L. N. G. Malbrain

Abbreviations

ACS	Abdominal compartment syndrome
AKI	Acute kidney injury
ALI	Acute lung injury
APP	Abdominal perfusion pressure
APV	Abdominal pressure variation
ATI	Abdomino-thoracic index of transmission
Cab	Abdominal compliance
CARS	Cardio-abdominal-renal syndrome
CO	Cardiac output
CP	Compartment pressure
CPP	Cerebral perfusion pressure
CS	Compartment syndrome
CSF	Cerebrospinal fluid
CVP	Central venous pressure
ECP	Extremity compartment pressure

A. Minini
Department of Intensive Care Medicine, University Hospital Brussels (UZB), Jette, Belgium

Department of Intensive Care Medicine and Anaesthesia, University of Insubria, Varese, Italy

M. M. Emara
Department of Anaesthesiology and Intensive Care, Faculty of Medicine, Mansoura University, Mansoura, Egypt

M. L. N. G. Malbrain (✉)

Department of Intensive Care Medicine, University Hospital Brussels (UZB), Jette, Belgium

Faculty of Medicine and Pharmacy, Vrije Universiteit Brussel (VUB), Jette, Belgium

President, International Fluid Academy, Lovenjoel, Belgium
e-mail: manu.malbrain@uzbrussel.be

© Springer Nature Switzerland AG 2021
F. Coccolini et al. (eds.), *Compartment Syndrome*, Hot Topics in Acute Care
Surgery and Trauma, https://doi.org/10.1007/978-3-030-55378-4_9

ECS   Extremity compartment syndrome
EVLW   Extravascular lung water
FG   Filtration gradient
GEDVI   Global end-diastolic volume index
HAPS   Hepato-abdominal-pulmonary syndrome
HARS   Hepato-abdominal-renal syndrome
IAH   Intra-abdominal hypertension
IAP   Intra-abdominal pressure
IAV   Intra-abdominal volume
ICP   Intracranial pressure
ITP   Intra-thoracic pressure
IVC   Inferior vena cava
MAP   Mean arterial pressure
PAOP   Pulmonary artery occlusion pressure
PCS   Polycompartment syndrome
PEEP   Positive end-expiratory pressure
PPV   Pulse pressure variation
ROSC   Return of spontaneous circulation
RPP   Renal perfusion pressure
RVEDVI   Right ventricular end-diastolic volume index
SVV   Stroke volume variation
TAI   Thoraco-abdominal index of transmission
TCS   Thoracic compartment syndrome
VPS   Ventriculo-peritoneal shunt

9.1   Summary

A compartment is a closed anatomic space within the human body. It is like a box with six walls that can be partially rigid or flexible. There are four major compartments in the human body: head, chest, abdomen, and extremities. Each compartment contains single or multiple organs with their blood perfusion systems.

A compartment syndrome (CS) is the pathological increase in the pressure within a compartment that impairs blood supply to the contents and threatens the viability of surrounding tissue. Within each compartment, an individual organ or a region with multiple organs can develop compartment syndrome.

Different body compartments can be differentiated according to the contained organs and the anatomical site but should not be considered physiologically isolated. Changes in one compartment can affect the adjacent one as well as remote ones, either upstream or downstream.

Scalea et al. first described the combination of increased compartmental pressures existing in multiple compartments: intra-abdominal pressure (IAP), intrathoracic pressure (ITP), and intracranial pressure (ICP) in traumatic brain injury patients [1]. He called this combination the multi- or multiple compartment syndrome. The term polycompartment syndrome was coined afterwards to stop confusion with multiple limb trauma and a compartment syndrome justifying decompressive fasciotomy.

The polycompartment syndrome (PCS) is a constellation of the physiological sequelae of increased compartment pressures in multiple compartments of the body. The abdomen plays a central role in the polycompartment syndrome, and the effects of IAH on different organ systems within and outside the abdomen are well recognized.

In this chapter, we will understand the pathophysiology, clinical presentation, and the management of the polycompartment syndrome.

9.2 Definitions

According to the Abdominal Compartment Society, formerly known as the World Society on Abdominal Compartment Syndrome (WSACS, www.wsacs.org) [2] consensus definitions, polycompartment syndrome is the condition in which two or more anatomical compartments have elevated compartment pressures.

9.2.1 Compartment Syndrome

A compartment syndrome (CS) exists when the increased pressure in a closed anatomic space threatens the viability of surrounding tissue. Within the body, there are four compartments, the head, the chest, the abdomen, and the extremities. Within each compartment, an individual organ or a region with multiple organs can develop a CS. A CS is not a disease, and as such, it can have many causes, and it can develop within many disease processes [3].

The increased compartment pressure (CP) will exert a direct force on the original compartment and its contents by increasing venous resistance and decreasing perfusion pressure, as well as on distant compartments.

9.2.2 Polycompartment Syndrome

The polycompartment syndrome is a pathophysiological disorder of two or more compartments in which acute or chronic dysfunction of one compartment may induce acute or chronic dysfunction in the other [4]. Table 9.1 lists some examples.

9.2.3 Classification

Classification of compartment syndrome can be primary or secondary [2, 3]:

– *Primary* compartment syndrome is the condition in which injury or disease originates in this compartment as development of an abdominal compartment syndrome (ACS) after a ruptured abdominal aorta aneurysm.
Secondary compartment syndrome occurs when the injury does not originate within the compartment itself as in the development of lower extremity compartment syndrome with ACS.

Table 9.1 Example of case scenarios

Case scenario	Polycompartment syndrome presence	Treatment
Case scenario 1	A patient with a car accident and blunt abdominal trauma developed intracranial hypertension and worsening neurologic function due to spleen rupture with ACS	Neurologic condition improved after abdominal decompression and splenectomy
Case scenario 2	A patient with burns developed ACS after placement of a subclavian central venous line (IAP > 20 mmHg on continuous tracing) followed by acute respiratory failure due to tension pneumothorax and subsequent ACS	Respiratory and hemodynamic function improved after placement of a chest tube, but moreover, IAP also returned to normal
Case scenario 3	A hematologic patient with graft versus host disease of the bowel developed abdominal hypertension related to infection with clostridium difficile and toxic megacolon	Finally, a total colectomy was performed resulting in reduction of IAV and normalization of IAP
Case scenario 4	A hematologic patient with chronic myeloid leukemia and splenomegaly developed signs and symptoms of dyspnea related to pulmonary hypertension on transthoracic cardiac ultrasound	After splenectomy, abdominal hypertension normalizes, and pulmonary hypertension disappeared
Case scenario 5	A patient with a ventriculoperitoneal shunt (VPS) developed headache due to shunt dysfunction because of obstipation and abdominal hypertension	After rectal enema and bowel evacuation, (with normalization of IAH), the VPS functioned again normally
Case scenario 6	A patient with morbid obesity had signs and symptoms of idiopathic intracranial hypertension (pseudotumor cerebri)	The symptoms disappeared after bariatric surgery and weight loss
Case scenario 7	A patient with COPD was treated with noninvasive ventilation via mask interface. When the physiotherapist puts him into the upright position, the patient suffered from a cardiac arrest due to aerophagia and gastric distension	Only after the placement of a nasogastric tube and evacuation of the air from the stomach, return of spontaneous circulation (ROSC) occurred
Case scenario 8	A patient with head trauma developed intracranial hypertension during colonoscopy	After colonic decompression, ICP normalized

9.2.4 Abdominal Compliance

Abdominal compliance (C_{ab}). Abdominal compliance plays a central role in the development of polycompartment syndrome. It is a measure of the ease of the abdominal expansion in response to an increase in the intra-abdominal volume (IAV). From the physics point of view, it is reciprocal to elasticity (E).

$$\text{Compliance } (C) = \Delta v$$

$$C_{ab} = \Delta \text{IAV}$$

where the IAV is the intra-abdominal volume. Normal C_{ab} is 250–450 mL/mmHg.

The compliance can be presented by a volume/pressure curve, where the slope of the curve represents C_{ab}. The C_{ab} is initially linear, and then at a particular "critical" volume, the pressure increases exponentially after exhaustion of the compensatory mechanisms from reshaping to stretching and pressurization of the abdominal cavity [5]. This is illustrated in Fig. 9.1.

Measurement of IAV may be cumbersome at the bedside; however, we need the change in IAV, not the resting or the static IAV, to calculate C_{ab}. Therefore, we can

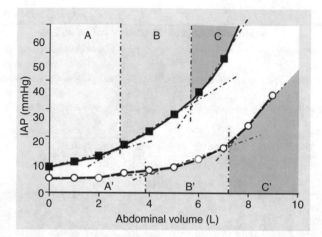

Fig. 9.1 The pressure–volume curve in the abdominal compartment. Schematic representation of different phases during increasing intra-abdominal volume (IAV) in two patients undergoing laparoscopy (CO_2—insufflation). Shaded areas represent in light gray the reshaping phase (A and A′), in mid-gray the stretching phase (B and B′), and in dark gray the pressurization phase (C and C′). The accent (′) indicates the patient with poor abdominal compliance. In the patient with poor compliance, the reshaping phase went from IAV of 0–2.8 L (vs 0–3,8 L when compliance was normal), the stretching phase from IAV of 2.8 to 5.6 L (vs 3.8–7.2 L, respectively), and the pressurization phase from IAV beyond 5.6 L in the patient with low vs 7.2 L in the patient with normal compliance. Adapted from Malbrain et al. with permission under the Open access CC BY License 4.0 [6]

obtain the ΔIAV during addition or removal of abdominal fluid (or fluid from the stomach as a surrogate) or abdominal gas following induced pneumoperitoneum during laparoscopic surgery. Abdominal pressure variation (APV) during continuous IAP monitoring is a useful estimate of the C_{ab}, and the higher the APV, the lower the C_{ab} and vice versa (Fig. 9.2). The APV can be defined as follows [7]:

$$APV = \Delta IAP/mean\ IAP$$

This chapter will discuss the different individual compartment syndromes from head till toe, as well as the different possible combinations (polycompartment syndrome) and how each compartment can affect others. Being apparently the most critical and the key to understanding *polycompartment syndrome*, we will discuss the abdominal compartment first.

9.3 Abdominal Compartment Syndrome (ACS)

9.3.1 Background

The abdominal compartment takes a central position among other compartments, and ACS can affect all other major compartments, head, chest, and extremity, along with the contained mini-compartments in the abdomen such as kidney, liver, and pelvis.

The IAP increases the ITP by a certain degree. This is called the abdomino-thoracic index of transmission (ATI). As the abdomen plays a central role, the IAP will also be transmitted to other compartments (Fig. 9.3).

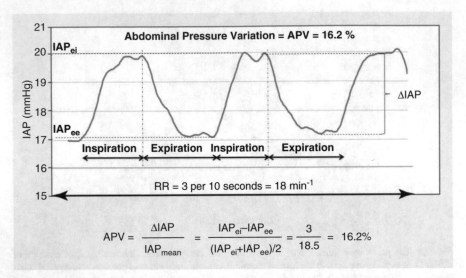

$$APV = \frac{\Delta IAP}{IAP_{mean}} = \frac{IAP_{ei} - IAP_{ee}}{(IAP_{ei} + IAP_{ee})/2} = \frac{3}{18.5} = 16.2\%$$

Fig. 9.2 Estimation of abdominal compliance with abdominal pressure variation. Smoothed average of a continuous IAP tracing, excluding the pulse pressure artifacts during BiPAP ventilation with a plateau pressure of 25 and PEEP of 10 cmH$_2$O. Mean IAP was 18.5 mmHg with IAP = 17 mmHg at end-expiration (IAPee) and IAP = 20 mmHg at end-inspiration (IAPei), resulting in an ΔIAP (defined as IAPei—IAPee) = 3 mmHg. The abdominal pressure variation (APV) can be calculated as ΔIAP divided by mean IAP (i.e., 3/18.5 = 16.2%). Higher APV values for a given ventilator setting correspond to lower abdominal wall compliance. The thoraco-abdominal index (TAI) of transmission can be calculated as ΔIAP divided by (Plateau pressure minus PEEP) or, thus, 3 mmHg = 4 cmH$_2$O/15 = 26.7%. Adapted from Malbrain et al. with permission according to the Open access CC BY License 4.0 [7]

For calculation of ATI, we will need continuous and simultaneous monitoring of central venous pressure (CVP) or pulmonary artery occlusion pressure (PAOP) and IAP. The application of external pressure on the abdominal wall during end-expiration will affect filling pressures. The change in CVP or PAOP during end-expiration is expected to be due to the change in the IAP (Fig. 9.4).

So, the

$$ATI = \Delta CVPee/\Delta IAPee \text{ or } = \Delta PAOPee/\Delta IAPee.$$

The ATI is always estimated roughly as 50% and is important when estimating trans-mural pressures. So that as a rule of thumb trans-mural can be calculated as follows:

$$CVP (CVP_{tm}) = CVPee - IAP/2.$$

The abdomino-thoracic effects are mainly pulmonary and cardiovascular. The index of transmission is affected by actions of the diaphragm, the rib cage, and the abdominal wall (Table 9.2).

9.3.2 Pulmonary Effects of ACS

9.3.2.1 Pathophysiology

High IAP affects the thoracic compartment both directly and indirectly.

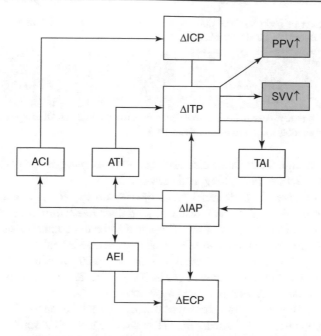

Fig. 9.3 Changes in intra-abdominal pressure (ΔIAP) will lead to concomitant changes in pressures of other compartments. Thoraco-abdominal pressure transmission can be seen with positive pressure ventilation, PEEP or auto-PEEP, or pneumothorax. *ACI* abdomino-cranial index of transmission, *AEI* abdomino-extremities, *ATI* abdomino-thoracic index of transmission, *ECP* extremity compartment pressure, *ICP* intrathoracic pressure, *ITP* abdomino-thoracic index of transmission, *PPV* pulse pressure variation, *SVV* stroke volume variation, *TAI* thoraco-abdominal index of transmission

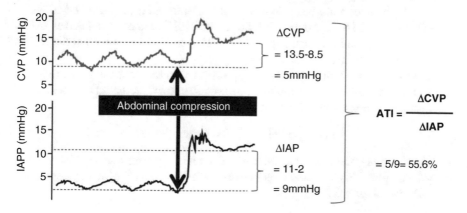

Fig. 9.4 Calculation of abdomino-thoracic index of transmission (ATI). The change in IAP from 2 to 11 mmHg results in a concomitant change in CVP from 8.5 to 13.5 mmHg. Hence the ATI can be calculated as the ΔCVPee/ΔIAPee, or thus 5/9 or 55.6%

Table 9.2 Effect of actions of the diaphragm, the rib cage, and the abdominal wall on intra-abdominal pressure (IAP) and intra-abdominal volume (IAV)

	Effect on IAP	Effect on IAV
Abdominal muscle contractions	↑	↓
Diaphragm movement (inspiration)	↑[a]	↑
Rib cage action (inspiration)	↓	↓

[a]The effect of diaphragm excursions on IAP depends on the abdominal wall compliance; in case of very good compliance, there will be no increase in IAP

Directly through the cephalic displacement of the diaphragm and compression of the thoracic structure (heart, lung, and vessels).

Indirectly where the abdominal pathology causes *capillary leak syndrome* as seen in abdominal sepsis or as a result of *fluid over-resuscitation* for initial treatment of hypotension caused by IAH. This can also be a secondary increase related to causes outside the abdomen and the chest (e.g., severe burns).

Lung compression causes decreased lung compliance, decreased functional residual capacity, and alveolar atelectasis. These effects will lead to ventilation-perfusion mismatch, hypercapnia, and hypoxemia.

In critically ill patients, these changes usually necessitate mechanical ventilation which, in turn, will further increase the ITP and IAP. Mechanical ventilation in these patients is problematic in dealing with these increased pressures.

9.3.2.2 Mechanical Ventilation During Raised IAP

Mechanical ventilation in IAH/ACS has special considerations [8]. The main issue is to set the ventilator pressure to counteract the increased IAP and ITP.

- Positive end-expiratory pressure (PEEP): The best PEEP should be set at least equal to the abdomino-thoracic index transmission (ATI) as calculated above. ATI is estimated to be around 50%. So, the best PEEP can be calculated as IAP/2. As a rule of thumb, we can adjust the PEEP in cmH_2O to counteract the IAP in mmHg where (cmH_2O = 1.36 mmHg).
- Plateau pressure (Pplat): During lung-protective strategy, plateau pressure is recommended to be kept <30 cmH_2O; however, in case of increased ITP, we should consider the trans-mural Pplat ($Pplat_{tm}$) < 30 cmH_2O.

$$Pplat_{tm} = Pplat - ITP = Pplat - IAP/2.$$

- Higher airway pressures may be acceptable and may arise due to reduced chest wall compliance. Corrected target plateau pressure = target plateau pressure − 7 + IAP (mmHg) * 0.7 [8].

9.3.3 Cardiovascular Effects of ACS

IAH worsens all cardiac functions in terms of contractility, preload, afterload, and diastolic function [9–12].

- Direct compression on the heart decreases contractility and diastolic function, primarily, of the low-pressure chambers.

- IAH compresses the infgerior vena cava (IVC) and the heart, hence reducing venous return and cardiac filling, thereby decreasing the cardiac preload.
- The increasing ITP compresses the aorta and the pulmonary circulation, thereby increasing the afterload.
- Coronary perfusion pressure (CoPP) can also be affected by the raised ITP as follows:

$$CoPP = DBP - PAOP = DBP - ITP$$

where DBP is the diastolic blood pressure.

9.3.3.1 Effects of IAH and ACS on Hemodynamic Monitoring

- IAH and the raised ITP makes the pressure-related preload measurements falsely high. The use of trans-mural filling pressures during end-expiration can correct for the increased outside pressure. The ATI can be used for this purpose as mentioned above.
- Volumetric preload measures as right ventricular end-diastolic volume index (RVEDVi) and global end-diastolic volume index (GEDVi) may be preferred over barometric preload indices during IAH.
- Pulse pressure variation (PPV) is preferred over stroke volume variation (SVV) with increasing the threshold for fluid responsiveness and fluid administration from 12 to 20%.

Venous return from the lower limbs is impaired by the raised IAP, so the passive leg raising test can be a false negative.

9.3.4 Central Nervous System Effects of ACS

IAH compresses the IVC and lumbar venous plexus, causing engorgement of the peri-spinal venous plexus that increases the spinal cord pressure and the intra-cranial pressure (ICP).

Raised ITP—resulting from the IAH—impairs the cerebral venous blood flow along with the usual accompanying hypotension with low mean arterial pressure (MAP). All of these combined factors can impair the cerebral and spinal cord perfusion accordingly:

- *Cerebral perfusion pressure (CPP) = MAP − (ICP or CVP) whichever is highest*
- *Spinal cord perfusion pressure (ScPP) = MAP − (ICP or IAP) whichever is highest*

9.3.5 Extremity Effects of ACS

Vascular supply of the lower limbs originates primarily in the abdominal compartment, so the IAP can compress arterial and venous system, causing ischemia and venous congestion. This will cause eventually lower extremity compartment syndrome as will be discussed further.

9.3.6 Renal Compartment Syndrome

The kidneys are especially prone to increases in IAP and are considered to be the canaries in the coalmine for IAH [4]. This will be discussed in a separate chapter on cardioabdominal-renal syndrome (CARS). Elevated IAP significantly decreases renal artery blood flow and compresses the renal vein leading to renal dysfunction and failure.

Oliguria develops when IAP > 15 mmHg and anuria when IAP is >20–25 mmHg in the presence of normovolemia and at lower levels of IAP in the patient with hypovolemia or sepsis. Renal perfusion pressure (RPP) and renal filtration gradient (FG) have been proposed as critical factors in the development of IAP-induced renal failure.

An increasing number of large clinical studies have identified that IAH (15 mmHg) is independently associated with renal impairment and increased mortality. The etiology of these changes is not entirely well established; however, it may be multifactorial:

- Reduced renal perfusion
- Increased venous congestion
- Reduced cardiac output
- Increased systemic vascular resistance
- Alterations in humoral and neurogenic factors

Within the capsule of the kidney itself, local hematoma formation (caused by trauma or bleeding diathesis) may have an adverse effect on tissue perfusion, causing local renal compartment syndrome [4].

9.3.7 Hepatic Compartment Syndrome

9.3.7.1 Pathophysiology

IAH-related liver dysfunction is probably caused by multiple factors through direct compression on hepatocytes, and the hepatic arterial, portal, venous, and microcirculation, causing decreased liver perfusion. It may also be related to the associated reduced cardiac output.

IAH-related liver dysfunction is associated with reduced mitochondrial function, disturbed glucose metabolism with an increase in lactate production and reduced lactate clearance.

Local hepatic compartment syndrome can occur after liver surgery, trauma (packing), and liver sub-capsular hematoma.

9.3.7.2 Hepato-Abdominal-Renal Syndrome (HARS)

The term HARS describes the pathophysiology of the *hepato-renal syndrome* by addressing the vital role of IAP [13].

Cirrhosis is associated with progressive vasodilatation, reduced the effective circulating volume and microcirculatory damage with glycocalyx shedding. Portal hypertension, along with hypo-albuminemia causes ascites that may increase IAP, which, in turn, impairs the renal function.

Reducing the IAP by paracentesis can restore the renal function as long as the patient is euvolemic.

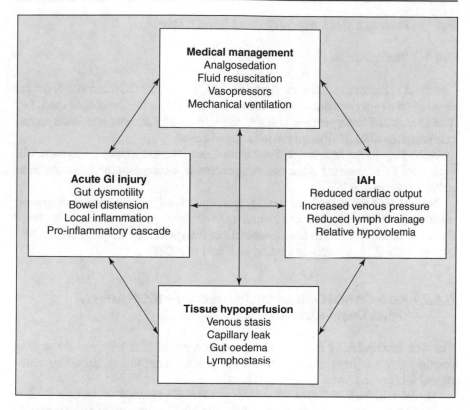

Fig. 9.5 Interactions between medical management, intra-abdominal hypertension (IAH), acute gastro-intestinal (GI) injury, and tissue hypoperfusion. Adapted with permission from Blaser et al. [14]

Hepatic congestion associated with cardiac failure may cause HARS and can be a contributing factor in developing CARS. This will be discussed in a separate chapter.

9.3.7.3 Hepato-Abdominal-Pulmonary Syndrome (HAPS)

The term HAPS is developed to emphasize the important role of IAP in the pathophysiology of dyspnea during liver disease.

Many causes of dyspnea during liver disease is associated with raised IAH. IAH causes basal lung atelectasis, reduced lymphatic drainage with interstitial edema, and fluid overload, which may be caused by CARS [15–17] as illustrated in Fig. 9.5.

9.3.8 Pelvic Compartment Syndrome

The pelvic compartment can be further divided into three regions: the gluteus medius-minimus, gluteus maximus, and the iliopsoas [18]. Local compartment syndromes would occur due to local hematoma and infection. Retroperitoneal hematoma (iliopsoas compartment) can cause pressure over the ureters leading to obstructive uropathy.

Massive retroperitoneal hematoma would itself cause an increase in the IAP and all the secondary effects, including renal dysfunction.

9.4   Intracranial Compartment Syndrome

9.4.1   Background

The brain is enclosed within the rigid bony skull. This puts the brain at risk for the development of a compartment syndrome, being within a low compliant space [4]. The intracranial compartment contains three main components: the brain tissue, cerebrospinal fluid (CSF), and the intracranial blood.

According to the Monroe-Kellie doctrine, any increase of one component will reciprocally decrease the other two components as a compensatory mechanism to prevent the rise in ICP.

Normal ICP should be <10 mmHg, and intracranial hypertension is diagnosed when ICP > 15 mmHg. ICP can be measured directly via the pressure in the brain tissue, or indirectly via the lateral ventricle or the spinal CSF in the lateral recumbent position if freely communicating with the brain CSF.

9.4.2   How Cranial Compartment Syndrome (CCS) Affects Other Compartments?

The first description of the relationship between raised ICP, IAP, and ITP was in traumatic brain injury patients by Scalea et al., who named this syndrome by multi- or multiple compartment syndrome [1].

To maintain the CPP (with CPP = MAP − ICP or CVP), we should reduce the ICP according to the cause and maintain sufficient MAP. Maintenance of MAP is usually accomplished by fluids or vasopressors. Fluids used to augment MAP can promote further brain edema (with higher ICP) and capillary leakage, causing ITP, IAP to rise.

The raised ITP and IAP themselves increase the CVP as mentioned before, causing further reduction of the CPP.

9.4.3   Orbital Compartment Syndrome

The acute form of this syndrome is rare [4]. Orbital pressure is difficult to measure, so the orbital pressure is used as a surrogate. It may happen in burn patients after 24 h of fluid resuscitation, peri-ocular burn, spine surgery, intra-orbital hematoma, or vascular disorders with the ophthalmic vessels. It will also compress the contained ocular compartment.

9.4.4   Ocular Compartment Syndrome

Primary ocular compartment syndrome can occur with glaucoma and tumors. Intraocular hypertension is defined as intraocular pressure (IOP) > 17 mmHg and ocular compartment syndrome as IOP > 25 mmHg.

9.5 Thoracic Compartment Syndrome

9.5.1 Background

Thoracic compartment syndrome (TCS) has traditionally been described in adult and pediatric patients undergoing cardiac surgical procedures [19, 20]. In the setting of substantial myocardial edema, acute ventricular dilatation, mediastinal hematoma, or noncardiogenic pulmonary edema, sternal closure may precipitate cardiac tamponade physiology leading to hemodynamic instability or collapse [19, 20]. TCS is rarely seen in patients with thoracic trauma due to the limited survival when injuries are significant enough to result in massive tissue edema after resuscitation, although traumatic cardiac tamponade due to bleeding can be seen as a hyperacute primary TCS. In the ICU, increased ITP is seen most commonly in relation to sepsis, capillary leak, fluid resuscitation, positive pressure ventilation with high PEEP or dynamic hyperinflation, pneumothorax, COPD with auto-PEEP, diminished chest wall compliance (e.g., morbid obesity or eschars), lung fibrosis, and ARDS. Due to the rising ITP, the resulting increased mean or peak inspiratory pressure during thoracic wall closure may serve as an early warning that the patient is at risk for TCS. The increased ITP (normal <5–7 mmHg) that can be measured via a balloon-tipped catheter positioned in the lower third of the esophagus will exert its effect on the lungs, the heart, and the brain (by limiting venous return).

Primary causes of the thoracic compartment syndrome are as follows:

1. Accumulation of air:
   - Pneumothorax, pneumo-mediastinum, and pneumo-pericardium
   - PEEP and alveolar pressure during MV, or auto-PEEP in COPD patients
2. Accumulation of fluid: as hydrothorax and pericardial effusion *OR* interstitial lung edema (extravascular lung water (EVLW)) in the setting of capillary leak and increased IAP with venous and lymphatic congestion.
3. Accumulation of blood: as hemo-thorax and hemo-pericardium
4. Decreased chest and/or lung compliance: as in the case of morbid obesity, chest deformities, chest wall burn, lung fibrosis, and ARDS.

There are special considerations for mechanical ventilation in patients with increased ITP and IAP to counteract their effects on pulmonary pressures. They were discussed above with the pulmonary effects of raised IAP.

9.5.2 How the Thoracic Compartment Affects Other Compartments?

The thoracic compartment is considered central in the *polycompartment model*. Just like the abdomen, it can affect all other compartments, and it contains the vital organs, the heart, and the lungs.

- *Cranial compartment:*
  As mentioned before, CPP = MAP − ICP or CVP, *which is higher.* Increased ITP decreases MAP and increases both ICP and CVP; therefore, intrathoracic hypertension (ITH) causes impairment of the CPP.
- *Abdominal compartment:*
  The interaction between the abdominal and thoracic compartment is complicated, but it is easily identified. The thoracic pressure is transmitted to the abdominal compartment by a certain degree, which is called the thoraco-abdominal index of transmission (TAI).

  Thoraco-abdominal index of transmission = ΔIAP/(Pplat − PEEP), where Δ IAP is the difference between the IAP in end-inspiration and in end-expiration, Pplat is the plateau alveolar pressure and PEEP is the positive end-expiratory pressure.

  Note: The *TAI* is the index of transmission of the thoracic pressure to the abdominal compartment, while the *ATI* is the index of transmission of abdominal pressure to the thoracic compartment.

9.5.3 Cardiac Compartment Syndrome

The cardiac compartment lies within the thoracic compartment. Cardiac compartment syndrome is well known as cardiac tamponade. Acute accumulation of fluid or air in the pericardium can compress the heart, impairing cardiac filling, increasing afterload by compressing the major vessels within the pericardium, and decreasing cardiac contractility due to ischemia and direct compression. This is manifested by tachycardia, low MAP, high CVP, and pulsus paradoxus.

As little as 250 mL of fluid can cause acute cardiac tamponade, whereas under chronic conditions, greater amounts of fluid can accumulate as the cardiovascular system can slowly adjust. The same effect on the heart can occur via the transmission of increased ITP either directly, as seen with TCS or indirectly, as seen with ACS, due to the cephalad movement of the diaphragm. In the case of increased ITP or IAP, coronary perfusion pressure (CoPP) is lowered as previously discussed.

The increase in ITP will also result in a problematic preload assessment because traditional filling pressures will be erroneously increased. When ITP or IAP rises above 10–12 mmHg, CO drops due to an increase in afterload (systemic vascular resistance) and a decrease in preload and left ventricular compliance [10–12]. Tachycardia may develop, mean arterial blood pressure will decrease, and a pulsus paradoxus (or increase in pulse pressure variation (PPV)) may occur. Cardiovascular dysfunction and failure (low CO, high SVR) are common in conditions of increased ITP or IAP [9]. Finally, hepatomegaly (backward failure) may develop in chronic cases so that cardiac tamponade may have indirect effects on other organs.

9.6 Limb/Extremity Compartment Syndrome

In extremity compartment syndrome (ECS), the pressure within a skeletal muscle compartment increases to the degree, which impairs the blood supply and tissue viability. Arteriolar and capillary pressures are usually 25–30 mmHg, so above this level, the blood supply to any compartment would reduce [4, 21].

ECS can occur due to increased pressure within the compartment due to tissue edema, hemorrhage, venous obstruction, and post-ischemic swelling or due to decreased compartment compliance due to tight dressings or casts, surgical closure, burn eschars, and extensive traction of fractures.

Trauma is the most common cause of ECS. It may cause compartment syndrome by causing tissue edema, hematoma, bone fracture, or by the treatment measures themselves as tight casts and dressings.

As mentioned before, IAH/ACS may result in lower limb ECS by compression of arterio-venous supply of the lower limb, or as a result of the capillary leak and fluid over-resuscitation.

Extremity compartment pressure can be diagnosed by measurement of ECP using a needle inserted in the compartment and connected to a fluid-filled pressure transducer. The pressure should be <20 mmHg, or the tissue viability will be threatened.

Fasciotomy cannot be delayed in lower limb ECS (>30 mmHg) except if the *DBP – compartment pressure is >30 mmHg* without complications. This would highlight the importance of compartment pressure monitoring concerning the general patient condition to guide the best treatment.

Risk factors for ECS that would necessitate invasive pressure measurement:

1. Males >35 years with tibia and/or radius/ulna fractures
2. High-energy injuries
3. Soft tissue injuries in male >35 years with bleeding disorders or on anticoagulants
4. Crush injuries
5. Prolonged limb compression

Effects of the ECS:

1. Local effects: it causes ischemia, muscle necrosis, and rhabdomyolysis.
2. Distant effects and effects on other compartments:
   • Rhabdomyolysis may cause acute kidney injury (AKI), capillary leakage, acute lung injury (ALI), and shock. This may cause other compartment syndromes.
   • Ischemia/reperfusion injury: Reperfusion of the ischemic regions may result in the production of oxygen-free radicals and washout of waste products into circulation. This also may cause ALI, AKI, and capillary leakage with possible development of ITH and IAH.

9.7 Diagnosis and Management of Polycompartment Syndrome

The diagnosis relies mainly on CP measurement. Within the polycompartment syndrome, the abdomen plays a central role, and the effect of IAH on different organ systems has been described, along with recommendations to compensate for these effects (Fig. 9.6). The ultimate goal of treatment is not only to decrease the CP but also to improve organ function and to decrease mortality (Table 9.3).

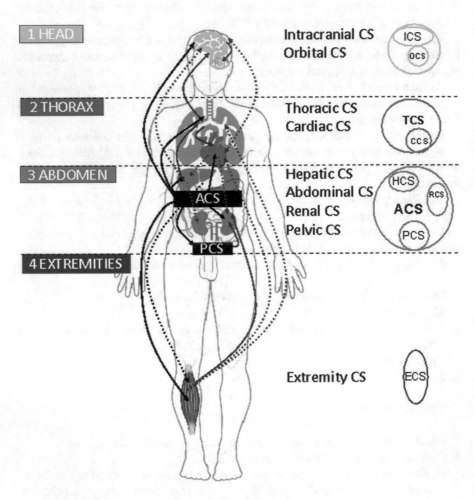

Fig. 9.6 Interactions between different compartments. Solid lines indicate direct effects by mechanical pressure forces. Dotted lines show the distant indirect effects between compartments. Arrow indicates the direction of effect. The abdominal compartment syndrome plays a central role

Table 9.3 Pathophysiology of the four major compartments

	Head			Chest		Abdomen	Extremities
	Brain	Eye	Thorax	Heart			
Primary physiologic parameter	Intracranial pressure (ICP)	Intra-orbital pressure (IOP)	Intrathoracic pressure (ITP)	Filling pressure (CVP, PAOP)	Intra-abdominal pressure (IAP)	Extremity compartment pressures (ECP)
Secondary parameter	Cerebral perfusion pressure (CPP) = MAP – ICP	Orbital perfusion pressure (OPP) = MAP – IOP	Peak, plateau, or mean airway pressure	Coronary perfusion pressure (CoPP) = DBP – PAOP = DBP – ITP	Abdominal perfusion pressure (APP) = MAP – IAP	Peripheral arterial perfusion pressure, tissue perfusion pressure (TPP) = capillary pressure – ECP
CP measurement	Fluid-filled ventriculostomy, air-filled balloon-tipped catheter, parenchymal solid-state microchip transducer	Orbital tissue tension manometry	Esophageal pressure measurement via a balloon-tipped catheter Palv (Ppeak, Pplat, Pmean)	Via deep venous or swan-Ganz catheter	Via bladder (Foley-Manometer, AbViser valve) Via stomach (Spiegelberg, Pulsion Medical Systems)	Via a needle connected to a fluid-filled pressure transducer system
Syndrome	Intracranial hypertension (ICH): ICP > 15 mmHg Intracranial compartment syndrome (ICS)—cerebral herniation: ICP > 25 mmHg	Intra-orbital hypertension (IOP > 17 mmHg) Orbital compartment syndrome (OCS): IOP > 30 mmHg	ITP > 15 mmHg Thoracic compartment syndrome (TCS): ITP > 25 mmHg	CVP > 20 mmHg PAOP >25 mmHg Cardiac compartment syndrome (CCS) – cardiac tamponade	Intra-abdominal hypertension (IAH): IAP > 12 mmHg Abdominal compartment syndrome (ACS): IAP > 20 mmHg	Extremity hypertension: ECP > 15 mmHg Extremity compartment syndrome: ECP > 30 mmHg
Etiology	Primary (tumor, hematoma, …) Secondary (auto-PEEP, hypoxia or hypercarbia, hypertension, ventilation, seizures, …) Postoperatively (edema, mass lesion,…)	Intrinsic (glaucoma) Extrinsic (traumatic retrobulbar hemorrhage) Combination (burn injury)	Post cardiac surgery, spontaneous mediastinal or pleural hemorrhage, tumor, COPD with dynamic hyperinflation, tension pneumothorax	Trauma, tumor, spontaneous bleeding, fluid resuscitation	Primary IAH: associated with injury or disease in the abdominopelvic region Secondary IAH: does not originate from the abdominopelvic region Recurrent IAH: chronic state of IAH	Crush injury Trauma with fractures Bleeding disorders Burns

Table 9.3 (continued)

| | Head | | Chest | | Abdomen | Extremities |
	Brain	Eye	Thorax	Heart		
Potential implication	Brain death	Blindness	Cardiopulmonary collapse	Cardiac collapse, electromechanical dissociation	Multiple organ dysfunction	Extremity loss
Therapeutic intervention	Lower ICP: CSF drainage	Lower IOP	Lower ITP	Evacuate pericardiac effusion	Lower IAP: ascites drainage	Lower ECP
	Increase CPP: vasopressors, fluids	Increase OPP	Escharotomy, chest tube	Pericardiac tube	Increase APP: vasopressors, fluids	Increase TPP
Resuscitative plan	Open compartment	Open compartment	Open compartment	Open compartment	Open compartment	Open compartment
	Decompressive craniectomy	Ocular decompression	Decompressive sternotomy	Decompressive pericardectomy	Decompressive laparotomy	Decompressive fasciotomy
Importance	Adaptation of ventilatory support essential	Recognition of syndrome can be eye saving	Recognition of syndrome can be life saving	Recognition of syndrome can be life saving	Prevention of bacterial translocation and MODS can be life saving	Recognition can be limb saving
Effect on	IOP, cardio-respiratory function (SVR, PVR)	–	Lung (Palv), ICP, IAP, CVP, PAOP	Lung, ICP	All other compartments (lung, ICP, ITP, CVP, PAOP, ...)	Kidney (rhabdomyolysis), lungs, heart
Affected by	Intracardiac pressures (CVP, PAOP), ITP, PEEP, and IAP	ICP, ITP, PEEP, IAP	IAP (abdomino-thoracic transmission 50% on average), mechanical ventilation (PEEP)	ITP, IAP (abdomino-thoracic transmission 50% on average), mechanical ventilation (PEEP)	ITP, mechanical ventilation (PEEP)	IAP (diminished venous return)

The management of the polycompartment syndrome (PCS) relies on three principles [18]:

1. *Specific procedures to reduce the compartment pressures:*

   The general principles of these interventions are to improve compliance of the compartment syndrome, reduce the compartment contents, optimize the fluid therapy by avoiding positive fluid balance and correction of the capillary leak (source control) and surgical decompression as rescue therapy.

2. *General Supportive therapy:*

   Management of critically ill patients with PCS may be challenging due to the complexity of the syndrome.

   Fluid resuscitation optimization, and especially the type, amount, and timing of fluids should be of special attention to optimize organ perfusion, avoiding over-resuscitation and the resultant secondary compartment syndromes that may arise.

3. *Optimization and prevention of surgical decompression:*

   Surgical decompression results in sudden release of the compartment pressure with the wash of the waste metabolites resulted from prolonged ischemia.

   Reperfusion or re-oxygenation of the ischemic tissue would result in the production of oxygen-free radicals.

   The release of these chemicals into the circulation causes immediate and late effects. Immediate effects are vasodilatation and hypotension with metabolic acidosis and hyperkalemia. Late effects may result in the capillary leak, AKI, and ALI.

Anesthesiologists and intensivists must be aware of the acute hemodynamic and metabolic consequences of reperfusion injuries (local; ischemia-reperfusion injury and systemic; post-reperfusion syndrome) during surgical decompression.

Take-Home Messages

- In this chapter, we presented the *abdominal polycompartment model* and presented how each compartment may affect or can be affected by other compartments.
- We emphasized the central role of the abdominal compartment in the polycompartment model, so cardio-abdominal-renal syndrome (CARS), hepato-abdominal-renal syndrome (HARS), and hepato-abdominal pulmonary syndrome (HAPS) may be more appropriate terms for cardio-renal, hepato-renal, and hepato-pulmonary syndromes, respectively.
- Every physician dealing with critically ill patients must have a high index of suspicion for ACS and PCS. They must be aware of the complex pathophysiology of PCS to optimize management in those difficult cases.

References

1. Scalea TM, Bochicchio GV, Habashi N, McCunn M, Shih D, McQuillan K, et al. Increased intra-abdominal, intrathoracic, and intracranial pressure after severe brain injury: multiple compartment syndrome. J Trauma. 2007;62(3):647–56; discussion 56.
2. Kirkpatrick AW, Roberts DJ, De Waele J, Jaeschke R, Malbrain ML, De Keulenaer B, et al. Intra-abdominal hypertension and the abdominal compartment syndrome: updated consensus definitions and clinical practice guidelines from the World Society of the Abdominal Compartment Syndrome. Intensive Care Med. 2013;39(7):1190–206.
3. Malbrain ML, Cheatham ML, Kirkpatrick A, Sugrue M, Parr M, De Waele J, et al. Results from the international conference of experts on intra-abdominal hypertension and abdominal compartment syndrome. I. Definitions. Intensive Care Med. 2006;32(11):1722–32.
4. Malbrain ML, Roberts DJ, Sugrue M, De Keulenaer BL, Ivatury R, Pelosi P, et al. The polycompartment syndrome: a concise state-of-the-art review. Anaesthesiol Intensive Ther. 2014;46(5):433–50.
5. Malbrain ML, Peeters Y, Wise R. The neglected role of abdominal compliance in organ-organ interactions. Crit Care. 2016;20:67. https://doi.org/10.1186/s13054-016-1220-x.
6. Malbrain ML, De Laet I, De Waele JJ, Sugrue M, Schachtrupp A, Duchesne J, Van Ramshorst G, De Keulenaer B, Kirkpatrick AW, Ahmadi-Noorbakhsh S, Mulier J, Pelosi P, Ivatury R, Pracca F, David M, Roberts DJ. The role of abdominal compliance, the neglected parameter in critically ill patients—a consensus review of 16. Part 2: measurement techniques and management recommendations. Anaesthesiol Intensive Ther. 2014;46(5):406–32. https://doi.org/10.5603/AIT.2014.0063.
7. Malbrain ML, Roberts DJ, De Laet I, De Waele JJ, Sugrue M, Schachtrupp A, Duchesne J, Van Ramshorst G, De Keulenaer B, Kirkpatrick AW, Ahmadi-Noorbakhsh S, Mulier J, Ivatury R, Pracca F, Wise R, Pelosi P. The role of abdominal compliance, the neglected parameter in critically ill patients—a consensus review of 16. Part 1: definitions and pathophysiology. Anaesthesiol Intensive Ther. 2014;46(5):392–405. https://doi.org/10.5603/AIT.2014.0062.
8. Regli A, Pelosi P, Malbrain MLNG. Ventilation in patients with intra-abdominal hypertension: what every critical care physician needs to know. Ann Intensive Care. 2019;9(1):52. https://doi.org/10.1186/s13613-019-0522-y.
9. Malbrain ML, De Waele JJ, De Keulenaer BL. What every ICU clinician needs to know about the cardiovascular effects caused by abdominal hypertension. Anaesthesiol Intensive Ther. 2015;47(4):388–99. https://doi.org/10.5603/AIT.a2015.0028.
10. Kashtan J, Green JF, Parsons EQ, Holcroft JW. Hemodynamic effect of increased abdominal pressure. J Surg Res. 1981;30(3):249–55.
11. Ridings PC, Bloomfield GL, Blocher CR, Sugerman HJ. Cardiopulmonary effects of raised intra-abdominal pressure before and after intravascular volume expansion. J Trauma. 1995;39(6):1071–5.
12. Richardson JD, Trinkle JK. Hemodynamic and respiratory alterations with increased intra-abdominal pressure. J Surg Res. 1976;20(5):401–4.
13. Mindikoglu AL, Pappas SC. New developments in hepatorenal syndrome. Clin Gastroenterol Hepatol. 2018;16(2):162–77.e1.
14. Blaser AR, Malbrain ML, Regli A. Abdominal pressure and gastrointestinal function: an inseparable couple?. Anaesthesiology Intensive Therapy. 2017;49(2):146–158.
15. Balogh Z, McKinley BA, Holcomb JB, Miller CC, Cocanour CS, Kozar RA, et al. Both primary and secondary abdominal compartment syndrome can be predicted early and are harbingers of multiple organ failure. J Trauma. 2003;54(5):848–59; discussion 59–61.
16. Goldman R, Zilkoski M, Mullins R, Mayberry J, Deveney C, Trunkey D. Delayed celiotomy for the treatment of bile leak, compartment syndrome, and other hazards of nonoperative management of blunt liver injury. Am J Surg. 2003;185(5):492–7.

17. Lawendy AR, Bihari A, Sanders DW, Badhwar A, Cepinskas G. Compartment syndrome causes systemic inflammation in a rat. Bone Joint J. 2016;98-B(8):1132–7.
18. Balogh ZJ, Butcher NE. Compartment syndromes from head to toe. Crit Care Med. 2010;38(9 Suppl):S445–51. https://doi.org/10.1097/CCM.0b013e3181ec5d09.
19. Rizzo AG, Sample GA. Thoracic compartment syndrome secondary to a thoracic procedure: a case report. Chest. 2003;124(3):1164–8.
20. Kaplan LJ, Trooskin SZ, Santora TA. Thoracic compartment syndrome. J Trauma. 1996;40(2):291–3.
21. Wall CJ, Lynch J, Harris IA, Richardson MD, Brand C, Lowe AJ, et al. Clinical practice guidelines for the management of acute limb compartment syndrome following trauma. ANZ J Surg. 2010;80(3):151–6.

Timing of Surgical Intervention for Compartment Syndrome

10

Mario Improta, Matteo Tomasoni, Paola Fugazzola, Andrea Lippi, Federico Coccolini, and Luca Ansaloni

Abbreviations

ACS	Abdominal compartment syndrome
CS	Compartment syndrome
DC	Decompressive craniectomy
DL	Decompressive laparotomy
ECS	Extremities compartmental syndrome
ICP	Intracranial pressure
mRS	Modified Rankin Score
OCS	Orbital compartment syndrome
TBI	Traumatic brain injury
TBSA	Total-body surface area

10.1 Introduction

When in a closed district of the body the pressure rapidly rises, some physiological changes that occur can be fatal. Three main factors define the ability to tolerate a rise in pressure of a body compartment: (1) expandability of the given district (e.g., the abdomen better tolerate pressure's rise than the unexpandable skull), (2) the presence of structures in that closed space that are likely to suffer from rise in pressure (e.g., nerves and blood vessels), and (3) the generalized effects that the increasing pressure generate on the global body homeostasis.

M. Improta · M. Tomasoni · P. Fugazzola · A. Lippi · L. Ansaloni (✉)
General, Emergency and Trauma Surgery Department, Bufalini Hospital, Cesena, Italy
e-mail: mario.improta@studio.unibo.it

F. Coccolini
General, Emergency and Trauma Surgery Department, Pisa University Hospital, Pisa, Italy

© Springer Nature Switzerland AG 2021
F. Coccolini et al. (eds.), *Compartment Syndrome*, Hot Topics in Acute Care
Surgery and Trauma, https://doi.org/10.1007/978-3-030-55378-4_10

Certain compartments can only briefly tolerate an acute rise in pressure, especially when this implies a sudden change in the ability to deliver efficient cardiac output as in tension pneumothorax or cardiac tamponade. Those scenarios require emergent surgical intervention, but the timing of intervention of more complex, still urgent compartmental syndromes, is a matter of debate.

10.2 Orbital Compartment Syndrome

OCS is a sight-threatening condition due to the optic nerve and retinal compromise secondary to retinal artery occlusion. Trauma, retrobulbar hemorrhage, and massive resuscitation after burn injuries are the most common causes [1]. Visual loss can occur after only 60 min of increased pressure within the orbit [2]. When suggestive clinical signs of OCS abruptly appear (proptosis, ocular pain, loss of sight, lateral gaze limitation, evident hematoma formation), decompression of ocular compartment by lateral canthotomy and cantholysis should be performed immediately. No further imaging studies should be addressed, oculist should be convoked and *immediate* treatment should be provided by an experienced physician. Delayed surgical intervention is the single factor affecting the rate of visual loss due to OCS [3] with a high rate of fully recovered vision in patients who are early decompressed.

10.3 Thoracic Compartment Syndrome

Various compartmental syndrome can occur within the chest wall, and most of them are immediately life-threatening.

Tension pneumothorax and cardiac tamponade are not officially recognized as a compartmental syndrome; furthermore, both share similar pathophysiology as other component syndromes such as abdominal, in term of the rise of pressure within a confined space that in healthy individuals bears different forces.

Tension PNX and cardiac tamponade are the cornerstones of the emergent treatment, and some extent of surgical interventions ranging from needle decompression, surgical drainage, emergency thoracotomy up to clamshell are always needed [4]. "Thoracic or mediastinal compartment syndrome" is itself a pathological entity; some case series reported in journals of cardio surgery [5] described how after cardiac surgery sternal closure was seldom associated with unexpectable hemodynamic instability. Open chest management was proposed to achieve good results in this population.

10.4 Extremities Compartment Syndrome

In limbs, longer periods of ischemia correlate with worst outcome, but definitive evidence of rapidity under which irreversible muscle damage will occur is lacking [6]. In a retrospective cohort analysis, it was noted that 37/76 of patient underwent surgery for ECS had some degree of muscle necrosis, with 37% of patients developing it after 3 h from injury. Once ECS is diagnosed, the only effective procedure is surgical decompression and still, trauma population experience delays in treatment up to 9 h although the time-dependent outcome related to this condition [7].

The assumption on how long can a muscle tolerate ischemia is derived from studies that took their data from tourniquet models. Those models assume muscle tissue to tolerate up to 6–8 h ischemia before necrosis occurs, nevertheless must be noted that the pathophysiology of the compartment syndrome in the setting of crush injury or long bone fractures (as seen in trauma population) may elicit cellular response different from one of the tourniquet, resulting in a shorter tolerated period [8].

Muscle necrosis can occur even faster than the historical 3 h burden, therefore the timing of intervention is based on disease model that underestimates the amount of damage that an injury-related ECS can provoke to the muscle belly. Recently, British Orthopaedic Association Standard for Trauma (BOAST 10) guidelines on ECS was released [9] and stated that decompressive surgery for ECS should occur *within an hour from the decision to operate*. If the absolute compartment pressure is greater than 40 mmHg in the presence of clinical symptoms, urgent surgical decompression should be considered unless other life-threatening conditions take priority. When a delay in diagnosis of more than 12 h occurs, or there is a late presentation in the E.D., ECS should be managed nonoperatively since surgical exploration can be harmful in this setting. Several cases of ACS who underwent fasciotomy in UK trauma centers had a delayed time to fasciotomy of 2 h, therefore, failing BOAST-10 goal of 1 h, supporting the idea that early decompression is uneasy to obtain in clinical practice, 34% of those patients suffered from major complications including limb loss [10].

The outcome of patients who undergo fasciotomy after vascular repair for lower extremity arterial injury (without other injuries) is different than in ECS: of 612 patients underwent early or delayed (<8 h or >8 h) intervention, there was a lower rate of limb amputation in the early group (8.5 vs 24.6% $p > 0.001$) [11]. Giving those results, authors suggested performing fasciotomy at the time of vascular repair for patients with arterial damages of limbs.

These findings were recently corroborated by recent series by Rothenberg et al. who investigated the relationship between the timing of fasciotomy and patient outcomes in patients undergoing fasciotomy for acute limb ischemia and revascularization [12]. Fasciotomy was classified as prophylactic (at the index operation of revascularization) or delayed. Prophylactic fasciotomy should be performed at the time of revascularization if there is suspect of longer than 6 h of ischemia or inadequate collateral flow or in the setting of trauma with a combined arterial and venous injury [13]. Postoperative LOS is predictably higher in patients undergoing prophylactic fasciotomy versus no intervention, but shorter in patients who eventually needed fasciotomy for developing CS and underwent delayed fashion intervention; moreover those who underwent delayed fasciotomy resulted in more major amputations at 30 days (50% vs 5.9%, $p = 0.002$).

Patients who underwent fasciotomy had a higher Rutherford classification score underling that surgeons prefer to perform in a prophylactic fashion in more severe cases of ALI. Interestingly, patients with coronary artery disease had a lower rate of fasciotomy, probably due to the systemic nature of the disease affecting also the peripheric circulation, thus producing more collateral circles, giving the surgeon the idea that revascularization could have safely performed without putting the leg at risk for reperfusion damage and subsequent compartment syndrome development.

It is reasonable to perform prophylactic fasciotomy in the setting of revascularization, with the anticipated "risk" of the leg of developing ECS being evaluated from expert surgeons. On the other hand, fasciotomy is not a benign procedure with some surgeons advocating its performance only when CS has developed, but the rate of amputation was observed to be higher when such threshold was chosen.

10.5   Abdominal Compartment Syndrome (ACS)

The effect of timely treatment of ACS has been recently investigated in a comparison between medical ICU and surgical ICU on nontraumatic population [14]. Mortality was 83% in the MICU vs. 12.5% in SICU with the only difference in the populations being the admission-to-diagnosis time; the authors concluded that prompt diagnosis and early intervention had a significant benefit. When a patient is diagnosed with ACS (abdominal pressure >20 mmHg in association with organ disfunction), decompressive laparotomy should be considered immediately and performed if medical treatment fails to improve symptoms [15].

In the guidelines of the World Society of Abdominal Compartment Syndrome (WSACS), Kirkpatric et al. recommend for decompressive laparotomy (DL) for patients with overt ACS (grade 1C); there is the suggestion to consider percutaneous drainage of peritoneal fluid when obviously present in order to avoid decompressive laparotomy (grade 2d), but they made no statement in regard to the timing of the decompression [16].

Observation of several studies investigating mortality in patients with ACS shows an interesting trend toward lowering mortality with advancing techniques and shortening of the time to diagnosis [17, 18]. Ke et al. in 2013 [19] conducted a study on a porcine model to evaluate the best timing for decompressive laparotomy for ACS due to severe acute pancreatitis and observed a survival benefit in those who were decompressed before 6 h. When applying to clinical practice, it must be remembered that decompressive laparotomy has several serious complications. It seems reasonable for pancreatitis causing ACS to use a step-up approach and consider all medical strategies to reduce intra-abdominal pressure before performing a decompressive laparotomy and proceed to it without further waiting if no effects are achieved with medical treatment.

In the setting of a secondary ACS (developed for a reason which is not primarily abdomino-pelvic, e.g., over resuscitation), it is reasonable that the timing of the DL should be different since the pathophysiology is different as well. Recently Ramirez et al. [20] retrospectively analyzed a group of 46 patients with burn injury and ACS to evaluate survival comparing the timing of DL. Three groups were created dividing patients according to the cause of ACS development: (1) initial injury resuscitation, (2) perioperative resuscitation, (3) sepsis. The group with the highest survival rate (up to 80%) was the one of immediate DL (within 1 h) after ACS due to initial injury resuscitation, and the difference in survival was not explained by TBSA. The authors noted increased survival rate in their population in respect of other series on ACS for a burn injury in which DL was used as the last resource, therefore concluded with the suggestion of *immediate DL* in ACS patients with burn injuries. The best outcome was seen in patients developing ACS immediately after resuscitation and that patient who developed ACS later in their hospital course had a worse outcome; this may be because those were sicker patient, but TBSA was similar if not lower in patients of the first group. Another explanation could be that best resuscitation with aggressive fluid intake was achieved in some patient, with the collateral effect of the development of ACS. In this setting, given that ACS is not due to a primary endo-abdominal pathology, it is possible that DL was curative and the benefit of the aggressive resuscitation overwhelmed the harm of ACS development. Further studies are needed to assess the relationship between resuscitation, ACS development, and survival.

10.6 Intracranial Pressure and Compartment Syndrome of the Brain

The skull is the compartment that less tolerate a rise in pressure. Since it is not-expansible, a rise in brain tissue (e.g., traumatic brain injury (TBI) edema) or unexpected presence of blood can rapidly deteriorate cellular permeability leading to edema and increased intracranial pressure (ICP) and to a compartment syndrome that, left untreated, points to brain herniation and death. 2016 Brain trauma foundation's guidelines declared that there should be a stair-chase approach to intracranial hypertension, with more aggressive therapies (up to surgery) if ICP is >22 mmHg in a comatose patient. No statement was done about the timing of the craniectomy in those cases where the elevated ICP did not respond to medical management [21].

Whether decompressive craniectomy is even indicated for TBI and elevated ICP is a matter of debate. It appears that DC does not result in better outcomes, but the short interval between TBI and surgery may have a positive impact on outcome [22], especially in younger patients undergoing intervention at 3–4 h after injury [23, 24].

Acute stroke can result in a dysregulation of ATP-dependent ionic-transporter, provoking brain edema, and is one of the most common indications for a decompressive craniectomy. The main difference between TBI and stroke, regarding indication for DC, is the timing. In TBI population, there could be a benefit in terms of survival from DC even if signs of brain herniation are present, whether in acute stroke after herniation has occurred, any treatment aimed to reduce ICP was found to be useless.

Three RCTs evaluated DC after a large ischemic stroke of the MCA (middle cerebral artery): all the trial showed a survival advantage in managing large MCA strokes with surgical decompression if craniectomy was performed before 48 h; those findings were also corroborated from a recent meta-analysis [25–28].

It is unclear if early decompression is beneficial itself or carries the survival improvement due to prevention of herniation; it seems that rate of herniation tends to be lower if decompression is performed within 24 h in patients with MCA infarction [29].

After an ischemic or hemorrhagic stroke, better outcomes were observed seen when DC was performed within 6 h despite herniation incidence seems similar: the benefit could rely on pathophysiology of the compartment syndrome itself more than just the prevention of herniation [30].

Clinical deterioration (e.g., worsening of Glasgow coma scale—GCS) is a factor that usually precipitates the decision to surgically decompress elevated ICP. A trial was conducted to assess if early decompression would have been beneficial over decompression based on the deterioration of GCS [31]. The group that was operated within 6 h despite GCS or radiological signs of deterioration showed better outcomes measured as mRS (modified Rankin scale). Data suggest that in acute stroke, most of the benefit from decompression is lost when brain herniation has already developed, thus aim to earlier decompression in selected patients should be encouraged especially in patients with large infarction ($>200cm^2$) or midline shift.

Many RTCs tried to extrapolate evidence for the use of DC in trauma settings. DECRA Trial [32] analyzed outcomes in TBI patients within 72 h from injury. Patients were randomized either to maximal medical management or DC after sustained (15 min within a 60 min period) elevated ICP (>20 mmHg) with a median time of DC from injury of 38 h. The DC group decreased ICP but had more unfavorable outcomes. Unfortunately the groups were irregular since patients who underwent DC were more likely to have signs of herniation at the time of intervention (27% vs 12% p: 0.04) therefore minimizing the potential beneficial effect of DC over medical management, besides the harm observed with DC was no longer evident when statistical analysis was conducted without taking into account patients with anisocoria or signs of herniation, as last criticism for the trial, the median time of intervention from injury was 38 h, leading to a loss of the potential benefit of an early decompression. To fulfill those questions, the RESCUEicp [33] trial was conducted. It compared patients with refractory elevated ICP (>25 mmHg for 1 h) managed by DC or medical therapy. The trial ultimately strengthened DECRA results without finding any substantial benefit in DC. Both trials were intended to evaluate DC and did not have analysis regarding the timing of the intervention that was at least 24 h after the injury. Effort was made to investigate the effect of early vs late decompression, but most studies were retrospective in nature showing a trend to higher survival in medical management group, although it is reasonable that given the retrospective nature, patients who were treated with DC were more severe and not amenable of management with medical therapy, therefore, a sicker subset of patients was identified. Only a retrospective series of 486 patients in a combat series noted an improvement in survival when performing DC within 5.30 h from TBI [34].

To date, a definitive conclusion on the appropriate timing of DC is lacking in stroke and TBI setting as well, although some preliminary evidence suggests that early decompression (within 24 h and in some series 6 h) may be beneficial in long-term outcome. In stroke, it appears that the ischemic insult prevents the brain to beneficiate from decompression after herniation has occurred, conversely, in some series of TBI some benefit can be observed from DC even after herniation has already occurred [35].

10.7 Timing of Intervention

We propose, based on current evidence, five categories of timely intervention: (1) immediate, for those compartmental syndromes which can rapidly lead to patient death or severe disability (e.g. life or sight-threatening conditions); (2) ultra-early, within 1 h period in ECS and ACS in the setting of burns and resuscitative ACS; (3) early with the time burden of 6–8 h and in any case before clinical signs of irreversible deterioration; (4) late decompression identified with decompression performed after 6–8 h or after signs of clinical deterioration has occurred (e.g., signs of cerebral herniation); (5) prophylactic decompression in those situations where high incidence of postoperative CS is expected (e.g., revascularization after acute limb ischemia, combined arterial/venous injury).

	Body district	Notes	References
Immediate	Ocular, sight-threatening	Lateral canthotomy and cantholysis	[1]
	Thorax, tension PNX, cardiac tamponade	A common cause of traumatic cardiac arrest	[4]
Ultra-early (within 1 h)	Abdomen (ACS)	Consider decompressive laparotomy within 1 h for ACS developed after burn injury secondary to aggressive resuscitation	[20]
	Extremities (ECS)	Decompression within 1 h of the decision to operate	[9]
Early (within 6–8 h)	Abdomen (ACS)	Decompression after ACS[a] development within 3–6 h from Dx if maximal medical management failed	[16, 17, 19]
	Brain (refractory elevated ICP)	Better outcomes in subgroups of younger patients, decompress before clinical signs of herniation	[23, 24, 29–31, 34]
Late (after 6–8 h)	Extremities (ECS)	Discouraged for ECS occurred >12 h, better outcomes with NOM	[9]
	Brain (refractory elevated ICP)	No advantage in DC after signs of herniation in stroke patients, some advantage in TBI patients even if herniated over nonsurgical management[b]	[24–28, 32]
Prophylactic	Thorax (after cardiac surgery)	Inability to tolerate closure of the sternum managed with "open chest" technique	[5]
	Extremities *with vascular injuries or acute limb ischemia*	Liberal use of prophylactic early fasciotomy (at index operation) leads to better outcomes	[11, 12]

[a]Abdominal pressure >20 *plus* signs of end-organ damage
[b]All benefits were lost in decompressive craniotomy performed after 48 h (Hamlet trial); no benefit was seen in trials while the median time of decompression was 38 h

10.8 Conclusions

Different compartment reacts with a variable degree of cellular injury and physiological deterioration to raised pressure, therefore, not all compartment syndrome would benefit in timely treatment at the same degree. Early decompression could be beneficial in some conditions, but physicians must be aware of the implied harm of decompression and relative procedural hazards, aiming to maximize the medical effort to diminish the rate of intervention when feasible, without delaying surgical intervention long till there is no longer opportunity for bettering outcomes.

References

1. Lima MD. Orbital compartment syndrome: the ophthalmic surgical emergency. Surv Ophthalmol. 2009;54:441–9.
2. Hayreh SS, Kolder WE, Weingeist TA. Central retinal artery occlusion and retinal tolerance time. Ophthalmology. 1980;87:75–8.
3. Hislop WS, Dutton GN. Retrobulbar hemorrhage: can blindness be prevented? Injury. 1994;25:663–5.
4. Subcommittee ATLS, and International ATLS Working Group. Advanced trauma life support (ATLS®): the ninth edition. J Trauma Acute Care Surg. 2013;74(5): 1363–66.
5. Christenson JT, Maurice J, Simonet F, et al. Open chest and delayed sternal closure after cardiac surgery. Eur J Cardiothorac Surg. 1996;10:305–11.
6. Cone J, Inaba K. Trauma Surg Acute Care Open 2017;2:1–6. https://doi.org/10.1136/tsaco-2017-000094; Vaillancourt C, Shrier I, Falk M, Rossignol M, Vernec A, Somogyi D. Quantifying delays in the recognition and management of acute compartment syndrome. Can J Emerg Med. 2001;3(1):26–30.
7. Haljamae H, Enger E. Human skeletal muscle energy metabolism during and after complete tourniquet ischemia. Ann Surg. 1975;182(1):9–14.
8. Heppenstall RB, Scott R, Sapega A, Park YS, Chance B. A comparative study of the tolerance of skeletal muscle to ischemia. Tourniquet application compared with acute compartment syndrome. J Bone Joint Surg [Am]. 1986;68(6):820–8.
9. British Orthopaedic Association BAoPRaAS, Royal College of Nursing. BOAST 10: Diagnosis and management of compartment syndrome of the limbs. Br Orthopaedic Assoc Stand Trauma. 2014. https://www.boa.ac.uk/publications/boa-standards-trauma-boasts.
10. Bodansky D, et al. Acute compartment syndrome: do guidelines for diagnosis and management make a difference? Injury. 2018;49:1699. https://doi.org/10.1016/j.injury.2018.04.020.
11. Farber, et al. Early fasciotomy in patients with extremity vascular injury is associated with decreased risk of adverse limb outcomes: a review of the national trauma data bank. Injury. 2012;43(9):1486–91. https://doi.org/10.1016/j.injury.2011.06.006.
12. Rothenberg KA, et al. Delayed fasciotomy is associated with higher risk of major amputation in patients with acute limb ischemia. Ann Vasc Surg. 2019;59:195–201.
13. Modrall CJ. Compartment syndrome. Rutherford's vascular surgery. 8th ed. Elsevier; 2014. p. 2544–54.
14. Nguyen J, et al. Expeditious diagnosis and laparotomy for patients with acute abdominal compartment syndrome may improve survival. Am Surg. 2018;84(11):1836–40.
15. Parsak CK, Seydaoglu G, Sakman G, et al. Abdominal compartment syndrome: current problems and new strategies. World J Surg. 2008;32:13–9.
16. Kirkpatric AW, et al. Intra-abdominal hypertension and the abdominal compartment syndrome: updated consensus definitions and clinical practice guidelines from the World Society of the Abdominal Compartment Syndrome. Intensive Care Med. 2013;39:1190–206. https://doi.org/10.1007/s00134-013-2906-z.

17. De Waele JJ, Kimball E, Malbrain M, Nesbitt I, Cohen J, Kaloiani V, Ivatury R, Mone M, Debergh D, Björck M. Decompressive laparotomy for abdominal compartment syndrome. Br J Surg. 2016;103(6):709–15.

18. De Waele JJ, Hoste EA, Malbrain ML. Decompressive laparotomy for abdominal compartment syndrome—a critical analysis. Crit Care. 2006;10:R51.

19. Ni HB, Tong ZH, Li WQ, Li N, Li JS. The importance of timing of decompression in severe acute pancreatitis combined with abdominal compartment syndrome. J Trauma Acute Care Surg. 2013;74:1060–6.

20. Ramirez JI, et al. Timing of laparotomy and closure in burn patients with abdominal compartment syndrome: effect on survival. J Am Coll Surg. 2018;226(6):1175–80.

21. Carney N, Totten AM, O'Reilly C, Ullman JS, Hawryluk GW, Bell MJ, ... Rubiano AM. Guidelines for the management of severe traumatic brain injury. Neurosurgery. 2017;80(1):6–15.

22. Barthélemy EJ, et al. Decompressive craniotomy for severe traumatic brain injury: a systematic review. World Neurosurg. 2016;88:411–20.

23. Girotto, et al. Efficacy of decompressive craniectomy in the treatment of severe brain injury. Coll Antropol. 2011;35(Suppl 2):255–8.

24. Shah A, Almenawer S, Hawryluk G. Timing of decompressive craniectomy for ischemic stroke and traumatic brain injury: a review. Front Neurol. 2019;10:11. https://doi.org/10.3389/fneur.2019.00011.

25. Vibbert M, Mayer SA. Early decompressive hemicraniectomy following malignant ischemic stroke: the crucial role of timing. Curr Neurol Neurosci Rep. 2010;10:1–3.

26. Vahedi K, et al. Sequential-design, multicenter, randomized, controlled trial of early decompressive craniectomy in malignant middle cerebral artery infarction (DECIMAL Trial). Stroke. 2007;38:2518–25.

27. Juttler E, Schwab S, Schmiedek P, Unterberg A, Hennerici M, Woitzik J, et al. Decompressive surgery for the treatment of malignant infarction of the middle cerebral artery (DESTINY): a randomized, controlled trial. Stroke. 2007;38:2518–25. https://doi.org/10.1161/STROKEAHA.107.485649.

28. Hofmeijer J, Kappelle LJ, Algra A, Amelink GJ, van Gijn J, van der Worp HB, et al. Surgical decompression for space-occupying cerebral infarction (the Hemicraniectomy After Middle Cerebral Artery infarction with Life-threatening Edema Trial [HAMLET]): a multicentre, open, randomized trial. Lancet Neurol. 2009;8:326–33. https://doi.org/10.1016/S1474-4422(09)70047-X.

29. Schwab S, Steiner T, Aschoff A, Schwarz S, Steiner HH, Jansen O, et al. Early hemicraniectomy in patients with complete middle cerebral artery infarction. Stroke. 1998;29:1888–93. https://doi.org/10.1161/01.STR.29.9.1888.

30. Cho DY, Chen TC, Lee HC. Ultra-early decompressive craniectomy for malignant middle cerebral artery infarction. Surg Neurol. 2003;60:227–32. https://doi.org/10.1016/S0090-3019(03)00266-0; discussion 232–23.

31. Elsawaf A, Galhom A. Decompressive craniotomy for malignant middle cerebral artery infarction: optimal timing and literature review. World Neurosurg. 2018;116:e71–8. https://doi.org/10.1016/j.wneu.2018.04.005.

32. Cooper DJ, Rosenfeld JV, Murray L, Arabi YM, Davies AR, D'Urso P, et al. Decompressive craniectomy in diffuse traumatic brain injury. N Engl J Med. 2011;364:1493–502. https://doi.org/10.1056/NEJMoa1102077.

33. The RESCUEicp trial. http://www.rescueicp.com/. Accessed 13 Aug 2015.

34. Shackelford SA, Del Junco DJ, Reade MC, Bell R, Becker T, Gurney J, et al. Association of time to craniectomy with survival in patients with severe combat-related brain injury. Neurosurg Focus. 2018;45:E2. https://doi.org/10.3171/2018.9.FOCUS18404.

35. Qiu W, Guo C, Shen H, Chen K, Wen L, Huang H, et al. Effects of unilateral decompressive craniectomy on patients with unilateral acute post-traumatic brain swelling after severe traumatic brain injury. Crit Care. 2009;13:R185. https://doi.org/10.1186/cc8178.

Abdominal Compartment Syndrome and Infection

11

Massimo Sartelli

11.1 Abdominal Compartment Syndrome in Patients with Intra-Abdominal Infections

A compartment syndrome is a condition of increased pressure in a confined anatomic space that adversely affects the circulation and threatens the function and viability of the tissues therein. This may arise in any closed compartment within the body.

Abdominal compartment syndrome (ACS) is a common consequence of severe intra-abdominal infections. Primary acute abdominal compartment syndrome occurs when an intra-abdominal injury or disease in the abdominopelvic region is directly responsible for the compartment syndrome. Secondary abdominal compartment syndrome occurs when sepsis and related-fluid resuscitation cause fluid accumulation in the abdomen in a scenario lacking primary intraperitoneal injury.

Abdominal sepsis is the host's systemic inflammatory response to bacterial or yeast peritonitis [1].

Sepsis from an abdominal origin is initiated by the outer membrane component of gram-negative organisms (e.g., lipopolysaccharide [LPS], lipid A, endotoxin) or gram-positive organisms (e.g., lipoteichoic acid, peptidoglycan), as well as toxins from anaerobic bacteria [1]. This leads to the release of proinflammatory cytokines such as tumor necrosis factor α (TNF-α) and interleukins 1 and 6 (IL-1, IL-6). TNF-α and interleukins lead to the production of toxic mediators [1], which may cause a complex, multifactorial syndrome that may evolve into conditions of varying severity and may lead to the functional impairment of one or more vital organs or systems.

Fluid therapy to improve microvascular blood flow is an essential part of the treatment of patients with sepsis. Crystalloid solutions should be the first choice because they are well tolerated and cheap. They should be infused rapidly to induce

M. Sartelli (✉)
Department of Surgery, Macerata Hospital, Macerata, Italy

a quick response but not so fast that an artificial stress response develops. They should be interrupted when no improvement of tissue perfusion occurs in response to volume loading [1].

However, in patient with abdominal sepsis, excessive infusion of fluids may become a counterproductive strategy [1].

The systemic inflammatory response syndrome, increased vascular permeability, and aggressive crystalloid resuscitation predispose to fluid sequestration with formation of peritoneal fluid. Patients with ongoing sepsis commonly develop shock bowel resulting in excessive bowel edema. These changes and associated forced closure of the abdominal wall may result in increased intra-abdominal pressure (IAP) ultimately leading to intra-abdominal hypertension (IAH).

Elevated IAP commonly causes marked deficits in both regional and global perfusion that may result in significant organ failure [2]. An uncontrolled IAH, with an IAP exceeding 20 mmHg and a new organ failure onset, leads to abdominal compartment syndrome (ACS). This in turn has further effects on intra-abdominal organs as well as indirect effects on remote organ(s) and system(s). ACS is a potentially lethal complication characterized by effects on splanchnic, cardiovascular, pulmonary, renal, and central nervous systems. Ventricular filling is reduced as a result of decreased venous return caused by the compression of the inferior vena cava or portal vein. Preload measurements such as central venous pressure (CVP) and pulmonary artery occlusion pressure (PAOP) may be falsely elevated. Critical clinical conditions play an important role in aggravating the effects of elevated IAP and may reduce the threshold of IAH that causes the clinical manifestations of ACS. In addition, IAH and ACS likely influence the clinical course of many critically ill patients with sepsis. This is a result of both primary intraperitoneal disease and the massive fluid resuscitation that is often required to stabilize hemodynamics in patients with ongoing sepsis or septic shock. The combination of IAH and the physiological effects of sepsis and septic shock may result in high morbidity and mortality rates. Especially in the case of severe peritonitis, the physiological effect of ACS to gastrointestinal tract may aggravate the abdominal sepsis. Specifically, the mucosal–barrier function is altered causing increased permeability and bacterial translocation.

11.2 Prevention of the Abdominal Compartment Syndrome in Patients with Abdominal Sepsis

Repeated intravesical measurements of intra-abdominal pressure should be frequently performed to identify patients at risk for intra-abdominal hypertension.

Although decompressive laparotomy historically constituted the standard method to treat severe IAH/ACS and to protect against their development in high-risk situations, it has been reported to result in an immediate decrease in IAP and improvements in organ function. However, decompressive laparotomy is associated with multiple complications and overall reported patient mortality is considerable (up to 50%), even after decompression [2].

In addition to decompressive laparotomy for ACS, numerous medical and minimally invasive therapies have been proposed or studied that may be beneficial for patients with IAH or ACS. Approaches or techniques of potential utility include adequate fluid resuscitation strategies, sedation and analgesia, neuromuscular blockade, body positioning, nasogastric/colonic decompression, promotility agents, diuretics, and continuous renal replacement therapies, percutaneous catheter drainage [3].

Presumptive decompression should be considered at the time of laparotomy in patients who demonstrate risk factors for IAH/ACS. The decision to perform a laparostomy in patients with severe intra-abdominal infections is usually based on the intraoperative judgment of the surgeon without IAP measurements during the operation. In these patients, the open abdomen (OA) procedure may be a useful option [3].

OA procedure may allow early identification and draining of any residual infection, control any persistent source of infection, and remove more effectively infected or cytokine-loaded peritoneal fluid, deferring definitive intervention until the patient is appropriately resuscitated and hemodynamically stable and thus better able to heal [2].

The OA concept is closely linked to damage control surgery and may be easily adapted to patients with ongoing sepsis. Patients may progress to septic shock having progressive organ dysfunction, hypotension, myocardial depression, and then coagulopathy. These patients are hemodynamically unstable and clearly not optimal for candidates for immediate complex operative interventions. After initial surgery, the patient is rapidly taken to the ICU for physiologic optimization. Early treatment with aggressive hemodynamic support can limit the damage of sepsis-induced tissue hypoxia and may limit the overstimulation of endothelial activity. Following the early hemodynamic support, in principle after 24–48 h, reoperation may be performed with or without final abdominal closure [4].

Following reexploration, the goal is early and definitive closure of the abdomen, in order to reduce the complications associated with an open abdomen, such as entero-atmospheric fistulas, fascial retraction with loss of abdominal wall domain, and development of massive incisional hernias. Early definitive closure is the basis for preventing or reducing the risk of these complications and should be the goal when the patient's physiological condition allows. The literature suggests a bimodal distribution of primary closure rates. Early closure depends on postoperative intensive care management, and delayed closure depends on the choice of the temporary abdominal closure technique. The first mode is to close within 4–7 days and achieve a high rate of primary closure, the second mode has a delay (20–40 days) having lower overall closure rate. Temporary closure of the abdomen may be achieved by using gauze and large, impermeable, self-adhesive membrane dressings, both absorbable and nonabsorbable meshes, and negative pressure therapy devices. The first and easiest method to perform a laparostomy was the application of a plastic silo (the "Bogota bag"). This system is inexpensive. However, it does not provide sufficient traction to the wound edges and allows the fascial edges to retract laterally, resulting in difficult fascial closure under significant tension, especially if the closure is delayed. At present, negative pressure techniques (NPT) have become the most extensively employed means of temporary closure of the abdominal wall [2].

OA strategy presents a clinical challenge that is associated with significant morbidity and should be used in the right patients at the right time. Even with the lack of strong evidence in international literature, OA may be an important option in the surgeon's strategy for the treatment of selected physiologically deranged patients with abdominal sepsis. Well-designed prospective and randomized studies are required to adequately define the role of OA and negative pressure in managing patients with abdominal sepsis.

11.3 Conclusions

Surgeons should be aware of physiopathology of sepsis and always keep in mind the pathophysiology of ACS. A correct prevention and management of ACS, when it occurs, is crucial to avoid severe complications.

In addition to decompressive laparotomy for ACS, numerous medical and minimally invasive therapies have been proposed or studied that may be beneficial for patients with IAH or ACS.

Despite lack of strong evidence in international literature, open abdomen may be an important option in the surgeon's armamentarium for the prevention of abdominal compartment syndrome. Well-designed prospective studies are required to better define the role of open abdomen in managing patients with abdominal sepsis.

References

1. Sartelli M, Catena F, Di Saverio S, Ansaloni L, Malangoni M, Moore EE, et al. Current concept of abdominal sepsis: WSES position paper. World J Emerg Surg. 2014;9(1):22.
2. Sartelli M, Abu-Zidan FM, Ansaloni L, Bala M, Beltrán MA, Biffl WL, et al. The role of the open abdomen procedure in managing severe abdominal sepsis: WSES position paper. World J Emerg Surg. 2015;10:35.
3. Kirkpatrick AW, Roberts DJ, De Waele J, Jaeschke R, Malbrain ML, De Keulenaer B, et al. Pediatric Guidelines Sub-Committee for the World Society of the Abdominal Compartment Syndrome. Intra-abdominal hypertension and the abdominal compartment syndrome: updated consensus definitions and clinical practice guidelines from the World Society of the Abdominal Compartment Syndrome. Intensive Care Med. 2013;39(7):1190–206.
4. Sartelli M, Catena F, Abu-Zidan FM, Ansaloni L, Biffl WL, Boermeester MA, et al. Management of intra-abdominal infections: recommendations by the WSES 2016 consensus conference. World J Emerg Surg. 2017;12:22.

Cardiac and Hemodynamic Consequences of Intra-abdominal Hypertension and the Abdominal Compartment Syndrome

12

Christopher James Doig, Kevin J. Solverson, and Kuljit (Ken) Parhar

C. J. Doig (✉)
Department of Critical Care Medicine, Cumming School of Medicine, University of Calgary, Calgary, AB, Canada

Department of Community Health Sciences, Cumming School of Medicine, University of Calgary, Calgary, AB, Canada

Department of Medicine, Cumming School of Medicine, University of Calgary, Calgary, AB, Canada

Multisystem Intensive Care Unit, Foothills Medical Centre, Calgary Zone, Alberta Health Services, Calgary, AB, Canada
e-mail: cdoig@ucalgary.ca, Chip.Doig@albertahealthservices.ca

K. J. Solverson
Department of Community Health Sciences, Cumming School of Medicine, University of Calgary, Calgary, AB, Canada

Multisystem Intensive Care Unit, Foothills Medical Centre, Calgary Zone, Alberta Health Services, Calgary, AB, Canada
e-mail: kjsolver@ucalgary.ca

K. (K.) Parhar
Department of Critical Care Medicine, Cumming School of Medicine, University of Calgary, Calgary, AB, Canada

Department of Medicine, Cumming School of Medicine, University of Calgary, Calgary, AB, Canada

Multisystem Intensive Care Unit, Foothills Medical Centre, Calgary Zone, Alberta Health Services, Calgary, AB, Canada

Cardiovascular Intensive Care Unit, Foothills Medical Centre, Calgary Zone, Alberta Health Services, Calgary, AB, Canada
e-mail: Kuljit.Parhar@albertahealthservices.ca

12.1 Illustrative Case

A 28-year-old female presented to the emergency department with severe pancreatitis. Her vital signs on arrival were heart rate 120 beats/min, respiratory rate 30 breaths/min, blood pressure of 80/50 mmHg, and a temperature of 38.1°C. Her abdomen was diffusely tender. Her blood work demonstrated a serum lipase >1000 U/L (0–80 U/L), hemoglobin of 144 g/L (137–180 g/L), and a white blood cell count of 11 × 10⁹/L (4.0–11.0 × 10⁹/L). In the emergency department, she received 6 L of normal saline over the first 3 h of her stay, with an increase in her blood pressure. A nasogastric tube provided gastric decompression and she was kept NPO. On the surgical floor, she received a total of an additional 12 L of intravenous normal saline over the next 24 h. Her vital signs slowly worsened. Her heart rate increased to 140 beats/min, her blood pressure dropped to 80/50 mmHg, her respiratory rate increased to 40 breaths/min. She required 60% inspired oxygen to maintain an oxygen saturation of 92%. She was afebrile. Her urine output decreased to <0.3 mL/Kg/h over consecutive hours. Her serum creatinine increased to 150 mmol/L (45–110 mmol/L). Her serum lactate increased to 5.0 mmol/L (0–2.0 mmol/L). She was admitted to the intensive care unit. She was intubated and started on invasive mechanical ventilation. A central line was placed and she was started on intravenous norepinephrine between 0.2 and 0.3 mcg/kg/min. A chest radiogram showed small lung volumes and bibasilar collapse. A CT scan of the abdomen showed progressive inflammatory change in her pancreas, free intra-abdominal fluid, but no other ominous intra-abdominal findings. Intra-abdominal pressures were recorded at 20 mmHg. Over the next 12 h, she became anuric, her norepinephrine requirements increased to 0.4–0.6 mcg/kg/min and her inspiratory ventilating pressures increased to maintain tidal volume of 6 mL/kg ideal body weight. A transthoracic echocardiogram demonstrated right ventricular enlargement, flattening of the ventricular septum, and a diminished left ventricular volume but with preserved systolic function, and a reduced IVC diameter. Her intra-abdominal pressure was recorded at 30 mmHg. She was maintained on intravenous neuromuscular relaxing agents (paralytics) and kept in a supine position. She was started on continuous venovenous hemodiafiltration with a neutral fluid balance after a negative fluid balance resulted in further increase in her norepinephrine dose. A percutaneous abdominal drain was placed and 500 mL was drained over the first hour without change in the abdominal pressure. A laparotomy was performed. During surgical incision, subcutaneous fluid "wept" from the surgical incision. Careful intra-abdominal exploration demonstrated no perforation or segment of ischemic bowel. A temporary vacuum-assisted abdominal closure was applied (ABTHERA™). Over the next few hours, with intra-abdominal pressures of 10 mmHg or less, her intravenous norepinephrine was decreased to 0.10–0.15 mcg/kg/min, her urine output increased to 1–1.5 mL/kg/min, and her inspiratory ventilating pressures decreased. Over 12 h, her serum lactate normalized. Her abdominal dressing was changed every 48 h with final closure on the fifth operation (8 days following laparotomy) after she had been off vasopressors for more than 24 h. She was discharged from the intensive care unit 14 days after admission and discharged home after 30 days in hospital.

12.2   Hemodynamic Effects of Abdominal Compartment Syndrome

12.2.1   Introduction and Definition

Multiple organ dysfunction syndrome has been described as the common final pathway to death in critically ill patients [1]. It was first described in the 1970s and the abdomen as the "motor of MOF" due to a combination of mucosal ischemia [2, 3], disruption of the intrinsic (mucosal) epithelial barrier [4–6], translocation of intraluminal bacteria or their byproducts [7], and activation of gastrointestinal associated lymphoid tissue with cytokine or other inflammatory mediator production and release [8, 9]. Despite extensive research on biological mechanisms, confirmation of the gut as the perpetrator—or conversely an alternative singular pathophysiologic process—has not been proven. Rather, it is likely that MODS is a final common pathway with multiple mechanisms which may precipitate its development. One such mechanism is elevated intra-abdominal pressure and the myriad consequences locally and systemically that result in multiple organ dysfunction [10]. Originally described more than 100 years ago, interest in the role of elevated intra-abdominal pressure and its systemic consequences was renewed in the 1970s and 1980s—in part due to observations associated with laparoscopic surgery and elevated intra-abdominal pressures associated with insufflation of the peritoneum [11]. It is now recognized as a potentially occult cause of increased morbidity and mortality in patients with primary intra-abdominal diseases or injuries or as a secondary complication of pathophysiologic abnormalities or their management in other diseases such as burns and severe sepsis [12–14].

In 2007 [15], and updated in 2013 [16], a standardized set of recommendations on the measurement of abdominal pressure and definitions of normal and abnormal pressures were published by the World Society of the Abdominal Compartment Syndrome. Intra-abdominal pressure in the critically ill can be measured by the use of an indwelling foley catheter with three-way stopcock [17–20]. Measurements should be performed in a supine patient with relaxed abdominal musculature. The transducer should be leveled to the mid-axilla. Twenty-five milliliters of fluid should be instilled into the bladder and measurements are taken at end expiration. The normal intra-abdominal pressure (IAP) is defined as 5–7 mmHg. The degree of elevated pressure or intra-abdominal hypertension (IAH) can be categorized: Grade 1—12–15 mmHg, Grade 2—16–20 mmHg, Grade 3—20–25 mmHg, and Grade 4—greater than 25 mmHg. Abdominal compartment syndrome (ACS) is defined as Grade 3 or IAH with concomitant new-onset organ dysfunction. Further, abdominal compartment syndrome (and hypertension) can be further classified into primary or secondary based on if there is a disease or injury that occurs in the abdominal–pelvic region [21].

12.2.2   Pathophysiology of Cardiovascular Consequences of IAH

The major cause of IAH and ACS is iatrogenic from overly exuberant fluid resuscitation with crystalloid solutions, particularly in the absence of careful monitoring of intra-abdominal pressures [22]. The abdominal compartment is a complex closed container closely integrated with intrathoracic pressure mediated through diaphragmatic position and by the compliance of the abdominal wall based on its elasticity and ability to distend [13, 23]. The remainder of the container is relatively static and noncompliant comprising the pelvic girdle and floor, and the vertebral column and paravertebral musculature and other structures. In critically ill patients, third spacing, or leakage of intravascular fluid into interstitial or nonvascular compartments, is common. Fluid may leak into subcutaneous tissues of the abdominal wall, into tissues of the abdominal organs such as the intestine or mesentery, into the peritoneal cavity, and into other cavities such as the pleural space. The result of this excess fluid is that the volume of structures within the abdominal cavity may increase, the walls of the container may become less elastic and compliant, and cephalad diaphragmatic excursion may occur: the sum total is as intra-abdominal volume increases, the overall system becomes less compliant, and intra-abdominal pressure increases, with an upward infection curve in pressure that may occur at a lower relative volume [24]. The relationship of the abdominal cavity, abdominal wall, and thoracic cavity may be further affected in patients with underlying chronic disease such as chronic obstructive pulmonary disease, diseases of the integument such as progressive systemic sclerosis, or due to the effect of acute injuries such as eschar and tissue edema associated with truncal burns (Table 12.1) [25]. What is not known is the appearance of volume pressure curves for the abdominal cavity and how these curves may be associated with intravenous fluid resuscitation.

The major hemodynamic consequence of IAH and ACS is a reduction in cardiac output, with the risk of subsequent ischemia to other organs. The level of elevated IAP which may affect cardiovascular performance is patient specific and may occur at relatively low levels of elevated IAP (e.g., 10 mmHg), or mean arterial blood pressure and cardiac output may be maintained despite significantly elevated IAPs [26, 27]. The mechanism of reducing cardiac output is multifactorial. The first and major cardiovascular consequence of IAH is cephalad displacement of the diaphragm, with elevation in intrathoracic pressure and subsequent reduction in venous return to the right heart [28]. These changes culminate in a direct effect on stroke volume and cardiac output [29]. Obviously, in individuals with reduced circulating volume, mild increases in IAP may have more significant reduction in venous return and cardiac output than in patients with normal or increased circulating volumes [30, 31]. Changes in diaphragmatic anatomy may also result in changes to the diaphragmatic foramen through which the IVC transits resulting in a partial physical obstruction further attenuating venous flow [32]. Elevation in intrathoracic pressure from diaphragmatic displacement will also cause pulmonary parenchymal and pulmonary vascular compression and an increase in pulmonary vascular resistance [33]. This may compromise left ventricular performance due to ventricular interdependence. Right ventricular dysfunction and dilatation results in septal shift, with a commensurate decrease in left ventricular end-diastolic volume and cardiac output. There may also be a direct effect of increased intrathoracic pressure decreasing cardiac compliance, attenuating ventricular expansion and end-diastolic volume,

Table 12.1 Factors contributing to elevated intra-abdominal pressures[a]

Abdominal wall and decreased compliance
• Tissue edema
• Pain and muscular contraction
• Prone positioning
• Burn eschar
• Abdominal dressings
• Obesity[b]
Intra-abdominal volume
• Luminal distension
– Gastroparesis
– Ileus
– Pseudo-obstruction
– Volvulus
– Intraluminal third spacing
• Intra-abdominal fluid
– Ascites
– Hemoperitoneum
– Abscesses
– Peritoneal dialysate
• Space occupying content
– Acute pancreatitis
– Intestinal wall and mesenteric edema
– Gravid uterus
– Tumor
– Excess air insufflation—laparoscopy
Impaired diaphragmatic excursion
• Intrapleural fluid/tissue
• Increased total lung volume from chronic obstructive pulmonary disease
• Higher positive end-expiratory pressure or lung volume during invasive mechanical ventilation
• Sitting position
Systemic factors
• Capillary fluid leak
– Massive fluid resuscitation
– Major trauma/burns/sepsis
– Acidosis/shock
• Age
• Systemic illnesses, e.g., progressive systemic sclerosis

[a]Adapted from Malbrain [21], Kirkpatrick [16]
[b]Obesity is associated with a slightly higher baseline intra-abdominal pressure [23]

and thereby causing a decrease in cardiac output, mimicking a tamponade-like effect. Finally, the effects of IAH on systemic vascular resistance are more complicated. Vasoconstriction may occur as the normal physiologic response to the underlying illness, in an attempt to maintain blood pressure in the face of a falling cardiac output, and related to intravenous vasoactive pharmacologic infusions. However, tissue edema as a consequence of third spacing of intravenous crystalloids may also increase peripheral vascular bed compression, and adversely increase systemic vascular resistance and local tissue perfusion.

Patients without preexisting cardiac dysfunction may have the physiologic reserve to respond to this myriad of insults. Whereas, patients with a diminished cardiac reserve from preexisting cardiac disease, or those patients with impaired circulating volume, may manifest more significant hemodynamic consequences. The hemodynamic consequence may not just be due to direct effects on the cardiovascular system [34]. Patients with ACS also demonstrate significant changes in blood flow to other organs and these ischemic changes may affect the propagation, circulation, or clearance of inflammatory humoral mediators [35]. For example, the gut may show attenuation of mesenteric arterial blood flow [36, 37]. As well, mesenteric venous pressure may be increased. Together, these blood flow changes may result in gut edema, mesenteric ischemia, and changes to gut integrity with damage to the intrinsic epithelial barrier, and subsequent translocation of bacteria or other intraluminal contents [38–40]. Hepatic blood flow may also be affected with subsequent effects on hepatic microcirculation and ischemic injury to the liver [41]. The regulatory function of the liver in processing materials absorbed or entering through the mesentery and damage to other biochemical processes such as lactic acid clearance may be affected [42]. Finally, IAH is associated with changes in renal blood flow, with a diminished renal arterial flow, raised renal venous pressures, shunting of blood away from the cortex, and a reduction in glomerular filtration [43]. Changes in hepatic and renal function may be associated with changes in circulating mediators which may further perpetuate changes in systemic hemodynamics.

12.2.3 Hemodynamic Assessment and Clinical Management

Hemodynamic management of abdominal compartment syndrome may be difficult. Furthermore, the risk of organ ischemia should be considered not only based on the absolute IAP but also in the context of the abdominal perfusion pressure (APP = MAP − IAP). High IAPs in the context of low MAPs (resulting in a low APP) are much more likely to lead to significant organ ischemia. A priority in the context of high IAP should be to raise the MAP in order to preserve the APP. Often time, simple intravascular pressure monitoring by either central venous pressure or pulmonary artery catheter may produce inaccurate results and be misleading. Prior work has demonstrated a very poor correlation between pulmonary arterial occluding pressure (PAOP)—or wedge pressure: an assessment of left ventricular end-diastolic pressure—or central venous pressure (CVP), and left ventricular cardiac output [44, 45]. Therefore, alternate methods of hemodynamic assessment should be considered. One of the most informative may be echocardiography [46]. Transthoracic echocardiography can be used for the assessment of vena cava size, left and right ventricular size and function, septal dyssynchrony and exaggerated interdependence, and noninvasive estimates of cardiac output. IVC diameter can be assessed with a subcostal view. Respiratory variation is present with significant reductions in venous return. Likewise, collapse of the abdominal IVC occurs when IAP exceeds right atrial pressure. Transthoracic echocardiography is routinely used for the assessment of ventricular chamber size and overall contractility. Transthoracic echocardiography is an effective and noninvasive diagnostic test that can be used serially to assess fluid responsiveness, right and left ventricular preload, as well as cardiac output and ongoing response to therapy.

Adequate intravascular volume is a cornerstone of the appropriate management of any critically ill patient. Unfortunately, there is no data to specifically guide what volume of crystalloid resuscitation is associated with a risk of IAP. Mildly elevated IAP may have more adverse consequences in an inadequately volume resuscitated patient. Whereas in the past, there was concern about inadequate volume resuscitation in many hypotensive patients, there is likewise now a similar concern about excessive volume resuscitation. In some patient populations, there is good clinical evidence that there are significant adverse consequences including an increased risk of death with excess fluid resuscitation particularly by crystalloids [44]. Raised IAP may be one consequence of excessive fluid resuscitation associated with mortality. Fluid resuscitation and hemodynamic support with vasopressors should be guided by careful clinical, hemodynamic, biochemical, and diagnostic/monitoring modalities. One of the most important measures should be ongoing monitoring of intra-abdominal pressures particularly in patients undergoing aggressive volume resuscitation, or in patients who require ongoing large volumes of crystalloids, or who have evidence of worsening organ function. The cornerstones of the appropriate hemodynamic assessment of elevated IAP are the cornerstones of overall management of elevated IAP [16]. First, there must be clinical awareness of the possibility of elevated IAP. Second, at minimum patients at higher risk of developing IAH should have routine measurement of IAP. Third, measures should be considered to minimize the risk of developing IAH by judicious but cautious volume resuscitation, particularly by indiscriminate use of crystalloid solutions or volume resuscitation not guided by hemodynamic monitoring and clear end points. Fourth, use of "volumetric" assessment of hemodynamics should be considered to guide decision-making on resuscitation and ongoing hemodynamic management. Finally, hemodynamic management should be considered in the wider context of overall IAH management including enteral decompression, intraperitoneal drainage, ventilator management, circulating fluid removal by diuresis or renal replacement therapy, and ultimately decisions to proceed with surgical decompression and temporary abdominal closure.

12.3   Conclusion

The hemodynamic consequences of IAH and ACS are significant. The cardiovascular consequences are multifactorial including direct effects on cardiac performance and indirect effects from regional organ or tissue ischemia. It is important to recognize the patient at risk of IAH and to monitor intra-abdominal pressure. Clinical management should be cognizant of intravascular volume and potential effects of IAP on venous return, and the necessity for clinical management to be guided by careful hemodynamic assessment.

References

1. Carrico CJ, Meakins JL, Marshall JC, Fry D, Maier RV. Multiple organ failure syndrome. Arch Surg. 1986;121:196–208.
2. Deitch EA, Morrison J, Berg R, Specian RD. Effect of hemorrhagic shock on bacterial translocation, intestinal morphology, and intestinal permeability in conventional and antibiotic-decontaminated rats. Crit Care Med. 1990;18:529–36.
3. Fink MP, Antonsson JB, Wang HL, Rothschild HR. Increased intestinal permeability in endotoxic pigs: mesenteric hypoperfusion as an etiologic factor. Arch Surg. 1991;126:211–8.
4. Deitch EA, Specian RD, Berg RD. Endotoxin-induced bacterial translocation and mucosal permeability: role of xanthine oxidase, complement activation, and macrophage products. Crit Care Med. 1991;19:785–91.
5. Harris CE, Griffiths RD, Freestone N, Billington D, Atherton ST, Macmillan RR. Intestinal permeability in the critically ill. Intensive Care Med. 1992;18:38–41.
6. Doig CJ, Sutherland LR, Sandham JD, Fick GH, Verhoef M, Meddings JB. Increased intestinal permeability is associated with the development of multiple organ dysfunction syndrome in critically ill ICU patients. Am J Respir Crit Care Med. 1998;158:444–51.
7. Mainous MR, Tso P, Berg RD, Deitch EA. Studies of the route, magnitude, and time course of bacterial translocation in a model of systemic inflammation. Arch Surg. 1991;126:33–7.
8. Haglund U. Systemic mediators released from the gut in critical illness. Crit Care Med. 1993;21:S15–8.
9. Johnston JD, Harvey CJ, Menzies IS, Treacher DF. Gastrointestinal permeability and absorptive capacity in sepsis. Crit Care Med. 1996;24:1144–9.
10. Sugerman HJ, Bloomfield GL, Saggi BW. Multisystem organ failure secondary to increased intra-abdominal pressure. Infection. 1999;27(1):61–6.
11. Van Hee R. Historical highlights in concept and treatment of abdominal compartment syndrome. Acta Clin Belg. 2007;62(Suppl 1):9–15.
12. Ball CG, Kirkpatrick AW, McBeth P. The secondary abdominal compartment syndrome: not just another post-traumatic complication. Can J Surg. 2008;51:399–405.
13. Cheatham ML. Abdominal compartment syndrome: pathophysiology and definitions. Scand J Trauma Resusc Emerg Med. 2009;17:10. https://doi.org/10.1186/1757-7241-17-10.
14. Balogh ZJ, Leppaniemi A. The neglected (abdominal) compartment: what is new at the beginning of the 21st century? World J Surg. 2009;33:1109.
15. Cheatham ML, Malbrain ML, Kirkpatrick A, et al. Results from the international conference of experts on intra-abdominal hypertension and abdominal compartment syndrome. II. Recommendations. Intensive Care Med. 2007;33:951–62.
16. Kirkpatrick AW, Roberts DJ, De Waele J, et al. Intra-abdominal hypertension and the abdominal compartment syndrome: updated consensus definitions and clinical practice guidelines from the World Society of the Abdominal Compartment Syndrome. Intensive Care Med. 2013;39:1190–206.
17. Malbrain ML. Different techniques to measure intra-abdominal pressure (IAP): time for a critical re-appraisal. Intensive Care Med. 2004;30:357–71.
18. Malbrain ML, Deeren DH. Effect of bladder volume on measured intravesical pressure: a prospective cohort study. Crit Care. 2006;10:R98.
19. Rao P, Chaudhry R, Kumar S. Abdominal compartment pressure monitoring—a simple technique. Med J Armed Forces India. 2006;62:269–70.
20. Cheatham ML, Fowler J. Measuring intra-abdominal pressure outside the ICU: validation of a simple bedside method. Am Surg. 2008;74:806–8.
21. Malbrain ML, Cheatham ML, Kirkpatrick A, et al. Results from the international conference of experts on intra-abdominal hypertension and abdominal compartment syndrome. I. Definitions. Intensive Care Med. 2006;32:1722–32.
22. Balogh Z, McKinley BA, Cocanour CS, et al. Supranormal trauma resuscitation causes more cases of abdominal compartment syndrome. Arch Surg. 2003;138:637–43.
23. De Keulenaer BL, De Waele JJ, Powell B, Malbrain ML. What is normal intra-abdominal pressure and how is it affected by positioning, body mass and positive end-expiratory pressure? Intensive Care Med. 2009;35:969–76.

24. Rogers WK, Garcia L. Intra-abdominal hypertension, abdominal compartment syndrome, and the open abdomen. Chest. 2018;153:238–50.
25. Malbrain MLNG, De Keulenaer BL, Oda J, et al. Intra-abdominal hypertension and abdominal compartment syndrome in burns, obesity, pregnancy and general medicine. Anaesthesiol Intensive Ther. 2015;47:228.
26. Cheatham ML, Malbrain MLNG. Cardiovascular implications of abdominal compartment syndrome. Acta Clin Belg. 2007;62(Suppl 1):98–112.
27. Kashtan J, Green JF, Parsons EQ, Holcroft JW. Hemodynamic effects of increased abdominal pressure. J Surg Res. 1981;30:249–55.
28. Pelosi P, Quintel M, Malbrain ML. Effect of intra-abdominal pressure on respiratory mechanics. Acta Clin Belg. 2007;62(Suppl):78–88.
29. Barnes GE, Laine GA, Giam PY, Smith EE, Granger HJ. Cardiovascular responses to elevation of intra-abdominal hydrostatic pressure. Am J Physiol. 1985;248(2 Pt 2):R208–13.
30. Schachtrupp A, Graf J, Tons C, Hoer J, Fackeldey V, Schumpelick V. Intravascular volume depletion in a 24-hour porcine model of intra-abdominal hypertension. J Trauma. 2003;55(4):734–40.
31. Ridings PC, Bloomfield GL, Blocher CR, Sugerman HJ. Cardiopulmonary effects of raised intra-abdominal pressure before and after intravascular volume expansion. J Trauma. 1995;39(6):1071–5.
32. Schein M, Wittmann DH, Aprahamian CC, Condon RE. The abdominal compartment syndrome: the physiological and clinical consequences of elevated intra-abdominal pressure. J Am Coll Surg. 1995;180(6):745–53.
33. Wauters J, Wilmer A, Valenza F. Abdomino-thoracic transmission during ACS: facts and figures. Acta Clin Belg. 2007;62(Suppl 1):200–5.
34. Malbrain ML, Marik PE, Witters I, et al. Fluid overload, de-resuscitation, and outcomes in critically ill or injured patients: a systematic review with suggestions for clinical practice. Anaesthesiol Intensive Ther. 2014;46:361–80.
35. Walker J, Criddle LM. Pathophysiology and management of abdominal compartment syndrome. Am J Crit Care. 2003;12:367–71.
36. Caldwell CB, Ricotta JJ. Changes in visceral blood flow with elevated intra-abdominal pressure. J Surg Res. 1987;43:14–20.
37. Friedlander MH, Simon RJ, Ivatury R, et al. Effect of hemorrhage on superior mesenteric artery flow during increased intra-abdominal pressures. J Trauma. 1998;45:433–9.
38. Diebel LN, Dulchavsky SA, Wilson RF. Effect of increased intra-abdominal pressure on mesenteric arterial and intestinal mucosal blood flow. J Trauma. 1992;33:45–9.
39. Diebel LN, Dulchavsky SA, Brown WJ. Splanchnic ischemia and bacterial translocation in the abdominal compartment syndrome. J Trauma. 1997;43:852–5.
40. Gargiulo NJ III, Simon RJ, Leon W, Machiedo GW. Hemorrhage exacerbates bacterial translocation at low levels of intra-abdominal pressure. Arch Surg. 1998;133:1351–5.
41. Diebel LN, Wilson RF, Dulchavsky SA, et al. Effect of increased intra-abdominal pressure on hepatic arterial, portal venous, and hepatic microcirculatory blood flow. J Trauma. 1992;33:279–83.
42. Nakatani T, Sakamoto Y, Kaneko I, Ando H, Kobayashi K. Effects of intra-abdominal hypertension on hepatic energy metabolism in a rabbit model. J Trauma. 1998;44:446–53.
43. De laet I, Malbrain M, Jadoul J, Rogiers P, Sugrue M. Renal implications of increased intra-abdominal pressure: are the kidneys the canary for abdominal hypertension? Acta Clin Belg. 2007;62(Suppl 1):119–30.
44. Malbrain ML, Ameloot K, Gillebert C, Cheatham ML. Cardiopulmonary monitoring in intra-abdominal hypertension. Am Surg. 2011;77(Suppl 1):S23–30.
45. Yang C, Yang Z, Chen X, et al. Inverted U-shaped relationship between central venous pressure and intra-abdominal pressure in the early phase of severe acute pancreatitis: a retrospective study. PLoS One. 2015;10:e0128493. https://doi.org/10.1371/journal.pone.0128493.
46. Mahjoub Y, Plantefeve G. Cardiac ultrasound and abdominal compartment syndrome. Acta Clin Belg. 2007;62(Suppl 1):183–9.

Liver Failure Associated to the Polycompartment Syndrome

13

Francesco Forfori, Francesco Corradi, and Giandomenico Biancofiore

13.1 Introduction

A compartment syndrome is defined as an increase in the compartmental pressure to such an extent that the viability of the tissues and organs within the compartment is threatened [1]. In particular, the term "polycompartment syndrome" is used when more than one compartment is affected (the head, the chest, the abdomen, and the extremities). The deleterious effects on organ function are directly related to the severity of the syndrome and the number of compartments involved. The abdomen plays a central role in the polycompartment syndrome and the effect of intra-abdominal hypertension (IAH) on different organ systems, not only within the abdomen, is well recognized [2]. Increased IAP induces organ dysfunction through two major pathways. Firstly, the pressure effect of increased IAP is transmitted directly to another body compartment and secondly, increased IAP influences systemic hemodynamic, decreasing perfusion pressure and increasing venous resistance [3].

The liver seems to be particularly susceptible to injury in the presence of elevated abdominal pressures, especially in case of IAH or ACS [4]. Abdominal compartment syndrome (ACS) can lead to liver injury either with a direct or indirect mechanism. In fact, both the increase in the intra-abdominal pressure (IAP) and the reduction of perfusion and oxygen delivery caused by the complex interplay of raised pressure between different compartments can be responsible for liver damage [5].

F. Forfori (✉)
Department of Surgical, Medical and Molecular Pathology and Critical Care Medicine, University of Pisa, Pisa, Italy

Azienda Ospedaliero Universitaria Pisana (AOUP), Pisa, Italy
e-mail: francesco.forfori@unipi.it, julia.wendon@kcl.ac.uk

F. Corradi · G. Biancofiore
Department of Surgical, Medical and Molecular Pathology and Critical Care Medicine, University of Pisa, Pisa, Italy

© Springer Nature Switzerland AG 2021
F. Coccolini et al. (eds.), *Compartment Syndrome*, Hot Topics in Acute Care Surgery and Trauma, https://doi.org/10.1007/978-3-030-55378-4_13

Furthermore, acute liver failure, decompensated chronic liver disease, and liver transplantation are frequently complicated by IAH and ACS [1, 6].

Deterioration of hepatic cell function and liver perfusion have been revealed by different animal and human studies even with reduced level of IAP (around 10 mmHg). Different studies described the adverse effects of increase intra-abdominal pressure on the hepatic blood flow and the subsequent dysfunction (or failure) related to the ischemia/reperfusion injury. Caldwell and Ricotta showed considerable changes in visceral blood flow correlated with intra-abdominal pressure [7]. In an animal experimental model, a significant decrease in liver blood flow has been evidenced using radiolabeled microspheres. The reduction of flow was more pronounced as the IAP rise, moving from 0.42 ± 0.09 cc/g/min at the baseline to 0.25 ± 0.01 cc/g/min with an IAP of 20 mmHg and ending to 0.15 ± 0.06 at an IAP of 40 mmHg. Moreover, the decrement in hepatic blood flow was more marked than the changes in the reduction of cardiac output suggesting that, in addition to decreased cardiac output and systemic perfusion, local control mechanisms may be further responsible for changes in blood flow. Diebel et al. observed, in a pig model, a progressive decrease in portal venous, hepatic arterial and hepatic microcirculatory blood flow when intra-abdominal pressure was increased, although MAP was kept constant [8]. Furthermore, the reduction in hepatic blood flow was also present for not significant reduction in cardiac output and even though pulmonary artery wedge pressure (PAWP) remained relatively constant. Of concern, the reduction in blood flow reached significant value compared to control at IAP of 10 mmHg, showing an earlier and more severe decrease in hepatic arterial blood flow compared to portal and microcirculatory level, suggesting a humoral basis for the hepatic perfusion changes observed [8]. When IAP is high, portal vein pressure rose steadily, reaching the same value of IAP (Table 13.1).

Hepatic perfusion may be even more impaired in the hypotensive hypovolemic patient. The increase of intra-abdominal pressure, in combination with mechanical positive pressure ventilation, may be extremely detrimental on splanchnic perfusion. Moreover, the observed compressive effect of high IAP on the inferior vena

Table 13.1 Effects of intraabdominal pressure (IAP) on systemic hemodynamic variables and hepatic blood flow

IAP (mmHg)	CO (L/min)	PAWP (mmHg)	MAP (mmHg)	HABF (% of baseline)	PVBF (% of baseline)	HMCBF (% of baseline)
Baseline	4.8 ± 0.6	6 ± 1	66 ± 9	100	100	100
10	4.7 ± 1.0	5 ± 1	77 ± 23	60.9 ± 16.7*	72.6 ± 23.9*	80.8 ± 12.6*
20	4.9 ± 1.2	7 ± 1	93 ± 23	45.4 ± 22.7*	65.5 ± 19.5*	71.1 ± 15.8*
30	4.4 ± 0.7	6 ± 1	91 ± 25	33.3 ± 19.0**	54.9 ± 21.8**	60.3 ± 15.9**
40	4.8 ± 0.4	8 ± 3	97 ± 26	30.1 ± 17.0**	47.8 ± 20.80**	48.4 ± 8.4**

*$p < 0.05$; **$p < 0.01$

Abbreviations: *CO* Cardiac output, *PAWP* Pulmonary artery wedge pressure, *MAP* Mean arterial pressure, *HABF* Hepatic artery blood flow, *PVBF* Portal venous blood flow, *HMCBF* Hepatic microcirculatory blood flow

Adapted from: Diebel LN et al. Effect of increased intra-abdominal pressure on hepatic arterial, portal venous, and hepatic microcirculatory blood flow. J Trauma. 1992 Aug;33(2):279–82

cava may lead to significant impairment with hepatic outflow resulting in further hepatic congestion [9]. The decrease in the hepatic arterial and venous portal flow and the following increase in the porto-collateral circulation exercise pathological effects on liver activity causing a decrease in the lactate clearance, an alteration in the glucose metabolism and the mitochondrial function [10]. The deleterious effects of increased IAP may be considered in terms of the hepatic circulation and of the biochemical dysfunction of the hepatocytes [11].

Despite monitoring hepatic blood flow and function might be fundamental during IAP, they remain difficult to assess at the bedside. Plasma concentrations of liver enzymes and laboratory parameters of liver synthesis offer partial and indirect information on actual liver function [12]. In an animal study of sustained raised IAP, Eleftheriadis and Kotzampassi compared healthy rats to those with induced cirrhosis, observed increased levels of alkaline phosphatase, alanine aminotransferase, and bilirubin concentrations in the latter, although these changes did not reach significance. The study does, however, suggest that patients with preexisting liver disease may be more susceptible to the effects of raised intra-abdominal pressure [13]. Noninvasive measurement of indocyanine green (ICG) plasma disappearance rate (PDR(ICG)) is supposed to be an accurate marker of liver function [14]. After intravenous injection, ICG is distributed via the bloodstream, excreted by hepatocytes into the bile, and then completely cleared by the gastrointestinal system without entering the enterohepatic recirculation [12]. Therefore, elimination of ICG is determined by cardiac output (CO), hepatic blood flow, and hepatocellular uptake; thus, PDR(ICG) has been shown to be a good surrogate marker for liver function and hepatosplanchnic perfusion. Different authors tried to assess the prognostic value of the indocyanine green plasma disappearance rate in critically ill patients. During liver transplantation, PDRICG has been demonstrated to reliably detect rapid variations in liver function caused by sudden changes in the hepatosplanchnic blood flow [13].

Kimura et al. identified PDR(ICG) as an early indicator of hepatocellular injury in the course of septic shock and assessed its predictive value of poor outcome [15]. Inal et al. showed in a retrospective analysis of 30 critically ill patients that IAP was significantly higher (21.5 ± 2 mmHg vs. 11.7 ± 1.5 mmHg) and PDRICG was significantly lower ($10.9 \pm 3.4\%$ vs. $24.5 \pm 6.8\%$) in non-survivors compared to survivors evidencing a superior sensitivity and specificity (AUROC = 0.78) of PDRICG compared to the APACHE-II score (AUROC = 0.64), SOFA score (AUROC = 0.56), and bilirubin (AUROC = 0.62) [16].

Malbrain et al. evidenced that PDR(ICG) correlated significantly with IAP and even more with APP (abdomen pressure perfusion), observing an important correlation between higher values of IAP and significantly lower values of APP and PDR(ICG) and mortality. The lower the PDRICG and APP, the higher the ICU and hospital mortality are [12]. In 40 critically ill patients, a PDR(ICG) $\geq 12\%$ had a sensitivity of 78.6% and a specificity of 80.8% for good outcome, while PDR(ICG) < 12% had significantly higher ICU and hospital mortality [12]. Sakka et al. classified patients according to their lowest ICG-PDR value and found that mortality was about 80% in patients with ICG-PDR lower than 8% per minute and survival was about 80% in patients with ICG-PDR greater than 16% per minute [17]. PDR(ICG) has been shown to be a good surrogate marker for liver function and hepatosplanchnic perfusion offering additional information always not "detected" by the classic liver function tests.

Liver injury during ACS may also be explained by the activation of the host's inflammatory cascade in a two steps model of postinjury MOF [18]. An initial insult (hemorrhage/trauma) primes the host's inflammatory cascade through an ischemia/reperfusion effect, creating a vulnerable milieu where a second insult (such as ACS) can provoke unbridled systemic hyperinflammation culminating in organ dysfunction and MOF [18]. The role of sequential insults to the organism (first hypovolemic shock and resuscitation and then IAH) may amplify the ill effects of IAP or lower the critical threshold for the development of severe IAH.

Rezende-Neto et al. showed that the development of ACS 8 h after resuscitation for hemorrhagic shock when there were already activated circulating neutrophils (PMNs) provoked acute lung and liver injury and resulted in a 33% mortality [18]. This model has direct clinical implications stressing the importance of promptly treating or controlling ACS after damage control resuscitation to prevent postinjury MOF in critically injured patients.

Moreover, it has been shown that in animal models of increased IAP there is a significantly higher *Escherichia coli* counts in the mesenteric lymph nodes, liver, and spleen 3 h later abdominal decompression [19]. It is generally accepted, that shock, major trauma, and thermal injury can cause mucosal disintegration contributing to distant organ failure either by the release of inflammatory mediators or gut mucosal barrier disruption leading to bacterial and endotoxin translocation [19].

These findings were an example of ischemia–reperfusion injury, and increased IAP caused significant intestinal ischemia, followed by reperfusion injury after abdominal decompression.

Moreover, high intra-abdominal pressure in critically ill unstable patients can exacerbate the other pathophysiological mechanisms of organ damage further worsening the multi-organ dysfunction associated with acute/chronic liver failure [11].

13.2   Hepato-Abdominal–Renal Syndrome (HARS)

Acute kidney injury (AKI) in critically ill cirrhotic patients is common and often multifactorial.

Hepatorenal syndrome likely reflects prerenal decrease of kidney function, occurs in patients with liver failure and ascites, and does not respond to volume loading. The pathophysiologic mechanism leading to hepatorenal syndrome is characterized by splanchnic arterial vasodilatation leading to renal vasoconstriction in the setting of a low flow state due to decreased systemic vascular resistance [20]. Although the incidence of HRS is unknown, especially in relation to other causes of renal failure, it is estimated to be 40% over a 5-year period in patients with cirrhosis and ascites [21].

Hepatorenal syndrome is one of the serious complications of cirrhosis and closely associated with increasing intra-abdominal pressure (IAP) [22].

Diagnosis of HRS involves the demonstration of low glomerular filtration rate in the absence of shock, infection, fluid losses, and nephrotoxic agents, with no improvement after discontinuation of diuretics and administration of 1.5 L fluid and proteinuria of less than 500 mg/day, with no ultrasonographic evidence of obstruction or intrinsic parenchymal disease [20].

The precise role of IAH in HRS remains incompletely understood. It can be argued that diminished glomerular perfusion due to venous congestion results in further decline of GFR coupled with reduction of cardiac output and elevated levels of catecholamines, renin, angiotensin, and inflammatory cytokines, leading to further renal dysfunction as IAP approaches the range of ACS [23]. The term HARS, hepato-abdominal–renal syndrome, succinctly describes this pathophysiological process, as increase in the IAP may be the missing link in the development of AKI in decompensated liver failure [24]. In patients with portal hypertension and esophageal varices, increases in IAP may have deleterious effects on variceal hemodynamic, markedly increasing the volume, pressure, and wall tension of the varices [25].

Paracentesis has been performed as treatment for hepatorenal syndrome, but generally was not advocated because of fears of inducing hypovolemia and further exacerbating kidney impairment [26].

However, several investigators have hypothesized that IAH may be an important contributing factor in the pathogenesis of hepatorenal syndrome, with observations in small studies that paracentesis and parenteral administration of albumin may lead to improved kidney function in critically ill patients with cirrhosis admitted with variceal bleeding, as well as in stable patients with hepatorenal syndrome [27].

Diuretics, albumin, or other treatments are often insensitive or ineffective to the recovery of renal function in the cirrhotic patients with ascites. However, it could be improved after the extraction of ascites. In clinical practice, IAP could be raised due to the increasing ascites in patients with cirrhosis. Early abdominal decompression, rather than late, is gaining more popularity with better outcomes.

Renal replacement therapies are not a treatment for HRS/cirrhosis-induced AKI but are often initiated as a bridge to either liver transplant or definitive decision [28].

13.3   Hepato-Abdominal–Pulmonary Syndrome (HAPS)

Pulmonary dysfunction is a common feature in patients with liver disease. Hypoxia has been found in one-third of patients with chronic liver disease [29]. Ascites, hepatopulmonary syndrome, extreme hepatomegaly, low albumin levels, anemia, increased closing volume, and respiratory muscle weakness are considered among the factors implicated in the pathogenesis of hypoxemia in cirrhosis [30].

The hepatopulmonary syndrome (HPS) is a rare lung complication of liver disease characterized by intrapulmonary vasodilation leading to a ventilation/perfusion mismatch with resultant hypoxemia that can be found in up to 40% of patients with end-stage liver disease. The clinical triad consists of: (1) liver disease and/or portal hypertension; (2) the presence of intrapulmonary vascular dilatations; and (3) increased alveolar-arterial gradient resulting in orthodeoxia (arterial hypoxemia in the upright position) and platypnoea (improved oxygenation in supine position) [31].

Diagnosis is based on identification of hypoxemia either through pulse oximetry or on arterial blood gas and the demonstration of an intrapulmonary shunt (which can usually be demonstrated with contrast echocardiography) if there is a normal chest X-ray and pulmonary function tests [32]. Portopulmonary hypertension is the presence of pulmonary arterial hypertension due to increased pulmonary vascular resistance and pulmonary vasoconstriction leading to right heart failure in the setting of advanced liver disease. Doppler echocardiography is a highly sensitive tool for detecting portopulmonary hypertension, using a right heart catheterization for confirmation and definitive diagnosis. The diagnosis is made if mean pulmonary arterial pressure is >25 mmHg or left ventricular end-diastolic pressure <15 mmHg in the setting of liver disease or portal hypertension. In general, the presence of portopulmonary hypertension is a poor prognostic sign in liver failure [32].

Moreover, pulmonary function can also be compromised by direct mechanical effects of hydrothorax and abdominal ascites on diaphragmatic movement. Hydrothorax is defined as a significant pleural effusion, usually >500 mL in a patient with end-stage liver disease. Various mechanisms have been proposed such as decreased osmotic pressure, leakage of plasma from azygous venous system, and lymph leakage from the thoracic duct, although the prevailing thought is direct transport into pleural space through diaphragmatic defects [21].

The new term HAPS, or hepato-abdominal-pulmonary syndrome, describes this clinical problem. Indeed the nitric oxide–induced vasodilation, the water and sodium retention coupled with the cirrotic hyperdynamic state, and the increased IAP will lead to expansion of systemic and central blood volumes resulting in interstitial fluid accumulation, triggering a vicious cycle [33].

Finally, the presence of an exaggerated inflammatory response, coupled with a relative immunocompromised state likely can predispose patients to acute lung injury. The risk of aspiration pneumonias also high because of altered consciousness, swallowing dysfunction, gastric stasis, increased intra-abdominal pressure due to ascites, and ileus resulting from infection and electrolyte abnormalities [34].

Medical treatment is generally indicated as a bridge to transplant and is based on the continuous infusion of a prostacyclin such as epoprostenol for mean pulmonary artery pressures >25 mmHg. As for HRS, the cornerstone of management remains albumin (1 g/kg initially followed by 20–40 g/day) and vasopressor therapy to mitigate splanchnic and systemic vasodilatation.

The only definitive treatment for HPS is liver transplantation, which will result in complete resolution in 80% of the cases. Other forms of medical therapy such as somatostatin, indomethacin, methylene blue, and plasma exchange have been used but remain unvalidated.

With regard to PPH, the diagnosis has specific transplant implications, as orthotopic liver transplant is classified as high risk if mean pulmonary artery pressure is between 35 and 50 mmHg and contraindicated if mean pulmonary artery pressure is >50 mmHg due to high mortality from acute right heart failure [35].

13.4 Conclusion

Polycompartment syndrome is a clinical severe condition generated by increased compartmental pressures in multiple compartments of the body and able to compromise tissue and organ perfusion. The abdomen plays a central role and the liver seems to be particularly susceptible to the effect of IAH. Deterioration of hepatic cell function and liver perfusion have been revealed by different animal and human studies associated with IAP and are more pronounced in acute/chronic failure. ACS exerts a role in the pathophysiology of cardiorenal and hepatorenal syndromes that are often worsened by the pathophysiological condition occurring during IAH. Close monitoring and adequate therapy aimed at lowering compartmental pressure and restoring organ perfusion preventing organ failure are necessary to improve outcome decreasing mortality.

References

1. Papavramidis TS, Marinis AD, Pliakos I, Kesisoglou I, Papavramidou N. Abdominal compartment syndrome—intra-abdominal hypertension: defining, diagnosing, and managing. J Emerg Trauma Shock. 2011;4(2):279–91.
2. Malbrain ML, Wilmer A. The polycompartment syndrome: towards an understanding of the interactions between different compartments! Intensive Care Med. 2007;33(11):1869–72.
3. De Waele JJ, De Laet I, Malbrain ML. Understanding abdominal compartment syndrome. Intensive Care Med. 2016;42:1068–70. United States.
4. Biancofiore G, Bindi ML, Boldrini A, Consani G, Bisa M, Esposito M, et al. Intraabdominal pressure in liver transplant recipients: incidence and clinical significance. Transplant Proc. 2004;36:547 9. United States.
5. Bodnar Z. Polycompartment syndrome—intra-abdominal pressure measurement. Anaesthesiol Intensive Ther. 2019;51(4):316–22. Poland.
6. Biancofiore G, Bindi ML, Romanelli AM, Boldrini A, Consani G, Bisa M, et al. Intra-abdominal pressure monitoring in liver transplant recipients: a prospective study. Intensive Care Med. 2003;29(1):30–6.
7. Caldwell CB, Ricotta JJ. Changes in visceral blood flow with elevated intraabdominal pressure. J Surg Res. 1987;43(1):14–20.
8. Diebel LN, Wilson RF, Dulchavsky SA, Saxe J. Effect of increased intra-abdominal pressure on hepatic arterial, portal venous, and hepatic microcirculatory blood flow. J Trauma. 1992;33(2):279–82; discussion 82–3.
9. Wachsberg RH. Narrowing of the upper abdominal inferior vena cava in patients with elevated intraabdominal pressure: sonographic observations. J Ultrasound Med. 2000;19(3):217–22.
10. Hernandez G, Regueira T, Bruhn A, Castro R, Rovegno M, Fuentealba A, et al. Relationship of systemic, hepatosplanchnic, and microcirculatory perfusion parameters with 6-hour lactate clearance in hyperdynamic septic shock patients: an acute, clinical-physiological, pilot study. Ann Intensive Care. 2012;2(1):44.

11. Cresswell AB, Wendon JA. Hepatic function and non-invasive hepatosplanchnic monitoring in patients with abdominal hypertension. Acta Clin Belg. 2007;62(Suppl 1):113–8.

12. Malbrain ML, Viaene D, Kortgen A, De Laet I, Dits H, Van Regenmortel N, et al. Relationship between intra-abdominal pressure and indocyanine green plasma disappearance rate: hepatic perfusion may be impaired in critically ill patients with intra-abdominal hypertension. Ann Intensive Care. 2012;2(Suppl 1):S19.

13. Eleftheriadis E, Kotzampassi K. Hepatic microcirculation after continuous 7-day elevated intra-abdominal pressure in cirrhotic rats. Hepatol Res. 2005;32:96–100. Netherlands.

14. Stehr A, Ploner F, Traeger K, Theisen M, Zuelke C, Radermacher P, et al. Plasma disappearance of indocyanine green: a marker for excretory liver function? Intensive Care Med. 2005;31(12):1719–22.

15. Kimura S, Yoshioka T, Shibuya M, Sakano T, Tanaka R, Matsuyama S. Indocyanine green elimination rate detects hepatocellular dysfunction early in septic shock and correlates with survival. Crit Care Med. 2001;29(6):1159–63.

16. Inal MT, Memis D, Sezer YA, Atalay M, Karakoc A, Sut N. Effects of intra-abdominal pressure on liver function assessed with the LiMON in critically ill patients. Can J Surg. 2011;54(3):161–6.

17. Sakka SG, Reinhart K, Meier-Hellmann A. Prognostic value of the indocyanine green plasma disappearance rate in critically ill patients. Chest. 2002;122(5):1715–20.

18. Rezende-Neto JB, Moore EE, Masuno T, Moore PK, Johnson JL, Sheppard FR, Cunha-Melo JR, Silliman CC. The abdominal compartment syndrome as a second insult during systemic neutrophil priming provokes multiple organ injury. Shock. 2003;20(4):303–8.

19. Doty JM, Oda J, Ivatury RR, Blocher CR, Christie GE, Yelon JA, Sugerman HJ. The effects of hemodynamic shock and increased intra-abdominal pressure on bacterial translocation. J Trauma. 2002;52(1):13–7.

20. Dundar HZ, Yılmazlar T. Management of hepatorenal syndrome World. J Nephrol. 2015;4:277–86.

21. DellaVolpe J, Garavaglia JM, Huang DT. Management of complications of end-stage liver disease in the intensive care unit. J Intensive Care Med. 2016;31:94–103.

22. Chang Y, Qi X, Li Z, Wang F, Wang S, Zhang Z, Xiao C, Ding T, Yang C. Hepatorenal syndrome: insights into the mechanisms of intra-abdominal hypertension. Int J Clin Exp Pathol. 2013;6(11):2523–8.

23. Mikami O, Fujise K, Matsumoto S, Shingu K, Ashida M, Matsuda T. High intra-abdominal pressure increases plasma catecholamine concentrations during pneumoperitoneum for laparoscopic procedures. Arch Surg. 1998;133:39–43.

24. Malbrain ML, De Laet I. A new concept: the polycompartment syndrome—part 2. Int J Intensive Care. 2009;16(1):24–31.

25. Escorsell A, Gines A, Llach J, Garcia-Pagan JC, Bordas JM, Bosch J, Rodes J. Increasing intra-abdominal pressure increases pressure, volume, and wall tension in esophageal varices. Hepatology. 2002;36:936–40.

26. De Waele JJ, De Laet I, Kirkpatrick AW, Hoste E. Intra-abdominal hypertension and abdominal compartment syndrome. Am J Kidney Dis. 2011;57(1):159–69.

27. Umgelter A, Reindl W, Wagner KS, et al. Effects of plasma expansion with albumin and paracentesis on haemodynamics and kidney function in critically ill cirrhotic patients with tense ascites and hepatorenal syndrome: a prospective uncontrolled trial. Crit Care. 2008;12:R4.

28. Karvellas CJ, Bagshaw SM. Advances in management and prognostication in critically ill cirrhotic patients. Curr Opin Crit Care. 2014;20:210–7.

29. Alkhayat K, Moustafa G, Zaghloul A, Elazeem AA. Pulmonary dysfunction in patients with liver cirrhosis. Arch Med. 2017;9:4.

30. Krowka MJ, Cortese DA. Severe hypoxaemia associated with liver disease: Mayo Clinic experience and the experimental use of almitrine bismesylate. Mayo Clinic Proc. 1987;62:164–73.

31. Malbrain MLNG, De laet I, De Waele J. The polycompartment syndrome: what's all the fuss about? In: Vincent J-L, editor. Yearbook of intensive care and emergency medicine. Berlin: Springer; 2010. p. 465–84.

32. Raevens S, Geerts A, Van Steenkiste C, Verhelst X, Van Vlierberghe H, Colle I. Hepatopulmonary syndrome and portopulmonary hypertension: recent knowledge in pathogenesis and overview of clinical assessment. Liver Int. 2015;35:1646–60.
33. Malbrain MLNG, Roberts DJ, Sugrue M, De Keulenaer BL, Ivatury R, Pelosi P, Verbrugge F, Wise R, Mullens W. The polycompartment syndrome: a concise state of the art review. Anaesthesiol Intensive Ther. 2014;46(5):433–50.
34. Olson JC, Wendon JA, Kramer DJ, et al. Intensive care of the patient with cirrhosis. Hepatology. 2011;54:1864–72.
35. Krowka MJ, Mandell MS, Ramsay MA, et al. Hepatopulmonary syndrome and portopulmonary hypertension: a report of the multicenter liver transplant database. Liver Transpl. 2004;10:174–82.

Kidney Failure Associated with Polycompartment Syndrome

14

Andrea Minini, Philippe Rola, and Manu L. N. G. Malbrain

Abbreviations

ACS	Abdominal compartment syndrome
ADHF	Acute decompensated heart failure
APP	Abdominal perfusion pressure
ARF	Advanced renal failure
BP	Blood pressure
CABG	Coronary artery bypass surgery
CARS	Cardio-abdominal-renal syndrome
CCU	Cardiac/coronary care unit
CrCl	Creatinine clearance
CVP	Central venous pressure
EVLWI	Extravascular lung water index
FG	Filtration gradient
GEDVI	Global end diastolic volume index
GFP	Glomerular filtration pressure
GFR	Glomerular filtration rate
HF	Heart failure

A. Minini
Department of Intensive Care Medicine, University Hospital Brussels (UZB), Jette, Belgium

Department of Intensive Care Medicine and Anaesthesia, University of Insubria, Varese, Italy

P. Rola
Division of Intensive Care, Santa Cabrini Hospital, Montreal, QC, Canada

M. L. N. G. Malbrain (✉)
Department of Intensive Care Medicine, University Hospital Brussels (UZB), Jette, Belgium

Faculty of Medicine and Pharmacy, Vrije Universiteit Brussel (VUB), Jette, Belgium

International Fluid Academy, Jette, Belgium
e-mail: manu.malbrain@telenet.be

© Springer Nature Switzerland AG 2021
F. Coccolini et al. (eds.), *Compartment Syndrome*, Hot Topics in Acute Care
Surgery and Trauma, https://doi.org/10.1007/978-3-030-55378-4_14

HJR   Hepatojugular reflux
IAH   Intra-abdominal hypertension
IAP   Intra-abdominal pressure
ICU   Intensive care unit
ITP   Intrathoracic pressure
IVCCI   Inferior vena cava collapsibility index
JVP   Jugular venous pressure
MAP   Mean arterial pressure
MV   Mechanical ventilation
PAOP   Pulmonary artery occlusion pressure
PAP   Pulmonary artery pressure
PTP   Proximal tubular pressure
RVP   Renal venous pressure
STEMI   ST-elevation myocardial infarction
WRF   Worsening renal function

14.1   Introduction

Intra-abdominal hypertension (IAH) and abdominal compartment syndrome (ACS) are closely associated with renal impairment. The detrimental effects of elevated intra-abdominal pressure (IAP) on kidney function have been known for centuries, however, only recently has there been an increasing focus on this subject. Critical care nephrology demands an in-depth understanding of the interactions and "cross-talks" that occur between the kidney and multiple other organ systems (heart, lungs, gut, brain), and there are many pathophysiological aspects still insufficiently elucidated.

This lack of understanding may explain the difficulty in treating patients where these multiple organ "cross-talks" lead to complex syndromes (i.e., acute kidney injury in decompensated heart failure), leading to a lack of clarity in therapeutic decision-making.

A potential role of venous congestion in the development of renal failure, through coexisting repercussions on the heart and abdominal compartment, has recently been proposed. In contrast with the traditional perception of worsening renal function due to hypoperfusion through low-flow states (i.e., low cardiac output), systemic congestion due to a backward failure is characterized by right ventricular dysfunction, increased central venous (CVP), and renal venous pressures (RVP), IAH and as a result worsening renal function.

This chapter discusses the pathophysiological insights on kidney injury induced by IAH and the role of IAP in worsening renal function in the setting of decompensated heart failure, introducing the new concept of "cardio-abdominal-renal syndrome" (CARS).

14.2   Clinical Case Conundrum

A 66-year-old man with a known history of hypertension, type 2 diabetes, hypercholesterolemia, and chronic kidney failure (CrCl 32 mL/min) was referred to our institution for a second opinion.

After a STEMI 40 years ago followed by CABG, he had an NSTEMI 15 years ago with a redo-CABG followed by another STEMI 4 years ago. His left ventricular ejection fraction was estimated at 29%. He falls within the criteria of heart failure with reduced ejection fraction (HFREF). He is referred because of progressive exertional dyspnea for the last 6 months. The last 5 days he had orthopnea, cough but no chest pain or fever. Upon clinical examination: weight 98 kg, height 168 cm, BP 102/58 mmHg, HR 104 bpm, sat 84% (RR 28) on room air, crepitations, JVP >10, a positive hepatojugular reflex, 4+ leg edema, an S3, a systolic murmur 4/6 with radiation to the apex. Blood gas analysis shows a shunt with pO_2 of 59 mmHg and pCO_2 43.6 mmHg while on room air. Chest X-ray shows cardiomegaly (Fig. 14.1).

The most important laboratory results showed: Urea 131 mg/dL, Creatinine 2.34 mg/dL, eGFR 27 mL/min, Potassium 6.1 meq/L, Troponin 0.035 ng/mL, CK 245 U/L, AST 34 U/L, LDH 597 U/L, Pro NT BNP 3100, CRP 126 mg/L.

His treatment consisted of ramipril 2.5 mg once daily po, spironolactone 25 mg once daily po, carvedilol 12.5 mg bid po, and bumetanide 2.5 mg bid po.

In summary, the patient has known chronic heart failure with now a history of acute decompensation and worsening renal function and inflammation. Fluid overload is apparent on clinical examination and he is grossly edematous.

He is admitted to CCU and given bumetanide 2 mg IV bolus and 1 mg/h infusion for 4 h, with little effect, diuresing only 650 mL in 24 h, clinically remaining congested. Lab: Creat 3.2, eGFR 22 mL/min, Na 131, K 5.4. His respiratory condition worsens and he is admitted to ICU where the patient needs to be intubated and mechanically ventilated. Low-dose dobutamine is started (5 µg/kg/min). His central venous pressure is 17 mmHg.

Transthoracic ultrasound (under dobutamine) shows: Moderate LV/RV dysfunction, high R/L filling pressures, PAP = 45 mmHg + CVP = 63 mmHg, E/e' = 15 (grade 2 diastolic dysfunction), and PAOP estimation of 20.7 mmHg, dilated atria, IVCCI = 0%, Tricuspid and mitral regurgitation (Fig. 14.2).

Fig. 14.1 Chest X-ray. Previous CABG and cardiomegaly present. Vascular hili is prominent and the left costodiafragmatic sinus is shaded. No B-lines

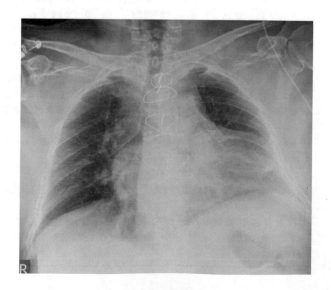

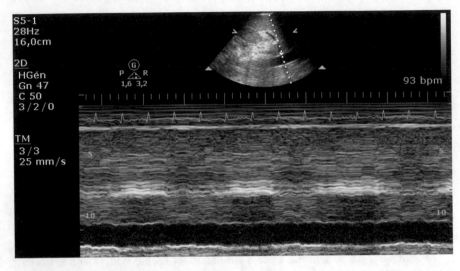

Fig. 14.2 Transesophageal cardiac ultrasound. Grade 4 inferior vena cava (IVC) congestion >20 mm with minimal or no respiratory variation

A transpulmonary thermodilution measurement is performed (with PiCCO$_2$, Getinge, Solna, Sweden) and shows a CI of 2.2 L/min/m^2, GEDVI 949 and EVLWI 15 mL/kg PBW. IV diuretics and dobutamine are increased. However, cumulative fluid balance remains positive at 3358 mL and urine output dropped to 79 mL over the last 24 h. We absolutely do not know how to treat these patients as we don't want to see the full picture. The IAP measured via the bladder was 21 mmHg, compatible with ACS. Treatment was intensified and focused on the reduction of venous congestion and lowering IAP. The IAP was lowered by improving abdominal wall compliance (with sedation and analgesia), reduction of intraluminal volume (with nasogastric suctioning, gastro- and colonoprokinetics, and rectal enemas), evacuation of free abdominal fluids (with ultrasound-guided paracenthesis), and avoiding further fluid overload combined with deresuscitation. This was done initially with a combination of diuretics: spironolactone, acetazolemide, thiazide (indapamide), and high-dose continuous loop diuretics in combination with salt and water restriction. Dobutamine was replaced by milrinone and CVVH with aggressive UF was started. The APP was maintained at 65 mmHg with a low dose of norepinephrine and IAP dropped below 15 mmHg. Cumulative fluid balance came back to normal with deresuscitation and urine output increased and kidney function was preserved at baseline levels (Fig. 14.3).

14.3 Definitions

14.3.1 Acute Decompensated Heart Failure (ADHF)

ADHF is a common and potentially fatal cause of acute respiratory distress. The clinical syndrome is characterized by the development of dyspnea, generally

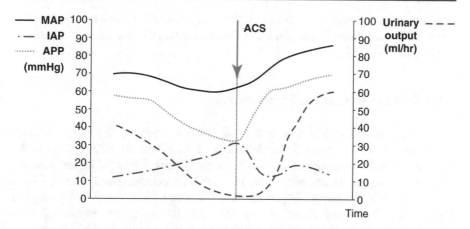

Fig. 14.3 Graphical illustration of the effects of elevated intra-abdominal pressure (IAP) and abdominal compartment syndrome (ACS) on abdominal perfusion pressure (APP) and urinary output (UO). Note the beneficial effects of reduced IAP levels due to deresuscitation

associated with rapid accumulation of fluid within the lung's interstitial and alveolar spaces, which is the result of acutely elevated cardiac filling pressures (cardiogenic pulmonary edema) [1]. ADHF can also present as elevated left ventricular (LV) filling pressures and dyspnea without pulmonary edema.

14.3.2 Acute Kidney Injury (AKI)

According to the KDIGO guidelines [2], acute kidney injury is defined by either an increase in serum creatinine ≥0.3 mg/dL within 48 h or an increase in serum creatinine ≥1.5 times baseline or an urine output ≤0.5 mL/kg/h for 6 h.

14.3.3 Worsening Renal Function (WRF)

Recent interest has focused on worsening renal function (WRF), a situation strongly related to mortality, but seemingly only when heart failure status deteriorates [3]. Worsening renal function (WRF) is defined as a 0.3–0.5 mg/dL rise in serum creatinine or a decrease in glomerular filtration rate (GFR) of 9–15 mL/min during hospitalization for acute decompensated heart failure. From the patients with acute decompensated heart failure that develop WRF, 66% die within 1 year [4].

14.3.4 Intra-Abdominal Pressure (IAP)

IAP is the steady-state pressure concealed within the abdominal cavity. It is measured at end expiration in the supine position excluding muscle contractions and with the zero-reference set at the level where the midaxillary line crosses the iliac crest. The gold standard method is via the bladder after instilling a maximal priming volume of 20–25 mL.

14.3.5 Intra-Abdominal Hypertension

IAH is defined as a sustained increased IAP equal to or above 12 mmHg. IAH is a strong independent risk factor for the development of AKI and the relationship between IAP and renal function appears to be linear, with a greater impact at higher pressure. Animal data suggest a clear relationship between IAP and renal resistive index [5].

Furthermore, the earliest important manifestation of increasing IAP is oliguria [6] and the detrimental effects on kidney perfusion have been associated with increased morbidity and mortality in critically ill patients [7, 8]. The kidneys are also considered as the canary in the coal mine for IAH and are usually the first organs visibly failing when IAP increases.

In the presence of normovolemia, oliguria usually develops when IAP increases above 15 mmHg and anuria at levels above 25 mmHg. In the setting of decreased heart function (advanced decompensated heart failure), oliguria may develop at lower levels of IAP (as low as 8–10 mmHg).

14.3.6 Cardiorenal Syndrome

Several articles in the literature discuss the interactions between the heart and kidneys. These two organs are involved in maintaining hemodynamic stability and organ perfusion. This relationship becomes fragile in case of organ dysfunction. Cardiorenal syndrome can be defined as a pathophysiological disorder of the heart and kidneys in which acute or chronic dysfunction of one organ may induce acute or chronic dysfunction in the other [9].

The cardiorenal syndrome may in fact have two opposite yet partly overlapping pathophysiological mechanisms presenting with AKI/WRF, the first being the commonly thought of "low-flow" state with the renal dysfunction predominantly due to a poor cardiac output, and the second, actually more prevalent where it is due to increased venous congestion [10]. The therapeutic approach to these is diametrically opposite, yet at the bedside, particularly without sonography, that may be impossible to differentiate. Even the commonly used urine sodium does not differentiate, as it will also be low in congestive states, as the nephron will only sense the low renal perfusion pressure and retain sodium as long as it is functioning. By direct compression of the kidney, renal veins and IVC, as well as by decreasing venous return and CO, IAP may cause both pathophysiological mechanisms, as will be discussed further below. Hence it is important to develop an approach based on physiology.

The pathophysiology of CRS is not fully understood, and it is a heterogeneous and complex clinical entity. It can present with heart and/or kidney failure that can be either acute or chronic and can be summarized as a complex symbiosis gone wrong.

It is now sufficiently clear that renal dysfunction occurs frequently in all pheno-
types of heart failure, and when present, it is associated with higher mortality and
morbidity. While the pathophysiology is multifactorial, the most important factors
are a reduced renal perfusion and venous congestion.

14.4   Incidence

The incidence of IAH in critically ill patients is 25% on admission and 50% within
the first week of stay. The most important risk factors for the development of IAH
are a positive cumulative fluid balance and fluid overload (defined as a 10% increase
in cumulative fluid balance from baseline body weight). IAH is a strong independent risk factor AKI, which in turn develops in approximately 30% of critically ill
patients with IAH [11].

In a study conducted by Dalfino et al. an IAP of 12 mmHg was identified to have
the best sensitivity to specificity ratio for predicting AKI [12]. Biancofiore et al.
identify an IAP ≥ 25 mmHg as an important factor for renal failure in patients who
underwent liver surgery [13]. In another prospective cohort of 83 ICU patients,
those with IAH had significantly higher mortality (53 vs. 27%) and higher incidence
of renal dysfunction by Sequential Organ Failure Assessment renal subscore (58 vs.
27%). This was also shown in the first multicenter epidemiologic study on the incidence of IAH [14] and an individual patient database meta-analysis [7].

Worsening renal function occurs in 30% of patients admitted for acute decompensated heart failure regardless of whether there is decreased or reduced (HFREF)
or preserved (HFPEF) systolic function. Worsening renal function typically occurs
early, within days after hospitalization, suggesting a direct causative effect of the
hemodynamic alterations that occur while treatment for acute decompensated heart
failure is optimized and in which IAP can play a significant role.

14.5   Impact of Increased IAP on Kidney Function in Patients
with Normal Heart Function

In the late nineteenth century, Wendt and Landois were the first to identify the harmful effect of elevated IAP on renal function and urinary output by reporting oliguria
in the presence of elevated IAP in animal models [15, 16]. Afterwards, Bradley and
Bradley performed the first study looking at the effects of increased IAP in humans
in 1947 [17].

Several mechanisms have been suggested as etiology for IAH-induced renal failure. Renal artery and vein compression coupled with renal tubule compression have
been suggested as the likely mechanism behind the kidney dysfunction and failure
accompanied by reduced cardiac output.

To explain this, we have to introduce a similar concept to cerebral perfusion pressure, namely abdominal perfusion pressure (APP). APP is a measurable parameter that
has been introduced to explain the circulatory compromise in the abdominal cavity in
the presence of IAH/ACS. The APP can be defined as the difference between the mean

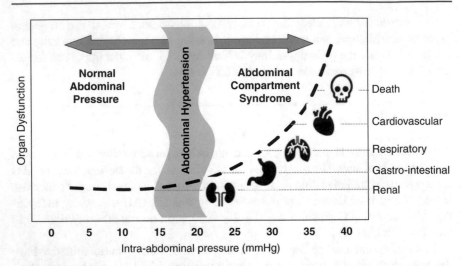

Fig. 14.4 Distinctions and interactions between normal intra-abdominal pressure (IAP), intra-abdominal hypertension (IAH), and abdominal compartment syndrome (ACS). The shaded area illustrating IAH may undergo shifts to the right or left depending on the clinical scenario (adapted from Malbrain et al. with permission [20])

arterial pressure (MAP) and the IAP, and implies that as the IAP rises, the perfusion of organs or vessels in or near the abdomen falls even in the absence of a drop in MAP.

$$APP = MAP - IAP$$

The compliance of the abdominal wall generally limits the increase in IAP as abdominal girth increases. However, once a critical volume is reached, compliance of the abdominal wall decreases abruptly. Further distension beyond this critical IAP results in rapid increases in IAP and resultant organ dysfunction [18, 19]. This is illustrated in Fig. 14.4.

Changes in IAP have a greater impact than changes in MAP on renal function and urine production.

$$FG = GFP - PTP$$
$$= (MAP - IAP) - IAP$$
$$= MAP - 2 \times IAP$$

The filtration gradient (FG) is the mechanical force across the renal glomerulus and equals the difference between the glomerular filtration pressure (GFP) and the proximal tubular pressure (PTP). In the presence of IAH, PTP may be assumed to equal IAP. GFP can be estimated as MAP minus IAP.

Moreover, an acute increase of IAP reduces the renal blood flow and triggers the autoregulatory mechanism, acutely rising glomerular filtration. But the integrity of the kidney response might be related to the patient's capability to maintain an adequate glomerular filtration rate during stressful conditions. When IAP overcomes the intrarenal autoregulation, glomerular hypoperfusion, and clinical AKI becomes manifest [21].

Since the kidneys are encapsulated organs located in the retroperitoneal space of the abdominal compartment, also a direct parenchymal compression is considered

Table 14.1 Primary intra-abdominal hypertension-induced effects on kidney function

Renal effects of IAH	
Renal parenchymal compression	▲
Renal perfusion pressure	▼
Filtration gradient	▼
Renal arterial blood flow	▼
Renal venous pressure	▲
Renal interstitial pressure	▲
Renal venous compression	▲
Tubular dysfunction	▲
Glomerular perfusion	▼
Diuresis (oliguria to anuria)	▼
Renin, angiotensin, aldosterone	▲
Compression of ureters	▲
Antidiuretic hormone	▲
Systemic hypertension in chronic IAH	▲
Corticomedullar shunting in renal plasma flow	▼
Sympathetic nervous system stimulation	▲

▲ increase, ▼ decrease

to have a role on kidney impairment, especially when a localized renal compartment syndrome develops. Interstitial edema follows AKI and can lead to ischemic lesions due to a reduction in the vascular flow and an increase of venous congestion due to the alteration on vascular permeability [22–24]. A study conducted on piglets showed that decapsulated kidneys displayed an effective reduction of intrarenal pressure, an increment of renal tissue oxygen pressure, and a better performance in the regional delivery consumption and extraction of oxygen after reperfusion. This regional effect resulted in a marked attenuation of acute kidney injury progression due to reduced structural damage and improved renal function [25] (Table 14.1).

Direct parenchymal compression may instigate the development of a "renal compartment syndrome" wherein renal arterial blood flow is diminished while renal venous pressure and renal vascular resistance are increased causing blood to be shunted away from the renal cortex and glomeruli leading to tubular dysfunction and subsequent renal failure.

Other etiological stimuli such as inflammatory end/or toxic exposures may induce kidney impairment and/or kidney dysfunction. In a rodent model study, IAH resulted in edema and neutrophil infiltration in the kidney.

Despite the increasing focus on the detrimental effects of elevated IAP in AKI, many pathophysiological aspects are not well characterized. Historically it is believed that the decrease in renal perfusion pressure is one of the most important, but this can explain only in part the pathophysiology of the syndrome. Also, studies with placement of ureter stent failed to overcome AKI in the setting of increased IAP and compression of ureters. On the other hand, renal decapsulation has proven beneficial in local renal CS [25].

In an animal model of IAH blood volume expansion corrected cardiac output but this did not restore renal blood flood or GFR above 25% of normal. Placement of ureteric stents did not influence renal response to raise IAP and was not protective to prevent AKI [26]. He concluded that the impairment in renal function produced by increased intra-abdominal pressure is a local phenomenon caused by direct renal compression and is not related to cardiac output.

14.6   Impact of Increased IAP on WRF in Patients with Decompensated Heart Failure

The hallmark feature of heart failure (HF) is characterized by the combination of low cardiac output (forward failure) and systemic venous congestion (backward failure), manifesting as elevated jugular venous pressure often leading to anasarca edema.

In HF, because of the backward failure and increased arteriolar vasoconstriction, a progressive shift of blood from the effective circulatory volume to splanchnic capacitance veins might be expected (Fig. 14.5). The total amount of this hidden volume (sometimes referred to as the third ventricle) can be estimated as high as 800 mL (intestines 400 mL + liver 300 mL + spleen 100 mL). Hence autotransfusion of 800 mL from abdomen into systemic circulation within seconds following increased abdominal sympathetic drive [27].

In addition, inefficient natriuresis and progressive volume overload may lead ultimately to a state of congestion with increased IAP if the splanchnic capacitance is unable to cope with congestion [28]. Analogous to the production of ANP and BNP (B-type natriuretic peptide) in the heart, in heart failure patients also natriuretic substances are produced in the gut such as the peptides uroguanylin and guanylin [29].

Recent studies focusing on kidney afterload have revived the interest in older studies which suggested that kidney dysfunction is a result of venous congestion transmitted to the renal venous compartment. Almost a century ago, it was indeed demonstrated than hypervolemia induced increase in RVP caused AKI [30]. Therefore the term "congestive kidney" was coined to describe a pathophysiological condition in which multiple and complex clinical patterns (such as cardiorenal and hepatorenal syndromes) converge to cause a common final state: an increase in renal venous pressure (RVP) [31].

An indirect assessment of renal venous hypertension may be the value of the central venous pressure (CVP). The CVP is the pressure recorded from the superior vena cava and is widely used as a surrogate of intravascular volume. CVP measurements therefore are often applied at the bedside to guide fluid administration in postoperative and critically ill patients. The normal value of CVP is 5–7 mmHg. Pressures above 12 mmHg indicate overhydration, heart failure, or pulmonary artery stenosis, which limit venous outflow and lead to venous congestion. A high CVP might impede venous return to the heart and disturb microcirculatory blood flow which may cause tissue congestion and organ failure. Hence pursuing high CVP levels has recently been challenged.

Furthermore, by imposing an increased "afterload" on the kidney, an elevated CVP will particularly harm kidney hemodynamics and promote acute kidney injury (AKI) even in the absence of volume overload. This is why maintaining the lowest possible CVP should become routine to prevent and treat AKI, especially when associated with septic shock, mechanical ventilation, and IAH [32].

Fig. 14.5 The forward failure (RED) hypothesis and net effects on salt and water homeostasis (in ORANGE). *MAP* mean arterial pressure, *RAAS* renin angiotensin aldosterone system, *RPP* renal perfusion pressure, *SAP* systolic arterial pressure

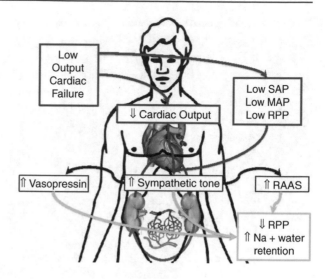

Fig. 14.6 Pathophysiological effect of heart failure (in RED forward failure) related venous congestion (in BLUE backward failure) on organ function and net effects on salt and water homeostasis (in ORANGE). *CVP* central venous pressure, *IAP* intra-abdominal pressure, *RAAS* renin angiotensin aldosterone system, *RH* right heart, *RPP* renal perfusion pressure

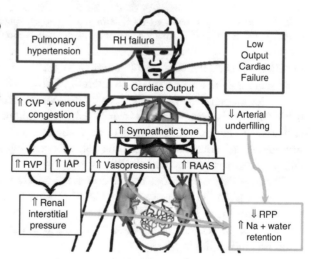

More precisely, CVP must be lower than RVP in order to allow an adequate venous return blood flow to the heart. Accordingly, the presence of a high CVP requires a much higher RVP to ensure this flow. Renal perfusion pressure (RPP) approximates the difference between renal arterial pressure and RVP. As such, a higher RVP lowers RPP. In analogy with cardiac physiology, this forms the basis for the renal afterload concept [33].

Evidence suggests that acute increases of CVP should be actively treated to avoid a deterioration of the renal function, particularly in patients with poor ventricular fraction. Besides, the practice of treating right heart failure with fluid loading should be avoided in favor of other ways to optimize hemodynamics in this setting, because of the detrimental effects on the kidney function [34]. Recent studies showed that in fact CVP seems more important than cardiac output as predictor for WRF in patients with ADHF [24]. Figure 14.6 explains the occurrence of WRF

Table 14.2 Grading table for assessment of venous congestion with point-of-care ultrasound

	Grade 0	Grade 1	Grade 2	Grade 3	Grade 4
VCI	<5 mm with respiratory variation	5–9 mm with respiratory variation	10–19 mm with respiratory variation	>20 mm with respiratory variation	20 mm with minimal or no respiratory variation
Hepatic vein	Normal S > D	S < D with antegrade S	S flat or inverted or biphasic trace		
Portal vein	<0.3 pulsatility index	0.3–0.49 pulsatility index	0.5–1.0 pulsatility index		
Renal Doppler	Continuous monophasic/pulsatile flow	Discontinuous biphasic flow	Discontinuous monophasic flow (diastole only)		
VEXUS score	IVC grade < 3, HD grade 0, PV "grade 0" (RD grade 0)	IVC grade 4, but normal HV/PV/RV patterns.	IVC grade 4 with mild flow pattern abnormalities in two or more of the following HV/PV/RV	IVC grade 4 with severe flow pattern abnormalities in two or more of the following HV/PV/RV	

VEXUS venous congestion assessment with ultrasound (adapted with permission from Rola P. et al. book "Bedside Ultrasound: a primer for clinical integration" [37])

in patients with ADHF via a combination of forward and backward failure. However, this model may not fully explain all alterations observed.

In addition, an increase in RVP can cause sodium retention by a direct action on the kidney: a rise in RVP could thereby initiate a vicious circle by causing sodium and water retention, expansion of plasma volume, and further increase in venous pressure. This sequence of events may an exacerbating factor in edematous states and polycompartment syndrome [35].

The importance of venous congestion in the development of WRF in ADHF can possibly explain the greatest improvement of the renal function after medical treatment for advanced HF in patients characterized by echocardiographic signs of the impact of right ventricular dysfunction on inferior vena cava, portal, hepatic, and renal veins [36] (Table 14.2).

14.7 CARS Cardio-Abdominal–Renal Syndrome

Only recently, it was shown that IAP is often raised in patients with ADHF. In a study of 40 patients, hospitalized for ADHF, more than 50% presented with raised IAP, mostly with minimal or no abdominal complaints [1]. Intriguingly, in ADHF—presumably because of low renal perfusion—the kidneys are extremely sensitive to even small elevations in IAP (8–10 mmHg) and CVP [1]. Interestingly, ascites could only be found in a small subset of cases, so the presence of raised IAP in ADHF is probably due to visceral (tissue) edema as a result of progressive whole-body fluid accumulation or systemic congestion [1, 38].

Elevated IAP seems to correlate with more impaired renal function in patients presenting with ADHF and reduction of IAP after tailored medical therapy is associated with improvement of the renal function [1]. Furthermore, in the subgroup of patients with ADHF where medical treatment failed to reduce IAP, prompt reduction in IAP following large-volume mechanical fluid removal with either paracentesis in case of ascites or ultrafiltration dramatically improved renal function [38].

Interestingly, increases in IAP and CVP also seem to be more important than decreases in CI [39] and this is also the case in sepsis [24].

Notably, while organ dysfunction in the intensive care literature has only been described when IAP exceeds 12 mmHg, patients with ADHF might already develop WRF with a much lower IAP [1]. This suggests that the underlying reserve of the kidneys to counteract an increased IAP is limited in this setting. It is also vital to emphasize that although the degree of renal dysfunction probably correlates with the degree of elevated IAP; there can be a wide range of IAPs in relation to serum creatinine levels at presentation. While we can only speculate why this discrepancy exists, other mechanisms including coexisting systemic congestion, preexisting renal insufficiency, as well as drugs used during the treatment of ADHF, may probably also play a role.

Because of the central role that IAP plays in cardiovascular and renal hemodynamics in critically ill patients, we believe that it may present the missing link between the heart and the kidney. Therefore, the term cardio-abdominal–renal syndrome (CARS) was coined for the first time in 2012 [40].

14.8   Prevention of IAH-Induced Kidney Injury

Successful prevention strategies for AKI are based on fluid administration. Fluid resuscitation can be helpful in the presence of IAH if aiming to increase the APP. However, a positive cumulative fluid balance increases the IAP linearly and may trigger a vicious cycle (Fig. 14.7). Diuresis is not a good parameter to guide fluid resuscitation in critically ill patients with IAH.

Fig. 14.7 The pathophysiological vicious cycle of fluid overload leading to CARS

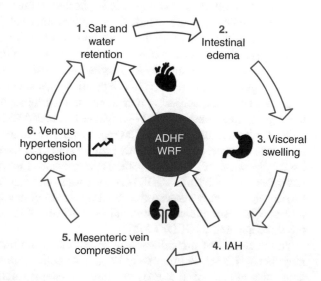

Therefore, clinicians should have a low threshold for measuring baseline IAP when two or more risk factors are present. Serial measurements of IAP are essential, as these patients are constantly changing physiologically, and isolated measurements are of little value. Continuous IAP monitoring via a balloon-tipped nasogastric probe or a 3-lumen Foley needs to be considered, especially if the patient demonstrates evidence of IAH and low APP.

Therefore, the best prevention relies on IAP monitoring as soon as the kidneys become dysfunctional and avoiding fluid overload (defined as 10% increased from baseline body weight).

14.9 Treatment of Patients with IAH-Induced AKI

Correcting positive fluid balance is critical and often requires limiting fluid administration. A fluid management based on fluid stewardship is recommended [41]. In analogy to the way antibiotics are handled we can consider four phases of fluid therapy: resuscitation phase, the optimization phase, the stabilization phase, and the evacuation phase. The last phase is the most important in case of systemic decongestion. A continuous infusion of loop diuretics may be effective although it is uncertain whether diuretics alone are sufficient to reach a neutral or negative cumulative fluid balance. Often combination therapy of different classes of diuretics is needed as shown in the clinical conundrum but often diuretics only allow 1 or 2 days of negative fluid balance and escalation to RRT may be needed. A recent, large, double-blind, randomized clinical trial could not prove a benefit for high versus low dosing or administration with bolus versus continuous infusions, although a trend toward more WRF was seen in the high-dose group [42].

There are several potential mechanisms through which diuretics could worsen heart failure progression and increase the risk of WRF. First, diuretics further stimulate the neurohormonal axis which is implicated in the progression of heart failure. Second, diuretics can cause marked electrolyte abnormalities such as potassium and magnesium depletion, as well as metabolic alkalosis, possibly resulting in lethal arrhythmias. Third, intravascular underfilling can occur if diuresis exceeds the plasma refilling time which is about 3–4 mL/kg/h. This causes decreased RBF and often provokes a significant decrease in GFR. Nevertheless, recent data suggest that in cases of clear hypervolemia, achieving hemoconcentration through extensive use of diuretic therapy—despite transient WRF—might be associated with a better prognosis [43].

RRT with net ultrafiltration can rapidly remove large amounts of fluids to optimize fluid balance. In a retrospective cohort study, De Laet et al. registered a significantly decrease of IAP in patients who were treated with either sustained low-efficiency dialysis (SLEDD) or continuous venovenous hemofiltration (CVVH). Moreover, this study showed that renal replacement therapy with net fluid removal lowers volumetric indices in critically ill patients, although EVLWI reduction was modest compared to GEDVI [44].

In the setting of a capillary leak syndrome, a multimodal restrictive approach may be considered. A pilot study in patients with acute lung injury (ALI) investigated the effects of the PAL treatment strategy: high levels of **PEEP**, small

Table 14.3 Therapeutic options in CARS to improve WRF in patients with ADHF

Treatment option	Description
1. Metabolic	• Limit fluid intake • Limit sodium intake
2. Combination therapy diuretics	• Loop diuretic: high dose and continuous furosemide or bumetanide • Acetazolemide: inhibition Na reabsorption proximal tubule • Thiazide/Indapamide: inhibition Na reabsorption distal tubule • Spironolactone: inhibition Na reabsorption proximal tubule
3. Vasodilators (calcium antagonists, ACE-I)	• Increase renal blood flow • Reduce filtration fraction • Reduce lymph flow
4. Inotropes	• Dobutamine • Milrinone (especially when right heart pressures increased)
5. Lower IAP	• Improve abdominal wall compliance • Reduce intraluminal volume (ileus) • Reduce intra-abdominal volume (ascites) • Optimize fluid administration • Optimize systemic regional perfusion
6. Increase APP	• APP = MAP − IAP • Vasopressors when needed, low-dose terlipressin, vasopressin or norepinephrine
7. Active de-resuscitation	• Combination therapy diuretics • Application of PEEP • Albumin 20% + diuretics • PAL treatment: PEEP (=IAP) + albumin 20% + Lasix • SLEDD with UF • CVVH with UF

ADHF advanced or acute decompensated heart failure, *APP* abdominal perfusion pressure, *CARS*: cardio abdominal renal syndrome, *CVVH* continuous venovenous hemofiltration, *IAP* intra-abdominal pressure, *MAP* mean arterial pressure, *Na* sodium, *PEEP* positive end-expiratory pressure, *SLEDD* slow extended daily dialysis, *UF* ultrafiltration, *WRF* worsening renal function

resuscitation with albumin and fluid removal with furosemide (Lasix®) or ultrafiltration. PAL-treated patients had a greater reduction of EVLWI, IAP, and cumulative fluid balance with minimum repercussions on cardiovascular and renal function; the intervention group required also fewer days on mechanical ventilation and had a lower 28-day mortality (28.1% vs. 49.1%, $p = 0.034$) [45].

Continuous RRT can provide a minute-to-minute control of the fluid balance and this may be an advantage in unstable patients.

Peritoneal dialysis is not an option in patients with IAH since the added intra-abdominal volume will further increase IAP, especially in presence of reduced abdominal compliance. Table 14.3 summarizes the different treatment options.

The use of a composite bedside ultrasound assessment for venous congestion may allow the clinician to determine the degree of importance of congestion in a given patient. The presence of a plethoric IVC along with marked abnormalities of splanchnic venous Doppler flow has been associated with a markedly increased risk of AKI on post-op cardiac surgery patients and general critically ill patients (unpublished data, personal communication, Rola, Spiegel, and Beaubien-Souligny). In IAH patients, the IVC, HV, and PV Doppler signals may be difficult to interpret, but the intrarenal venous Doppler flow, if found to be markedly abnormal, should point to IAH as a significant cause of AKI. Further studies on this are needed but this may be a powerful bedside tool for the clinician facing therapeutic dilemmas.

Take-Home Messages

- Normal IAP is around 5–7 mmHg.
- IAH (sustained IAP > 12 mmHg) is frequently associated with AKI.
- The cause of AKI in IAH is multifactorial (fluid overload, low perfusion, neurohumoral, ...)
- The kidneys are often the first organs failing in IAH (canary in the coal mine).
- Already small elevations in IAP (at levels of 8–10 mmHg) can cause WRF.
- IAP is considered the missing link in patients with congestive heart failure and worsening kidney function and this is termed CARS.
- Multimodal monitoring is indicated: (continuous) IAP, CVP, cardiac output, ultrasound, venous congestion.
- Treatment should focus on improvement on Caw, lowering IAP and fluid removal.
- Diuretic combination therapy offers a good first choice but often (C)RRT with UF is needed.
- Hepatorenal syndrome needs to be considered in patients with cirrhosis and worsening kidney function.
- Bedside ultrasound of the intrarenal venous flow may provide important clinical information.

References

1. Mullens W, Abrahams Z, Skouri HN, Francis GS, Taylor DO, Starling RC, et al. Elevated intra-abdominal pressure in acute decompensated heart failure: a potential contributor to worsening renal function? J Am Coll Cardiol. 2008;51(3):300–6.
2. Kellum JA, Lameire N. Diagnosis, evaluation, and management of acute kidney injury: a KDIGO summary (part 1). Crit Care. 2013;17(1):204.
3. Damman K, Testani JM. The kidney in heart failure: an update. Eur Heart J. 2015;36(23):1437–44.
4. Metra M, Ponikowski P, Dickstein K, McMurray JJ, Gavazzi A, Bergh CH, et al. Advanced chronic heart failure: a position statement from the Study Group on Advanced Heart Failure of the Heart Failure Association of the European Society of Cardiology. Eur J Heart Fail. 2007;9(6–7):684–94.
5. Kirkpatrick AW, Roberts DJ, De Waele J, Jaeschke R, Malbrain ML, De Keulenaer B, et al. Intra-abdominal hypertension and the abdominal compartment syndrome: updated consensus definitions and clinical practice guidelines from the World Society of the Abdominal Compartment Syndrome. Intensive Care Med. 2013;39(7):1190–206.
6. Mohmand H, Goldfarb S. Renal dysfunction associated with intra-abdominal hypertension and the abdominal compartment syndrome. J Am Soc Nephrol. 2011;22(4):615–21.
7. Malbrain ML, Chiumello D, Cesana BM, Reintam Blaser A, Starkopf J, Sugrue M, et al. A systematic review and individual patient data meta-analysis on intra-abdominal hypertension

in critically ill patients: the wake-up project. World initiative on Abdominal Hypertension Epidemiology, a Unifying Project (WAKE-Up!). Minerva Anestesiol. 2014;80(3):293–306.

8. Vidal MG, Ruiz Weisser J, Gonzalez F, Toro MA, Loudet C, Balasini C, et al. Incidence and clinical effects of intra-abdominal hypertension in critically ill patients. Crit Care Med. 2008;36(6):1823–31.

9. Ronco C, Di Lullo L. Cardiorenal syndrome. Heart Fail Clin. 2014;10(2):251–80.

10. Mullens W, Abrahams Z, Francis GS, Sokos G, Taylor DO, Starling RC, et al. Importance of venous congestion for worsening of renal function in advanced decompensated heart failure. J Am Coll Cardiol. 2009;53(7):589–96.

11. Sugrue M, Jones F, Deane SA, Bishop G, Bauman A, Hillman K. Intra-abdominal hypertension is an independent cause of postoperative renal impairment. Arch Surg. 1999;134(10):1082–5.

12. Dalfino L, Tullo L, Donadio I, Malcangi V, Brienza N. Intra-abdominal hypertension and acute renal failure in critically ill patients. Intensive Care Med. 2008;34(4):707–13.

13. Biancofiore G, Bindi ML, Romanelli AM, Bisa M, Boldrini A, Consani G, et al. Postoperative intra-abdominal pressure and renal function after liver transplantation. Arch Surg. 2003;138(7):703–6.

14. Malbrain ML, Chiumello D, Pelosi P, Bihari D, Innes R, Ranieri VM, et al. Incidence and prognosis of intraabdominal hypertension in a mixed population of critically ill patients: a multiple-center epidemiological study. Crit Care Med. 2005;33(2):315–22.

15. Wendt E. Uber den einfluss des intraabdominalen druckes auf die absonderungsgeschwindig-keit des harnes. Arch Physiologische Heilkunde. 1876;57:525–7.

16. Landois L. Increase in IAP decreased BP, pulse and urine output. Lehrbuch der physiologie des Menschen. 1st Halfe. 1899. p. 218.

17. Bradley SE, Bradley GP. The effect of increased intra-abdominal pressure on renal function in man. J Clin Invest. 1947;26(5):1010–22.

18. Doty JM, Saggi BH, Blocher CR, Fakhry I, Gehr T, Sica D, et al. Effects of increased renal parenchymal pressure on renal function. J Trauma. 2000;48(5):874–7.

19. Malbrain ML, Peeters Y, Wise R. The neglected role of abdominal compliance in organ-organ interactions. Crit Care. 2016;20:67.

20. Malbrain MLNG, Deeren D, De Potter TJR. Intra-abdominal hypertension in the critically ill: it is time to pay attention. Curr Opin Crit Care. 2005;11(2):156–71.

21. Villa G, Samoni S, De Rosa S, Ronco C. The pathophysiological hypothesis of kidney damage during intra-abdominal hypertension. Front Physiol. 2016;7:55.

22. Basile DP. The endothelial cell in ischemic acute kidney injury: implications for acute and chronic function. Kidney Int. 2007;72(2):151–6.

23. Le Dorze M, Legrand M, Payen D, Ince C. The role of the microcirculation in acute kidney injury. Curr Opin Crit Care. 2009;15(6):503–8.

24. Legrand M, Dupuis C, Simon C, Gayat E, Mateo J, Lukaszewicz AC, et al. Association between systemic hemodynamics and septic acute kidney injury in critically ill patients: a retrospective observational study. Crit Care (London, England). 2013;17(6):R278.

25. Cruces P, Lillo P, Salas C, Salomon T, Lillo F, Gonzalez C, et al. Renal decapsulation prevents intrinsic renal compartment syndrome in ischemia-reperfusion-induced acute kidney injury: a physiologic approach. Crit Care Med. 2018;46(2):216–22.

26. Harman PK, Kron IL, McLachlan HD, Freedlender AE, Nolan SP. Elevated intra-abdominal pressure and renal function. Ann Surg. 1982;196(5):594–7.

27. Fallick C, Sobotka PA, Dunlap ME. Sympathetically mediated changes in capacitance: redistribution of the venous reservoir as a cause of decompensation. Circ Heart Fail. 2011;4(5):669–75.

28. Verbrugge FH, Dupont M, Steels P, Grieten L, Malbrain M, Tang WH, et al. Abdominal contributions to cardiorenal dysfunction in congestive heart failure. J Am Coll Cardiol. 2013;62(6):485–95.

29. Carrithers SL, Eber SL, Forte LR, Greenberg RN. Increased urinary excretion of uroguanylin in patients with congestive heart failure. Am J Physiol Heart Circ Physiol. 2000;278(2):H538–47.

30. Winton FR. The influence of venous pressure on the isolated mammalian kidney. J Physiol. 1931;72(1):49–61.

31. Di Nicolo P. The dark side of the kidney in cardio-renal syndrome: renal venous hypertension and congestive kidney failure. Heart Fail Rev. 2018;23(2):291–302.

32. Chen X, Wang X, Honore PM, Spapen HD, Liu D. Renal failure in critically ill patients, beware of applying (central venous) pressure on the kidney. Ann Intensive Care. 2018;8(1):91.

33. Honore PM, Jacobs R, Hendrickx I, Bagshaw SM, Joannes-Boyau O, Boer W, et al. Prevention and treatment of sepsis-induced acute kidney injury: an update. Ann Intensive Care. 2015;5(1):51.

34. Gambardella I, Gaudino M, Ronco C, Lau C, Ivascu N, Girardi LN. Congestive kidney failure in cardiac surgery: the relationship between central venous pressure and acute kidney injury. Interact Cardiovasc Thorac Surg. 2016;23(5):800–5.

35. Firth JD, Raine AE, Ledingham JG. Raised venous pressure: a direct cause of renal sodium retention in oedema? Lancet. 1988;1(8593):1033–5.

36. Testani JM, Khera AV, St John Sutton MG, Keane MG, Wiegers SE, Shannon RP, et al. Effect of right ventricular function and venous congestion on cardiorenal interactions during the treatment of decompensated heart failure. Am J Cardiol. 2010;105(4):511–6.

37. Beaubien-Souligny W, Rola P, Haycock K, et al. Quantifying systemic congestion with Point-Of-Care ultrasound: development of the venous excess ultrasound grading system. Ultrasound J. 2020;12(1):16. https://doi.org/10.1186/s13089-020-00163-w.

38. Mullens W, Abrahams Z, Francis GS, Taylor DO, Starling RC, Tang WH. Prompt reduction in intra-abdominal pressure following large-volume mechanical fluid removal improves renal insufficiency in refractory decompensated heart failure. J Card Fail. 2008;14(6):508–14.

39. Tang WH, Mullens W. Cardiorenal syndrome in decompensated heart failure. Heart. 2010;96(4):255–60.

40. Verbrugge FH, Mullens W, Malbrain MLNG. Worsening renal function during decompensated heart failure: the cardio-abdomino-renal syndrome. In: Annual update in intensive care and emergency medicine 2012. Berlin: Springer; 2012. p. 577–88.

41. Malbrain M, Van Regenmortel N, Saugel B, De Tavernier B, Van Gaal PJ, Joannes-Boyau O, et al. Principles of fluid management and stewardship in septic shock: it is time to consider the four D's and the four phases of fluid therapy. Ann Intensive Care. 2018;8(1):66.

42. Felker GM, Lee KL, Bull DA, Redfield MM, Stevenson LW, Goldsmith SR, et al. Diuretic strategies in patients with acute decompensated heart failure. N Engl J Med. 2011;364(9):797–805.

43. Testani JM, Chen J, McCauley BD, Kimmel SE, Shannon RP. Potential effects of aggressive decongestion during the treatment of decompensated heart failure on renal function and survival. Circulation. 2010;122(3):265–72.

44. De Laet I, Deeren D, Schoonheydt K, Van Regenmortel N, Dits H, Malbrain ML. Renal replacement therapy with net fluid removal lowers intra-abdominal pressure and volumetric indices in critically ill patients. Ann Intensive Care. 2012;2(Suppl 1):S20.

45. Cordemans C, De Laet I, Van Regenmortel N, Schoonheydt K, Dits H, Martin G, et al. Aiming for a negative fluid balance in patients with acute lung injury and increased intra-abdominal pressure: a pilot study looking at the effects of PAL-treatment. Ann Intensive Care. 2012;2(Suppl 1):S15.

Compartment Syndromes in Children and Adolescents

15

Torsten Kaussen

Compartment syndromes are characterized by a discrepancy between the size of a limitedly compressible mass and the amount of space into which it is to be integrated. When a level of critical compliance is not reached, compensation mechanisms fail, leading to a decline in local or systemic perfusion. This resulting deficiency in perfusion is accompanied by hypoxemia and usually causes a switch to anaerobic energy production. It is at this point (at the latest) that an additional inflammatory stimulus is potentially induced, possibly contributing to a further triggering of the respective pressure gradients via capillary leak syndrome and extravasation. The smaller or younger the patient, the greater the risk of a size and space discrepancy accompanied by—when compared to adults—significantly lower blood pressure and tissue perfusion pressure.

In clinical practice, four types of compartment syndrome play a relevant role in children and adolescents:

1. Fascial/muscle compartment syndrome
2. Cerebral compartment syndrome
3. Thoracic compartment syndrome
4. Abdominal compartment syndrome

Evidence-based data on the first three types is limited. They do not differ from adults with regard to pathogenesis, diagnosis, and therapy [1–4]. There is no reliable epidemiological information on how frequently they occur in children and adolescents.

The lack of data becomes clear simply in that the respective suggested pressure limits vary greatly; moreover, they were set at 20–25 mmHg regardless of patient

T. Kaussen (✉)
Department of Pediatric Cardiology and Intensive Care Medicine, Hannover Medical School, Hannover, Germany
e-mail: kaussen.torsten@mh-hannover.de

© Springer Nature Switzerland AG 2021
F. Coccolini et al. (eds.), *Compartment Syndrome*, Hot Topics in Acute Care Surgery and Trauma, https://doi.org/10.1007/978-3-030-55378-4_15

age (i.e., for adults as well as children) until only a few years ago. From the pediatric perspective, such pressure levels are unreasonable when tissue perfusion pressure (TPP = MAP − Compartment pressure) is considered in relation to blood pressure adapted for age. In the case of a regular MAP level of 40 mmHg for an infant, a compartmental pressure of 20 mmHg would be an effective perfusion pressure of 20 mmHg, i.e., half the norm for blood and perfusion pressure in this age group. In recent years, the respective norms for upper limits in pediatric patients have been revised downwards incrementally. Currently, a tissue pressure below 13–16 mmHg is acceptable for cerebral and muscular compartments; up to 10 mmHg is a standard pressure value for intra-abdominal compartments. Knowledge about these new limits, which are adapted to pathophysiological conditions, can be considered neither widespread nor extensive.

Thus far, there has not been any useful data for thoracic compartment syndrome in children and adolescents. Elevated intrathoracic pressure in connection with cardiac surgery is clinically relevant. The decision to leave the thorax open perioperatively is made regardless of the definite pressure values and based on the surgeon's subjective impression as well as cardiorespiratory stability when the patient is taken off the heart-lung machine.

This chapter does not provide a detailed description of the first three types of compartment syndrome named and refers readers to the respective adult-focused chapter in this book.

Only in connection with abdominal compartment syndrome in children and adolescents is evidence continually growing. This is a result of increased attention and scientific research. In spite of this growth, a great lack of knowledge and considerable ambiguities remain.

Due to the significantly better evidence, the author limits himself to a more detailed description of abdominal compartment syndrome.

15.1 Abdominal Compartment Syndrome in Children and Adolescents

15.1.1 Background

Although intra-abdominal hypertension (IAH) and abdominal compartment syndrome (ACS) should be diagnosed especially often in neonatal (NICU) and pediatric intensive care units, both pathologies are still considered too seldom and barely actually diagnosed. This is astounding insofar as the so-called prototypes of high-risk illnesses, and procedures, potentially leading to IAH and/or ACS are to be found original in pediatrics [5]: In this case, there is the existence, and the closure, of a congenital abdominal wall defect (gastroschisis, omphalocele, congenital diaphragmatic hernia) and the transplantation of parenchymatous organs that can differ in size, making their volume a critical issue. Besides these prototypes, there are numerous other combinations of risks (in addition to those known in adult medicine) that can lead to an increase in intra-abdominal pressure (IAP). Through inflammation and capillary leak syndrome, a critical illness per se preordains the development of increased abdominal pressure. This is reflected in the fact that the likelihood of developing ACS along its associated likelihood of morbidity and mortality increases by 22 times when the PRISM-III-Score (PRISM: Pediatric Risk of Mortality [6, 7]) is above 17 [8].

By definition one speaks of ACS when organ dysfunction occurs or is aggravated in addition to intra-abdominal hypertension (IAH; present when intra-abdominal pressure [IAP] is ≥10 mmHg) [9, 10]. In a healthy child, IAP is between 0 and 5 mmHg; in a mechanically ventilated child (without IAH), one usually finds an IAP of around 7 mmHg [11]. In cases of delayed diagnosis or inadequate therapy, an ACS regularly leads to multi-organ failure and death as a result of mutually triggering organ dysfunction and increasing inflammatory cascades.

15.1.2 Epidemiology

Despite an ever-increasing body of evidence from more and more published studies and profound reviews, only few reliable statements on the epidemiology of ACS in children can be made. Depending on the spectrum of the clinic and severity of the underlying diseases managed and treated in the respective neonatal (NICU) or pediatric intensive care unit (PICU), the *prevalence* of ACS ranges between 0.6 and 4.7% in PICUs [8, 12–15] and 7 and 18% in NICUs [16, 17]. When grouped according to risk, the prevalence figures were from 27% (gastroschisis [18]), 37% (burn [19], pancreatitis [20]), and up to 74% (after liver transplantation [21]). All of these figures could still be rather underestimated since they are partially based on the data available at the time of their publication, i.e., when IAP limits were still significantly higher than the standard pediatric maximum of 10 mmHg issued by the WSACS in 2013. For instance, some previously applied standard maximums were at 25–30 mmHg [9].

That premature and newborn babies tend to develop an ACS more often can on the one hand be explained by the miniaturized anatomical conditions and pathophysiological consequences as well as limited compliance regarding intra-corporal increases in volume. On the other hand, the "prototype" [5] diseases named above are the ones primarily affecting premature and newborn babies. There are also typical abdominal complications related to premature and critical newborn births, for example necrotizing enterocolitis (NEC), ileus, volvulus, and intussusception. Due to their primary and secondary damage mechanisms, these are extremely often accompanied by IAH and ACS, which contributes significantly to the morbidity and mortality of abdominal complications in this age group [17].

The only figures estimating *incidences* of ACS in children come from a yet-to-be-published 2016–2018 surveillance study of all 530 children's clinics and departments in Germany [22, 23]. According to this study, ACS occurs in at least approximately 0.2% of children in intensive care. This figure may underestimate the actual circumstances, as there are massive signs of extensive underreporting due to failure to diagnose and failure to report (caused by the increased workload in intensive care) [22, 24]. Difficulties performing diagnoses did not occur due to the still somewhat little known WSACS criteria and definitions (ACS = IAH plus new or aggravated organ dysfunction). Only every fifth NICU, and PICU, even reported measuring IAP (at least in individual cases) [25]. Thus, it can be assumed that at least 80% of NICUs and PICUs are not (cannot be) considering the diagnostic criteria in a way that is true to definition. In approximately 18–20% of cases, even organ dysfunctions were not recognized correctly and in time—regardless of the organ system that was concretely affected [22].

Although neonatal patients are affected more often by IAH and ACS than older children, almost all case reports were made by PICUs (and barely by NICUs) in the framework of the surveillance study mentioned above as well as in that of two prevalence studies from 2010 and 2016, respectively [25]. It is even more astounding that—in spite of this—a peak in cases could be found at a median age of 7 months [22]. If neonatal intensive care stations were more thorough in their diagnostics and reporting, this peak would probably shift further towards an even younger class of infants. In contrast to adults, girls and boys appear to be almost equally affected by the development of ACS (no predominance in boys) [22].

That cases of ACS are almost only observed and reported by large departments and university clinics can be due to the on average greater complexity of diseases often treated in large hospitals. However, the data gathered speaks quite clearly for the idea that knowledge and trust in the ability to apply definitions, recommendations, and therapy options associated with IAP can be described as proportional to the size of the clinics, and a great need for training in small clinics and nonuniversity departments can be recognized. Although familiarity with and knowledge of IAP, IAH, and ACS has spread in recent years, it is still far from being sufficient across the board [25–27].

Lethality varies as well depending on the patient clientele and experience of the intensive care unit. It lies between 21 and 80% [8, 13, 17, 21–23, 28, 29], with specific combinations of risks being associated with a significantly higher lethality (above all pancreatitis, burns, NEC) [19, 20, 29, 30].

Risk of death is nine times higher when IAH and/or ACS occur [8]. According to Ejike et al., a 30% and 50% higher mortality rate can be predicted simply when the dynamic of an increase in IAP and "reaching" of the peak IAP value are observed.

The prognosis for the patient appears to essentially depend on doctors' openness to courageous and if necessary invasive but above all timely therapeutic intervention: when a conservative (noninvasive) therapy approach was applied in German-speaking (D-A-CH) NICUs and PICUs, the average likelihood of *survival* was 40–60%; meanwhile, the likelihood of survival following decompressive laparotomy proved to be at least 83% [25]. In cases of a significant IAP increase and dynamic as well as ACS that is either impending or already occurring, a rash reduction in pressure and with this usually an invasive procedure can be decisive for survival. In spite of this, there is often a fatal lapse in action before adequate therapy is introduced in daily clinical practice.

In this case there were also relevant differences depending on the academic background of care providers: whereas university pediatric clinics stated that they perform a yearly average of 2.4 laparotomies for decompression in cases of ACS, nonuniversity departments reported only 0.3 per year. Thus, outcome data differ depending on the size of the intensive care unit, and its academic nature/background [25].

15.1.3 Classification and Pathophysiology

Depending on the origin of the disease leading to an increase in IAP, there are primary, secondary, and recurring (previously tertiary) geneses [9].

Neonatal patients and infants tend to develop a *primary ACS* (from a disease of/ originating from an organ/tissue in the abdominal cavity) that is often associated with necrotized enterocolitis, intestinal perforation, or (meconium) ileus as well as volvulus [25]. In contrast, older pediatric and adolescent patients tend to develop a *secondary ACS* (due to an extra-abdominal pathology). This is related to their larger personal sphere of activity and increasing independence, which exposes them to greater traumatic, thermal, as well as inflammatory influences.

Secondary forms are often unexpected in this context and appear in connection with the surface activation of immunocompetent cells and to a certain extent in connection with every form of extracorporeal circulation (following a heart-lung machine operation, in the context of extracorporeal membrane oxygenation (ECMO), dialysis, etc.). Recently several research papers have described a compression of venal ECMO cannulas that is associated with IAH and results in an ECMO dysfunction or even ECMO failure, especially in pediatric patients [31–34]. As early as 2001, Beck et al. emphasized that—in contrast to those diagnosed in adult patients—secondary forms of IAH and ACS are more prevalent in pediatric patients [35].

Aside from this etiologically/pathogenetic classification, acuity is used as a basis for differentiating among acute, subacute, and chronic processes.

In general, there are four levels of IAH that differ from those in adults in regard to the respective pressure levels:

- Grade I: IAP 10 up to 12 mmHg
- Grade II: IAP >12 up to 15 mmHg
- Grade III: IAP >15 up to 18 mmHg
- Grade IV: IAP >18 mmHg [25]

Contrary to still commonly held opinions among active pediatricians, an ACS is not the same as an elevated or highly elevated IAH (see WSACS definitions). Interestingly, the mortality rate is almost identical in all four levels and—despite widespread beliefs—does not increase with the level [22, 23]. One explanation for this is that neonatal and infant patients often become severely ill and die at an IAH level of no more than one or two.

As known to animal experts and proven by yet-to-be-published in vivo study data taken from children and adolescents, there is an increased distribution of abdominal and mesenterial tissue perfusion that results from IAP-related mobilization of abdominal pooling reserves (so-called autotransfusion) in IAH grades I and II [21, 36]. In spite of a cardiac output that tends to increase under optimal intensive care treatment management with a sufficient increase in volume and individually adapted catecholamine therapy, the microcirculation in the liver, intestines, and kidneys can decrease to the benefit of the spleen and pancreas (redistribution of organ perfusion with "net winners" (spleen and pancreas) as well as "net losers" (liver, intestines, kidneys)) in this phase [21].

Starting at grade III (IAP >15 mmHg), the compromising pressure components are predominant, above all in diastolic, venal, and lymphatic flow. This is also in regard to spleen and pancreas perfusion. In spite of cardiac output being maintained where appropriate, microcirculation in all abdominal organs and tissue falls rapidly and massively (also because the abdominal pooling reserves are usually used up due to IAH). It is here at the latest that these pathophysiological changes are clinically observable via a decrease in spontaneous diuresis [37]. Due to the increasing liberal use of loop diuretics in pediatric intensive care medicine, oliguria and anuria are barely still detectable early cardinal symptoms of an ACS. This is fatal insofar as—contrary to the WSACS criteria and definitions—the traditional school of thought maintains that an ACS is a clinical diagnosis that can only be determined when there is a concurrence of the cardinal symptoms "abdominal distension," "oliguria/anuria," and "cardiorespiratory failure."

The changes in and redistribution of perfusion mentioned above are barely detectable when using traditional intensive care monitoring. This is where somatic (= abdominal) near-infrared spectroscopy (NIRS) could gain increased significance (Fig. 15.1). In contrast to conventional monitoring, it appears to be able to unmask these subclinical changes [38–41]. According to yet-to-be-published research results from a collection of 350 critically ill children, somatic tissue saturation (NIRS) decreases by about 10% points in cases of IAH (IAP ≥10 mmHg) [21]. If there is a new or aggravated organ dysfunction in the sense of a complete ACS, middle tissue saturation falls again by further 10% points in comparison to the non-IAH control group (composed of critically ill children in intensive care). The alarming extent of desaturation within parenchymatic tissue detected in this context points to the extent of IAH-associated cell and organ damage. This makes it no surprise that multi-organ failure, sepsis, and death can occur when therapy is delayed.

Similarly, there are promising study results on the use of micro-dialysis catheters, e.g., in the musculus rectus abdominis. With their help, an IAH-related hypoperfusion can be monitored in real time by measuring the increasing lactate concentrate associated with the resulting transition into an anaerobic metabolic state. Due to the invasiveness of the procedure, micro-dialysis has yet to enter clinical practice in adult medicine [42–45].

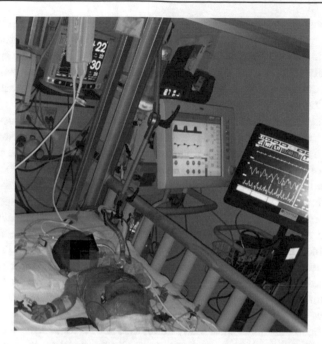

Fig. 15.1 Image of a 10-month-old infant with advanced hemodynamic monitoring following abdominal compartment syndrome with normalization of intra-abdominal pressure after a decompressive laparotomy and transient laparostomy. On the ventilator there is a gastric pressure monitor that indirectly measures an intra-abdominal pressure of 8.7 mmHg. On the right side of the screen, there is an impedance cardiography monitor for the noninvasive quantification of cardiac output, peripheral resistance, stroke volume, and intrathoracic fluid index. Above the head is a near-infrared spectroscopy (NIRS) monitor, which measures somatic tissue saturation right and left paravertebrally over the spleen-kidney or liver-kidney lodge. NIRS allows an indirect statement to be made on the histological restriction of perfusion as a function of intra-abdominal pressure via the course observation of tissue oxygenation

15.1.4 Measurement Methodology and Behavior

The measurement methodology in children does not differ from that in adults and is primarily based on the measurement of bladder pressure first described by Kron et al. [46, 47] and since then repeatedly modified. This is considered the gold standard for indirectly measuring IAP in children and adolescents. After one has carefully ensured that the bladder is completely empty, 1 mL/kg body weight of saline (warmed to body temperature) is inserted into the bladder under sterile conditions. It should be neither below 3 mL nor above 25 mL [11].

Semi-continual bladder pressure measurement via an AbViser®-Valve-System [11, 48, 49] as well as continual measurement of gastric pressure (Spiegelberg®-System, Fig. 15.1) [50–52] are establishing themselves as equally if not more valuable alternatives to measuring bladder pressure manually and have been validated for use in the field of pediatrics [21]. In addition to continual monitoring, the latter system stands out for its especially user-friendly, user-independent, and hygienic advantages.

In individual cases ventilator peak pressure is used to estimate IAP transmitted thoracically via the diaphragm. It is known from animal studies that around 30% of trans-diaphragmal IAP can be further transferred [53, 54]. The method appears to be less clinically feasible and is used for few indications (e.g., when "minimal handling" is necessary and/or in cases of injuries, and diseases, to the gastrointestinal and urogenital tract).

Measuring femoral vein pressure (FVP), and inferior vena cava pressure (IVCP), has proven to be not useful in children. For years this method of measurement was considered a reliable monitoring procedure. However, more and more publications in the field of adult medicine began to either dispute FVP's, and IVCP's, every ability to be used for the indirect quantification of pressure or only spoke for its at least justifiable tendency to estimate real IAP values once IAP has surpassed 18 mmHg [55, 56]. The data collected (but not yet published) recently in the framework of our work group was able to show that there is no justifiable correlation and that FVP, and IVCP, measurement must be rejected as a way of measuring IAP [21].

Direct methods of measurement only have an experimental character and—due to their invasive nature—no importance in the daily routine of pediatric clinics. In the mid to long term, a direct and continuous measurement system would, however, be desirable.

According to the surveillance study mentioned above, routine monitoring of IAP is usually part of the daily routine in pediatric clinics, above all in regard to operative closure of congenital abdominal wall and diaphragmatic hernias; liver failure and/or ascites; following parenchymatous organ transplantations; and following volume/transfusions as well as laparotomies in connection with polytraumatic events and/or larger pediatric abdominal surgical procedures [23].

Standardizing IAP monitoring in cases of specific combinations of risks and/or diseases is without a doubt correct and important [9]; however, this has been the absolute exception and only occurs in few clinics that generally have academic interests.

15.1.5 ACS Defining Organ Dysfunctions

Until the publication of the WSACS definitions in 2013, "new or aggravated" organ dysfunction was not necessarily a criterion considered for diagnosing ACS [9]. Published by Goldstein et al. in 2005, the criteria (depending on the standard values that sometimes vary remarkably among the different age groups within pediatrics) of the International Pediatric Sepsis Consensus Conference (IPSCC) consider static as well as dynamic criteria for assessing the function of every organ system and have proved to be helpful and sensible in standardizing the criteria used to define organ dysfunction [57] (Table 15.1):

Using these IPSCC criteria, a scientifically verifiable respiratory dysfunction in connection with the diagnosis of an ACS can be found in almost all pediatric patients (detectable in more than 90% of affected ACS patients). This dysfunction can be explained above all by the IAH-related elevation of the diaphragm with the

Table 15.1 Criteria for organ dysfunction, modified according to [57]

Cardiovascular	Despite intravenous application of ≥40 mL/kg isotonic volume in 60 min persisting:
	• Hypotension with BP <5th percentile for age or systolic BP <2 SD below normal for age
	   OR
	• Vasoactive drug therapy to keep BP in normal range (dopamine >5 µg/kg/min or epinephrine, norepinephrine, or dobutamine at any dose)
	   OR
	• Two of the following:
	   – Arterial lactate >2 times upper limit of normal
	   – Prolonged capillary refill >5 s
	   – Oliguria: urine output <0.5 mL/kg/h
	   – Metabolic acidosis (base deficit >5 mmol/L)
	   – Core to peripheral body temperature difference >3 °C

Hematologic	• Thrombocyte count <80,000/mm³ or decline of 50% in thrombocyte count from highest value recorded over the past 3 days (for chronic hematology/oncology patients) OR • International Normalized Ratio >2
Hepatic	• Total bilirubin ≥ 4mg/dL (not applicable for newborn) OR • ALT 2 times upper limit of normal age
Renal	• Serum creatinine ≥2 times upper limit of normal for age or twofold rise in baseline creatinine

Respiratory	• Oxygenation index <300 in the absence of cyanotic heart disease or preexisting lung disease
	   OR
	• $PaCO_2$ >65 mmHg or increase of >20 mmHg over baseline
	   OR
	• Proven need or FiO_2 >0.5 in order to maintain saturation ≥92%
	   OR
	Need for nonelective mechanical ventilation (invasive or noninvasive)

Table displays diagnostic criteria for cardiovascular, hematologic, hepatic, renal, and respiratory dysfunction according to the International Pediatric Sepsis Consensus Conference
BP blood pressure, *ALT* alanine aminotransferase

successive development of dys- and atelectasis in the basal lobes of the lung. The second most widely made observation is that of cardiocirculatory impairment, and then kidney and liver dysfunction [23].

Neurological impairments are excluded as ACS defining organ dysfunctions, because the majority of ACS patients require an intubation and mechanical respiration with the corresponding analgosedation, resulting in the neurological criteria generally only being viewed and assessed with reservation. Regardless of this, it is debatable whether—depending on the amount of intra-abdominal pressure—this pressure is distributed intracranially after spreading to the thorax and whether—depending on the extent of the resulting stasis—there is also relevant impairment of and damage to intracranial structures in the course of the disease [58–63].

In accordance with IPSCC criteria, there are massive changes in the corresponding vital and laboratory parameters in the case of ACS. However, they do not show any kind of specificity and cannot be interpreted as chemical biomarkers of an ACS [23]. Various work groups have been looking for such promising biomarkers for years now [64–66], because the transition from a "simple" IAH to ACS begins slowly and is usually recognized (too) late—but then with seriously deleterious results quoad vitam [64–66]. Just recently it was possible to identify and quantify a promising microRNA as well as diverse neuronal guidance proteins [21] that are detectable in significantly higher concentrations in patients' blood only after the transition from IAH to ACS [67, 68]. Furthermore, promising biomarkers include fatty acid-binding proteins [69–71], D-lactate [72], citrulline [73], and circulating tight-junction proteins of the enteral mucosa [74]. Considering the current state of research, it cannot be said how far these laboratory parameters can actually be used as biomarkers in daily clinical practice. Further studies are necessary.

15.1.6 Therapy Options and Goals

On average an ACS diagnosis is made too late. A retrospective investigation of adult patients found that the average diagnosis occurs with a latency of 18 h [75]. The goal of adequate therapy has to be to ensure sufficient perfusion of all tissue and organs, and reestablish it as quickly as possible—at the latest when ACS has been determined but more preferably once IAH has been recognized. Analogous to the surgical maxim with the ileus, the sun should not set and rise between when ACS is diagnosed and the therapeutic objective is reached (prose version of the max. 6-h ischemia rule). For estimation, determining abdominal perfusion pressure (APP) can be useful. Similar to cerebral perfusion pressure, APP = MAP − IAP (with MAP: mean arterial pressure; IAP: intra-abdominal pressure) [76, 77] [in the past by some authors (synonymous) also referred to as splanchnic perfusion pressure (SPP) [78, 79]]. Individual authors describe perfusion pressure instead as the difference in pressure between diastolic pressure and IAP. Considered in contrast to MAPs—but also considering the damaging components of stasis when diastolic pressure is exceeded—this form of calculation has yet to take hold. As long as the data available refer more to MAP, the methods first mentioned, and formulas, should be applied in an evidence-based way.

   The goal of adequate therapy should be for MAP as well as APP to be oriented towards the standard blood pressure range that corresponds with the patient's age (see Table 15.2 [80]). An iatrogenic increase in MAP via forced catecholamine therapy with the goal of achieving an age-appropriate normalization of APP is neither useful nor sustainable and, thus, obsolete. In the neonatal age, for example, the goal MAP level is the number of weeks that have passed since conception (in mmHg). Accordingly, a newborn delivered in the 36th week of pregnancy should have an average MAP of 36 mmHg. Considering their cardiovascular condition in cases of even moderate increases in IAP as well as the impairment of their microcirculation due to IAH, a neonatal or infant patient is at a significantly greater risk than an almost grown adolescent with age-adapted MAP standard limit of 70 or 80 mmHg.

Table 15.2 Age-appropriate standard value areas of mean arterial pressure [mmHg]; modified according to [80]

Age group limits [in months]		Mean arterial pressure (MAP) [mmHg]		
Lower limit	Upper limit	−2 SD	Average	+2 SD
1	3	40	50	60
>3	6	45	60	75
>6	12	50	70	90
>12	47	50	75	90
>47	83	55	75	95
>83	131	60	75	95
>131	167	65	80	95
>167	216	70	83	95

Abbreviation: *SD* standard deviation

For risk stratification of quantified IAPs, it is necessary to be aware of age-appropriate blood pressure values (with ±2 standard deviations [SD], see Table 15.2).

The recommendations published by the WCACS regarding medical, interventional, and emergency surgical therapy options in cases of a relevant IAH or ACS are also valid for children [9]. If using a feeding tube and purgative measures in addition to creating a negative balance with the help of diuretic therapeutics and emergency dialysis procedures is not enough, sufficiently deep analgosedation and even relaxation following previous intubation and mechanical ventilation are necessary [9]. Ascites that can be punctured or other effusions should be relieved generously [81]. Should a decompression be unavoidable due to the IAP dynamic, the clinical and above all intraoperative development of IAP should be used to consider the necessity of a laparostomy (synonym: open abdomen management, abdomen apertum, surgical enlargement of the abdominal wall, etc.). In the framework of the surveillance study mentioned above [23], a decompressive laparotomy was performed on 2/3 of the children studied; the abdomen was left open a median of 7.5 days (mean 9.9 ± 5.5) in 44%. A median of 4.0 (on average 3.2 ± 2.2) operations were necessary to reclose the abdomen. In 76% of the cases, open abdomen management was not associated with any complications. In the remaining cases, infectious septic events were more dominant than wound-healing disorders, adhesions, and failure of foreign materials that had been introduced. Enterocutaneous fistulas, the most common complication following open abdomen management in adults, were not observed in this pediatric study [23].

While a total of 83% of the patients on whom operative decompression was performed survived, 58% of children in whom there was an indication for temporary abdominal wall surgery survived. Thus, when a temporary surgical enlargement of the abdominal wall was implemented, the probability of pediatric patient survival was on average higher than when conservative therapy was administered (survival 40–60%) [23].

The median length of stay for pediatric intensive care patients with ACS who survived was 25.5 days in the ICU (mean 42.9 ± 42.2), and a total of 42.5 days in the hospital (mean 59.6 ± 49.5). Patients who did not survive ACS died medianly after 12 days (average 25.2 ± 35.5). In 74% of these cases, multi-organ failure that could not be controlled via organ replacement procedures was the cause [23]. In the remaining cases, it was incontrollable pulmonal arterial hypertonia, cardiovascular failure, bleeding complications due to impaired coagulation, and therapy-resistant tumor growth [23].

15.2 Conclusion

Thorough training appears to make it possible to create a sensitization for this topic and accelerate the application of adequate, and courageous, therapy options. Standard operating procedures with flowcharts on age-appropriate and problem-oriented diagnosis as well as therapy should increase the willingness to also act invasively and choose heretofore unpopular methods and options that can massively influence and ensure survival in pediatric patients. Initial outcome data are motivating and suggest that invasive therapy possibilities can be beneficial to survival in cases of abdominal compartment syndrome.

Only this seems to be the way to reduce morbidity and mortality in the mid to long term among the smallest patients.

References

1. von Keudell AG, Weaver MJ, Appleton PT, Bae DS, Dyer GSM, Heng M, et al. Diagnosis and treatment of acute extremity compartment syndrome. Lancet. 2015;386(10000):1299–310.
2. Kochanek PM, Tasker RC, Carney N, Totten AM, Adelson PD, Selden NR, et al. Guidelines for the management of pediatric severe traumatic brain injury, third edition: update of the brain trauma foundation guidelines, executive summary. Neurosurgery. 2019;84(6):1169–78.
3. Villalobos MA, Hazelton JP, Choron RL, Capano-Wehrle L, Hunter K, Gaughan JP, et al. Caring for critically injured children: an analysis of 56 pediatric damage control laparotomies. J Trauma Acute Care Surg. 2017;82(5):901–9.
4. Kayhanian S, Young AMH, Ewen RL, Piper RJ, Guilfoyle MR, Donnelly J, et al. Thresholds for identifying pathological intracranial pressure in paediatric traumatic brain injury. Sci Rep. 2019;9(1):3537.
5. Watson RA, Howdieshell TR. Abdominal compartment syndrome. South Med J. 1998;91(4):326–32.
6. Pollack MM, Patel KM, Ruttimann UE. PRISM III: an updated pediatric risk of mortality score. Crit Care Med. 1996;24(5):743–52.
7. Pollack MM, Ruttimann UE, Getson PR. Pediatric risk of mortality (PRISM) score. Crit Care Med. 1988;16(11):1110–6.
8. Ejike JC, Humbert S, Bahjri K, Mathur M. Outcomes of children with abdominal compartment syndrome. Acta Clin Belg Suppl. 2007;1:141–8.
9. Kirkpatrick AW, Roberts DJ, De Waele J, Jaeschke R, Malbrain ML, De Keulenaer B, et al. Intra-abdominal hypertension and the abdominal compartment syndrome: updated consensus definitions and clinical practice guidelines from the World Society of the Abdominal Compartment Syndrome. Intensive Care Med. 2013;39(7):1190–206.
10. Thabet FC, Ejike JC. Intra-abdominal hypertension and abdominal compartment syndrome in pediatrics. A review. J Crit Care. 2017;41:275–82.
11. Ejike JC, Bahjri K, Mathur M. What is the normal intra-abdominal pressure in critically ill children and how should we measure it? Crit Care Med. 2008;36(7):2157–62.

12. Beck R. Abdominal compartment syndrome in children. Pediatr Crit Care Med. 2001;2(1):51–6.
13. Diaz FJ, Fernandez Sein A, Gotay F. Identification and management of abdominal compartment syndrome in the pediatric intensive care unit. P R Health Sci J. 2006;25(1):17–22.
14. Pearson EG, Rollins MD, Vogler SA, Mills MK, Lehman EL, Jacques E, et al. Decompressive laparotomy for abdominal compartment syndrome in children: before it is too late. J Pediatr Surg. 2010;45(6):1324–9.
15. Thabet FC, Bougmiza IM, Chehab MS, Bafaqih HA, AlMohaimeed SA, Malbrain ML. Incidence, risk factors, and prognosis of intra-abdominal hypertension in critically ill children: a prospective epidemiological study. J Intensive Care Med. 2016;31(6):403–8.
16. Akhobadze GR, Chkhaidze MG, Kanjaradze DV, Tsirkvadze I, Ukleba V. Identification, management and complications of intra-abdominal hypertension and abdominal compartment syndrome in neonatal intensive care unit (a single centre retrospective analysis). Georgian Med News. 2011;192:58–64.
17. Kaussen T, Otto J, Steinau G, Hoer J, Srinivasan PK, Schachtrupp A. Recognition and management of abdominal compartment syndrome among German anesthetists and surgeons: a national survey. Ann Intensive Care. 2012;2(Suppl 1):S7.
18. Lao OB, Larison C, Garrison MM, Waldhausen JH, Goldin AB. Outcomes in neonates with gastroschisis in U.S. children's hospitals. Am J Perinatol. 2010;27(1):97–101.
19. Greenhalgh DG, Warden GD. The importance of intra-abdominal pressure measurements in burned children. J Trauma. 1994;36(5):685–90.
20. Dmytriiev DV. Intra-abdominal hypertension in children with acute pancreatitis. Acta Clin Belg Suppl. 2007;62:292–M25.
21. Kaussen T. pedACS study. 2015–2019 at the PICU of Hannover Medical School.
22. Gerner P, Gerstl L, Hoffmann F, Kallinich T, Kaussen T, Kidszun A, von Kries R, Liese J, Machaelis K, Rosenbauer J, Rostasy K, Staufner C. Abdominelles Kompartmentsyndrom bei Kindern und Jugendlichen. ESPED-Jahresbericht. 2017.
23. Fernandez Rodriguez S, Fischer M, Hoffmann F, Kallinich T, Kaussen T, Kidszun A, von Kries R, Liese J, Michaelis K, Müller H, Rosenbauer J, Rostásy K, Staufner C. Abdominelles Kompartmentsyndrom (AKS) bei Kindern und Jugendlichen. ESPED-Jahresbericht. 2018. p. 39–46.
24. Della Marina A, Gerstl L, Kallinich T, Kaussen T, von Kries M, Lee-Kirsch A, Liese J, Meyer S, Rosenbauer J, Schielke A, Staufner C, Tenenbaum T. Abdominelles Kompartmentsyndrom (AKS) bei Kindern und Jugendlichen. ESPED-Jahresbericht. 2016. p. 7.
25. Kaussen T, Steinau G, Srinivasan PK, Otto J, Sasse M, Staudt F, et al. Recognition and management of abdominal compartment syndrome among German pediatric intensivists: results of a national survey. Ann Intensive Care. 2012;2(Suppl 1):S8.
26. Ejike JC, Newcombe J, Baerg J, Bahjri K, Mathur M. Understanding of abdominal compartment syndrome among pediatric healthcare providers. Crit Care Res Pract. 2010;2010:876013.
27. Newcombe J, Mathur M, Bahjri K, Ejike JC. Pediatric critical care nurses' experience with abdominal compartment syndrome. Ann Intensive Care. 2012;2(Suppl 1):S6.
28. Steinau G, Kaussen T, Bolten B, Schachtrupp A, Neumann UP, Conze J, et al. Abdominal compartment syndrome in childhood: diagnostics, therapy and survival rate. Pediatr Surg Int. 2011;27(4):399–405.
29. Neville HL, Lally KP, Cox CS Jr. Emergent abdominal decompression with patch abdominoplasty in the pediatric patient. J Pediatr Surg. 2000;35(5):705–8.
30. Hobson KG, Young KM, Ciraulo A, Palmieri TL, Greenhalgh DG. Release of abdominal compartment syndrome improves survival in patients with burn injury. J Trauma. 2002;53(6):1129–33; discussion 33–4.
31. Mugford M, Elbourne D, Field D. Extracorporeal membrane oxygenation for severe respiratory failure in newborn infants. Cochrane Database Syst Rev. 2008;(3):CD001340.
32. Nagaya M, Kato J, Niimi N, Tanaka S. Extracorporeal membrane oxygenation for newborns with gastric rupture. Pediatr Surg Int. 2001;17(1):35–8.

33. Prodhan P, Imamura M, Garcia X, Byrnes JW, Bhutta AT, Dyamenahalli U. Abdominal compartment syndrome in newborns and children supported on extracorporeal membrane oxygenation. ASAIO J. 2012;58(2):143–7.
34. Okhuysen-Cawley R, Prodhan P, Imamura M, Dedman AH, Anand KJ. Management of abdominal compartment syndrome during extracorporeal life support. Pediatr Crit Care Med. 2007;8(2):177–9. PMID: 17273121.
35. Beck R, Halberthal M, Zonis Z, Shoshani G, Hayari L, Bar-Joseph G. Abdominal compartment syndrome in children. Pediatr Crit Care Med. 2001;2(1):51–6.
36. Schachtrupp A, Hoer J, Schumpelick V, Töns C. Extensive fluid resuscitation can preserve cardiac output and functional organ parameters in a porcine model of the abdominal compartment syndrome. Langenbecks Arch Chir. 2001;386:470.
37. Patel DM, Connor MJ Jr. Intra-abdominal hypertension and abdominal compartment syndrome: an underappreciated cause of acute kidney injury. Adv Chronic Kidney Dis. 2016;23(3):160–6.
38. Di Nardo M, Cecchetti C, Stoppa F, Pirozzi N, Picardo S. Abdominal compartment syndrome in childhood: the role of near infrared spectroscopy for the early detection of the organ dysfunction. Pediatr Surg Int. 2012;28(1):111–2.
39. Kaufman J, Almodovar MC, Zuk J, Friesen RH. Correlation of abdominal site near-infrared spectroscopy with gastric tonometry in infants following surgery for congenital heart disease. Pediatr Crit Care Med. 2008;9(1):62–8.
40. Varela JE, Cohn SM, Giannotti GD, Dolich MO, Ramon H, Wiseberg JA, et al. Near-infrared spectroscopy reflects changes in mesenteric and systemic perfusion during abdominal compartment syndrome. Surgery. 2001;129(3):363–70.
41. Widder S, Ranson MK, Zygun D, Knox L, Laupland KB, Laird P, et al. Use of near-infrared spectroscopy as a physiologic monitor for intra-abdominal hypertension. J Trauma. 2008;64(5):1165–8.
42. Meier C, Contaldo C, Schramm R, Holstein JH, Hamacher J, Amon M, et al. Microdialysis of the rectus abdominis muscle for early detection of impending abdominal compartment syndrome. Intensive Care Med. 2007;33(8):1434–43.
43. Maddison L, Karjagin J, Tenhunen J, Kirsimagi U, Starkopf J. Moderate intra-abdominal hypertension leads to anaerobic metabolism in the rectus abdominis muscle tissue of critically ill patients: a prospective observational study. Biomed Res Int. 2014;2014:857492.
44. Maddison L, Karjagin J, Tenhunen J, Starkopf J. Moderate intra-abdominal hypertension is associated with an increased lactate-pyruvate ratio in the rectus abdominis muscle tissue: a pilot study during laparoscopic surgery. Ann Intensive Care. 2012;2(Suppl 1):S14.
45. Benninger E, Laschke MW, Cardell M, Holstein JH, Lustenberger T, Keel M, et al. Early detection of subclinical organ dysfunction by microdialysis of the rectus abdominis muscle in a porcine model of critical intra-abdominal hypertension. Shock. 2012;38(4):420–8.
46. Kron IL. A simple technique to accurately determine intra-abdominal pressure [letter]. Crit Care Med. 1989;17(7):714–5.
47. Kron IL, Harman PK, Nolan SP. The measurement of intra-abdominal pressure as a criterion for abdominal re-exploration. Ann Surg. 1984;199(1):28–30.
48. Basterra Longas A, Arizcun Gonzalez S, Erdozain Rios B. [Abviser Kit intra-abdominal pressure monitoring]. Rev Enferm. 2008;31(10):43–4.
49. De Waele JJ, De Laet I, De Keulenaer B, Widder S, Kirkpatrick AW, Cresswell AB, et al. The effect of different reference transducer positions on intra-abdominal pressure measurement: a multicenter analysis. Intensive Care Med. 2008;34(7):1299–303.
50. Hilgendorff V, Spiegelberg A, Affeld K. Der Luftkapselkatheter- eine Methode zur Messung geringer intrakorporaler Drücke. Biomed Tech Berl. 1986;31:72–3.
51. Malbrain ML, De laet I, Viaene D, Schoonheydt K, Dits H. In vitro validation of a novel method for continuous intra-abdominal pressure monitoring. Intensive Care Med. 2008;34(4):740–5.
52. Schachtrupp A, Biermann A, Toens C, Schwab S, Becker HP, Schumpelick V. An air-capsule probe for the direct measurement of IAP in patients after abdominal surgery. Intensive Care Med. 2004;30(Suppl 1):566.

53. Regli A, Mahendran R, Fysh ET, Roberts B, Noffsinger B, De Keulenaer BL, et al. Matching positive end-expiratory pressure to intra-abdominal pressure improves oxygenation in a porcine sick lung model of intra-abdominal hypertension. Crit Care. 2012;16(5):R208.
54. Regli A, Pelosi P, Malbrain M. Ventilation in patients with intra-abdominal hypertension: what every critical care physician needs to know. Ann Intensive Care. 2019;9(1):52.
55. Howard AE, Regli A, Litton E, Malbrain MM, Palermo AM, De Keulenaer BL. Can femoral venous pressure be used as an estimate for standard vesical intra-abdominal pressure measurement? Anaesth Intensive Care. 2016;44(6):704–11.
56. De Keulenaer BL, Regli A, Dabrowski W, Kaloiani V, Bodnar Z, Cea JI, et al. Does femoral venous pressure measurement correlate well with intrabladder pressure measurement? A multicenter observational trial. Intensive Care Med. 2011;37(10):1620–7.
57. Goldstein B, Giroir B, Randolph A, International Consensus Conference on Pediatric Sepsis. International pediatric sepsis consensus conference: definitions for sepsis and organ dysfunction in pediatrics. Pediatr Crit Care Med. 2005;6(1):2–8.
58. Youssef AM, Hamidian Jahromi A, Vijay CG, Granger DN, Alexander JS. Intra-abdominal hypertension causes reversible blood-brain barrier disruption. J Trauma Acute Care Surg. 2012;72(1):183–8.
59. Rosenthal RJ, Friedman RL, Kahn AM, Martz J, Thiagarajah S, Cohen D, et al. Reasons for intracranial hypertension and hemodynamic instability during acute elevations of intra-abdominal pressure: observations in a large animal model. J Gastrointest Surg. 1998;2(5):415–25.
60. Rosenthal RJ, Hiatt JR, Phillips EH, Hewitt W, Demetriou AA, Grode M. Intracranial pressure. Effects of pneumoperitoneum in a large-animal model. Surg Endosc. 1997;11:376–80.
61. Rosenthal RJ, Friedman RL, Chidambaram A, Khan AM, Martz J, Shi Q, et al. Effects of hyperventilation and hypoventilation on PaCO2 and intracranial pressure during acute elevations of intra-abdominal pressure with CO2 pneumoperitoneum: large animal observations. J Am Coll Surg. 1998;187(1):32–8.
62. Liu D, Zhang HG, Zhao ZA, Chang MT, Li Y, Yu J, et al. Melanocortin MC4 receptor agonists alleviate brain damage in abdominal compartment syndrome in the rat. Neuropeptides. 2015;49:55–61.
63. Depauw P, Groen RJM, Van Loon J, Peul WC, Malbrain M, De Waele JJ. The significance of intra-abdominal pressure in neurosurgery and neurological diseases: a narrative review and a conceptual proposal. Acta Neurochir (Wien). 2019;161(5):855–64.
64. Kowal-Vern A, Ortegel J, Bourdon P, Chakrin A, Latenser BA, Kimball D, Casey LC, et al. Elevated cytokine levels in peritoneal fluid from burned patients with intra-abdominal hypertension and abdominal compartment syndrome. Burns. 2006;32(5):563–9. (0305-4179 (Print)).
65. Oda J, Ivatury RR, Blocher CR, Malhotra AJ, Sugerman HJ. Amplified cytokine response and lung injury by sequential hemorrhagic shock and abdominal compartment syndrome in a laboratory model of ischemia-reperfusion. J Trauma. 2002;52(4):625–31.
66. Rezende-Neto JB, Moore EE, Melo de Andrade MV, Teixeira MM, Lisboa FA, Arantes RM, et al. Systemic inflammatory response secondary to abdominal compartment syndrome: stage for multiple organ failure. J Trauma. 2002;53(6):1121–8.
67. Korner A, Schlegel M, Kaussen T, Gudernatsch V, Hansmann G, Schumacher T, et al. Sympathetic nervous system controls resolution of inflammation via regulation of repulsive guidance molecule A. Nat Commun. 2019;10(1):633.
68. Schlegel M, Korner A, Kaussen T, Knausberg U, Gerber C, Hansmann G, et al. Inhibition of neogenin fosters resolution of inflammation and tissue regeneration. J Clin Invest. 2019;129(5):2165.
69. Edelson MB, Sonnino RE, Bagwell CE, Lieberman JM, Marks WH, Rozycki HJ. Plasma intestinal fatty acid binding protein in neonates with necrotizing enterocolitis: a pilot study. J Pediatr Surg. 1999;34(10):1453–7.
70. Pelsers M, Morovat A, Alexander GJM, Hermens WT, Trull AK, Glatz JFC. Liver fatty acid-binding protein as a sensitive serum marker of acute hepatocellular damage in liver transplant recipients. Clin Chem. 2002;48(11):2055–7. (0009-9147 (Print)).

71. Sonnino R, Ereso G, Arcuni J, Franson R. Human intestinal fatty acid binding protein in peritoneal fluid is a marker of intestinal ischemia. Transplant Proc. 2000;32(6):1280.

72. Duzgun AP, Gulgez B, Ozmutlu A, Ertorul D, Bugdayci G, Akyurek N, et al. The relationship between intestinal hypoperfusion and serum d-lactate levels during experimental intra-abdominal hypertension. Dig Dis Sci. 2006;51(12):2400–3.

73. Fagoni N, Piva S, Marino R, Chiarini G, Ferrari D, Grespi E, et al. The IN-PANCIA study: clinical evaluation of gastrointestinal dysfunction and failure, multiple organ failure, and levels of citrulline in critically ill patients. J Intensive Care Med. 2020;35(3):279–83. https://doi.org/10.1177/0885066617742594.

74. Cheng JT, Xiao GX, Xia PY, Yuan JC, Qin XJ. [Influence of intra-abdominal hypertension on the intestinal permeability and endotoxin/bacteria translocation in rabbits]. Zhonghua Shao Shang Za Zhi. 2003;19(4):229–32.

75. De Waele JJ, Hoste EA, Malbrain ML. Decompressive laparotomy for abdominal compartment syndrome—a critical analysis. Crit Care. 2006;10(2):R51.

76. Cheatham ML, White MW, Sagraves SG, Johnson JL, Block EF. Abdominal perfusion pressure: a superior parameter in the assessment of intra-abdominal hypertension. J Trauma. 2000;49(4):621–6.

77. Horoz OO, Yildizdas D, Sari Y, Unal I, Ekinci F, Petmezci E. The relationship of abdominal perfusion pressure with mortality in critically ill pediatric patients. J Pediatr Surg. 2019;54(9):1731–5.

78. McGuigan RM, Azarow KS. Is splanchnic perfusion pressure more predictive of outcome than intragastric pressure in neonates with gastroschisis? Am J Surg. 2004;187(5):609–11.

79. McGuigan RM, Mullenix PS, Vegunta R, Pearl RH, Sawin R, Azarow KS. Splanchnic perfusion pressure: a better predictor of safe primary closure than intraabdominal pressure in neonatal gastroschisis. J Pediatr Surg. 2006;41(5):901–4.

80. Nicolai T. Kardiozirkulatorische Variablen, Blutdrucktabelle. In: Nicolai T, editor. Pädiatrische Notfall- und Intensivmedizin. Vol. 5. Springer International; 2014.

81. Latenser BA, Kowal-Vern A, Kimball D, Chakrin A, Dujovny N. A pilot study comparing percutaneous decompression with decompressive laparotomy for acute abdominal compartment syndrome in thermal injury. J Burn Care Rehabil. 2002;23(3):190–5.

How to Handle Compartment Syndrome in Resource-Limited Settings

16

Alain Chichom Mefire

16.1 Introduction

Compartment syndrome is the dysfunction of organs or tissues within a closed body part usually limited by fascia with little or no possibility of expansion. Following various mechanisms including but not limited to injury, the pressure within a body compartment increases and hinders appropriate blood supply to tissues within the compartment, thus compromising their survival. This phenomenon could be primary when the etiology of the increased pressure is internal to the compartment or secondary when increased pressure results from external compression. It could be acute or chronic and frequently affects limbs, abdomen, thorax, or even the cranium. A recently described form of this syndrome is referred to as the "multiple compartment syndrome" and often results from massive fluid resuscitation [1]. There also seems to be a strong relation between increased pressure in different body compartments: a raised abdominal pressure could result in raised intrathoracic and intracranial pressure [2].

Literature on compartment syndrome in low- and middle-income countries is extremely scarce [3, 4]. Consequently, it is a special challenge in these countries because of the low awareness of workers which makes it often pass unnoticed. The consequences of missing it could be dramatic as it is a frequent source of major complications such as limb amputations, major ventilation problems, permanent irreversible damage to intra-compartmental organs, and sometimes death depending on the location. The care of patients at risk of compartment syndrome is based on various strategies of reducing pressure within the body part involved. The major difficulty in countries with limited technical background is the extreme scarcity of intra-compartmental pressure measuring devices and probes as many gold standard treatment protocols depend on these measurements. There is a need to propose a specific approach to be used in the absence of such devices and equipment to assist

A. Chichom Mefire (✉)

Department of Surgery, Faculty of Health Sciences, University of Buea, Buea, Cameroon

© Springer Nature Switzerland AG 2021

F. Coccolini et al. (eds.), *Compartment Syndrome*, Hot Topics in Acute Care Surgery and Trauma, https://doi.org/10.1007/978-3-030-55378-4_16

health workers practicing under such conditions in reducing the burden and consequences of this situation.

We deliberately choose to limit our analysis to acute compartment syndrome (ACS) of two key body regions (extremities and abdomen) because they are usually immediately life or limb-threatening and seem to be the most frequently encountered.

16.2   Acute Compartment Syndrome of the Limb

16.2.1 Think About It!

What is likely to happen if a compartment syndrome, say the leg, is unrecognized or identified late? In a systematic review recently proposed by Glass et al., it was demonstrated that delayed compartment decompression (6–120 h) resulted in an overall amputation rate of over 37%! Two patients even died and most surviving limbs exhibited functional deficits such as foot drop or sepsis [5]. These are unacceptable outcomes often observed in sub-Saharan African countries for a problem that can be solved with a simple fasciotomy.

The difficulty in settings with limited technical background and more specifically in the absence of pressure measuring devices is to design a protocol permitting to reduce the risk of such morbid and deadly delay while avoiding excessive aggressive action and unnecessary surgical decompression which is associated with a specific morbidity as well. This is true for both the upper and the lower limbs.

16.2.2 Who Is a Suspect?

The first step is to be well aware of clinical situations considered as the highest providers of limb compartment syndrome. Every patient with a tibial fracture (closed or open), blunt soft tissue injury, circumferential burn or dressings, a cast immobilization, traction, or snake bite is a possible candidate for limb compartment syndrome and must be monitored clinically until he is considered out of danger [6–8]. The initial belief that in open fractures, the associated disruption of skin and fascia decompresses compartments and prevents compartment syndrome seems logical but is not supported by any evidence [8]. Particular attention must be paid to tibial fractures as they are the most frequent providers accounting for more than one-third of all cases of compartment syndrome [8]. It is also suspected (but not clearly established) that younger patients are at a higher risk [8]. Patients with comorbidities such as diabetes, hypothyroidism (a frequent and often unrecognized situation in the tropics), and the increasing number of patients under anticoagulation therapy also deserve special monitoring. These comorbidities often occur in combination: the young diabetic patient under anticoagulant therapy with a tibial fracture is the ideal candidate for leg ACS!

It is important to remember that in lower limb injuries, a fracture is not necessary before ACS occurs. Any injury to soft tissue (especially closed crush injuries) is enough to create the conditions for increased compartment pressure! This is particularly true for the legs, thighs, and gluteal regions [6].

Finally, there is absolute need to suppress the dogma according to which compartment syndrome does not affect the upper limb! Numbers of practitioners in limited settings have surely seen a patient with iatrogenic ulnar claw following a simple cast immobilization of the forearm.

16.2.3 How to Identify Compartment Syndrome in the Absence of Pressure Measuring Devices?

One thing must be said very clearly: the gold standard for diagnosis of compartment syndrome of the limb is the measurement of intra-compartmental pressure! In the absence of pressure measuring devices and equipment, the only way to reduce the consequences of compartment syndrome of the limb is to be able to recognize it early and define new criteria for decision-making, bearing in mind the increased risk of taking unnecessary action and performing fasciotomy that is not needed.

But despite its shortcomings, clinical assessment is still the cornerstone of the diagnosis of compartment syndrome of the limb [8–10]. It is known that it can present with a variety of findings, including pain, paresthesia, tenderness with passive stretch, tenseness or firmness of the compartment, focal motor or sensory deficits, or decreased pulse or capillary refill time. Pain is typically the earliest finding in patients with ACS. It is usually described as severe and out of proportion to the injury, increasing in intensity, and resistant to analgesics [8]. This progression of the characteristics of the pain can only be identified through repeated clinical assessment. The presence of nerve symptoms such as paresthesia and tingling should be considered the beginning of a countdown as irreversible damage could occur as early as 12 h following the unset with its dramatic and often definitive consequences. The presence of blisters is often a sign of such irreversible damage.

16.2.4 When to Decide to Perform a Fasciotomy?

Two schools of taught currently oppose the partners of aggressive surgical treatment and those who advocate for continuous monitoring of compartmental pressure to guide decision-making whenever possible. The contribution of fasciotomy in the reduction of the consequences of ACS of the limb has been proven beyond doubt [11]. But fasciotomy itself carries a number of short- and long-term risks, especially in settings with limited technical background where surgical safety is still a concern.

In the absence of pressure measuring devices, the decision should in our opinion be guided by the following principle: in the absence of decompression of the limb in a patient with ACS of the limb, there is a danger of permanent disability and even death! Consequently, fasciotomy to reduce pressure and restore perfusion must be considered with no delay upon strong clinical suspicion: the patient with increasing pain out of proportion to the injury combined with tenderness on passive stretch and/or sensory/motor deficit [12].

The absence of pulse is not a major diagnostic criterion of ACS of the limb as it has been demonstrated that pulse can be preserved even when a high-pressure ACS is diagnosed [8]. Fasciotomy could thus be decided in a limb with preserved pulse in the presence of other strong clinical arguments.

Initially, one should start by considering simple methods such as reduction of pressure by removing constricting dressings and casts and this sometimes suffices. Fighting hypotension and optimizing tissue perfusion by all possible means are also sometimes useful and surgical decompression should only be considered after all these measures have failed [13].

16.3   Acute Abdominal Compartment Syndrome (AACS)

16.3.1 What Is It and Why Is It a Problem?

Abdominal compartment syndrome has been defined as a continuous intra-abdominal pressure above 20 mmHg (2.67 kPa) with coexisting organ dysfunction or failure.

Abdominal compartment syndrome (ACS) is the end point of a process whereby massive interstitial swelling in the abdomen or rapid development of a space-filling lesion in the abdomen (such as ascites or a hematoma) leads to pathologically increased pressure. This results in so-called intra-abdominal hypertension (IAH), causing decreased perfusion of the kidneys and abdominal viscera and possible difficulties with ventilation and maintenance of cardiac output. These effects contribute to a cascade of ischemia and multiple organ dysfunctions with high mortality [14]. This makes IAH and ACS of the abdomen a frequent and potentially deadly condition. The mortality of patients with recognized abdominal compartment syndrome may be as high as 42–100% [15, 16].

IAH is a largely underestimated problem with a high prevalence [17]. The two main providers are known to be abdominal injuries and emergency laparotomy [18, 19]. Its occurrence could be as high as 80% after emergency laparotomy for whatever indication [20]. The problem seems to be of less importance after elective laparotomy [21]. Other providers of IAH/AACS include abdominal circumferential burns and aggressive fluid resuscitation [4]. The typical patient in our settings would be the one with a diffuse purulent peritonitis secondary to a peptic ulcer perforation that undergoes massive fluid resuscitation before and after emergency laparotomy.

Luckily IAH does not always result in abdominal ACS and it is estimated that only 10% of patients with IAH will develop ACS [22]. But there is a specific morbidity related to increased abdominal pressure itself after laparotomy: it was suggested that IAH has a direct influence on suture tension in midline laparotomy wounds in porcine model [23].

Primary AACS is a known complication of damage control surgery. Recently secondary ACS has been reported in patients without abdominal injury who require aggressive resuscitation.

Consequently, while the diagnosis of AACS is still based on measurement and protocolized monitoring of intra-abdominal pressure [24] and sometimes on indirect radiological means [25], in the absence of pressure measuring devices, every patient undergoing damage control laparotomy for trauma and non-trauma causes must be considered an AACS patient and managed accordingly!

16.3.2 How to Go About It?

Hecker et al. categorized therapeutic measures in IAH/AACS if five columns: intra-luminal evacuation, intraabdominal evacuation, improvement of abdominal wall compliance, fluid management, and improved organ perfusion. The general rule is that emergency decompressive laparotomy should be considered when all conservative measures fail to restore basic vital signs suggestive of reducing pressure [26]. Such conservative measures would include sedation and analgesia, neuromuscular blocking, prokinetic agents to encourage natural transit, gastric and enteral decompression tube placement, reduction of fluid administration to what is necessary after careful estimation, percutaneous drainage, and so forth [26]. These simple, cheap measures have proven to significantly improve patient survival [27].

However, surgeons working in low- and middle-income countries should never hesitate to take back the patient for a re-laparotomy within 24 h of the onset of the AACS as it has proven to be protective against mortality [28].

16.4 Other Compartment Syndromes

As mentioned earlier, it must be remembered that other body compartments are also prone to developing ACS. These include the thorax and the cranium.

Thoracic compartment syndrome (TCS) could be responsible for a major respiratory distress and has been reported predominantly in the pediatric and adult cardiac surgery populations, where this phenomenon has been described as a syndrome of "mediastinal tightness" following prolonged cardiac surgery. However, it could be exceptionally observed in thoracic injury cases especially when mediastinal organs are involved [29]. Circumferential thoracic burns could also result in such distressing situations. The management would depend on the specific situations.

Intracranial ACS if often the result of head injury, stroke, or brain tumors. Raised intracranial pressure (ICP) due to brain swelling within the closed compartment of the skull leads to death or severe neurological disability if not effectively treated. This sometimes warrants a decompressive craniectomy (part of the skull is removed and the underlying dura opened to reduce brain swelling-related raised ICP) which is neurosurgical intervention with complex and often controversial indications best decided and performed by the neurosurgeon [30, 31]. In such cases, the management in remote areas should be limited to supportive measures intended to provide support until the patient is referred to appropriate settings, except for life-threatening situations such as an acute epidural hematoma. It was recently suggested that a laparotomy could be effective in ensuring intracranial decompression [32, 33] but such decision should be taken with a lot of caution in the absence of a neurosurgeon.

16.5   Conclusions

Low-income countries in general and African countries in particular are characterized by the scarcity of pressure-measuring devices and equipment for various anatomical areas which are prone to developing compartment syndrome. This is explained by the extremely low level of awareness of the problem of compartment syndrome and explain the difficulties in documenting them, hence the extreme scarcity of literature on the problem. While encouraging decision makers on the need to provide for appropriate devices, the challenge is to be able to identify cases and make decisions purely on a clinical background. The management ACS in its various forms still has to rely very largely on preventive measures and early identification of cases for aggressive intervention or referral.

The burden of ACS of the limbs can only be reduced by a high suspicion index and repeated clinical assessment with particular attention to the patient whose pain is increasing and is out of proportion to the injury or tissue damage. In such patients, in the absence of pressure-measuring devices, the decision of performing a fasciotomy could reasonably be taken solely on strong clinical arguments.

Every patient undergoing emergency laparotomy must be considered to have IAH/AACS and treated accordingly. This means that the five principles of abdominal decompression must be systematically applied and decompressive laparotomy considered as a live-saving procedure.

References

1. Balogh ZJ, Butcher NE. Compartment syndromes from head to toe. Crit Care Med. 2010;38(9 Suppl):S445–51. https://doi.org/10.1097/CCM.0b013e3181ec5d09.
2. Bloomfield GL, Ridings PC, Blocher CR, Marmarou A, Sugerman HJ. A proposed relationship between increased intra-abdominal, intrathoracic, and intracranial pressure. Crit Care Med. 1997;25(3):496–503.
3. Kuteesa J, Kituuka O, Namuguzi D, Ndikuno C, Kirunda S, Mukunya D, Galukande M. Intra-abdominal hypertension; prevalence, incidence and outcomes in a low resource setting; a prospective observational study. World J Emerg Surg. 2015;10:57. https://doi.org/10.1186/s13017-015-0051-4. eCollection 2015.
4. Mbiine R, Alenyo R, Kobusingye O, Kuteesa J, Nakanwagi C, Lekuya HM, Kituuka O, Galukande M. Intra-abdominal hypertension in severe burns: prevalence, incidence and mortality in a sub-Saharan African hospital. Int J Burns Trauma. 2017;7(6):80–7. eCollection 2017.
5. Glass GE, Staruch RM, Simmons J, Lawton G, Nanchahal J, Jain A, Hettiaratchy SP. Managing missed lower extremity compartment syndrome in the physiologically stable patient: a systematic review and lessons from a Level I trauma center. J Trauma Acute Care Surg. 2016;81(2):380–7. https://doi.org/10.1097/TA.0000000000001107.
6. Roberts CS, Gorczyca JT, Ring D, Pugh KJ. Diagnosis and treatment of less common compartment syndromes of the upper and lower extremities: current evidence and best practices. Instr Course Lect. 2011;60:43–50.

7. Stella M, Santolini E, Sanguineti F, Felli L, Vicenti G, Bizzoca D, Santolini F. Aetiology of trauma-related acute compartment syndrome of the leg: a systematic review. Injury. 2019;50(Suppl 2):S57–64. https://doi.org/10.1016/j.injury.2019.01.047. Epub 2019 Feb 2.
8. Shadgan B, Menon M, Sanders D, Berry G, Martin C Jr, Duffy P, Stephen D, O'Brien PJ. Current thinking about acute compartment syndrome of the lower extremity. Can J Surg. 2010;53(5):329–34.
9. Long B, Koyfman A, Gottlieb M. Evaluation and management of acute compartment syndrome in the emergency department. J Emerg Med. 2019;56(4):386–97. https://doi.org/10.1016/j.jemermed.2018.12.021. Epub 2019 Jan 23.
10. Sellei RM, Andruszkow H, Weber C, Damen TO, Pape HC, Hildebrand F. Diagnostics and treatment decisions in acute compartment syndrome. Results of a survey in German hospitals. Unfallchirurg. 2016;119(2):125–32. https://doi.org/10.1007/s00113-014-2609-0.
11. von Keudell AG, Weaver MJ, Appleton PT, Bae DS, Dyer GSM, Heng M, Jupiter JB, Vrahas MS. Diagnosis and treatment of acute extremity compartment syndrome. Lancet. 2015;386(10000):1299–310. https://doi.org/10.1016/S0140-6736(15)00277-9.
12. Walters TJ, Kottke MA, Hargens AR, Ryan KL. Noninvasive diagnostics for extremity compartment syndrome following traumatic injury: a state-of-the-art review. J Trauma Acute Care Surg. 2019;87(1S Suppl 1):S59–66. https://doi.org/10.1097/TA.0000000000002284.
13. Donaldson J, Haddad B, Khan WS. The pathophysiology, diagnosis and current management of acute compartment syndrome. Open Orthop J. 2014;8:185–93. https://doi.org/10.217 4/1874325001408010185. eCollection 2014.
14. Rogers WK, Garcia L. Intraabdominal hypertension, abdominal compartment syndrome, and the open abdomen. Chest. 2018;153(1):238–50. https://doi.org/10.1016/j.chest.2017.07.023. Epub 2017 Aug 2.
15. Onichimowski D, Podlińska I, Sobiech S, Ropiak R. Measurement of the intra abdominal pressure in clinical practice. Anestezjol Intens Ter. 2010;42(2):107–12.
16. Hecker A, Hecker B, Hecker M, Riedel JG, Weigand MA, Padberg W. Acute abdominal compartment syndrome: current diagnostic and therapeutic options. Langenbecks Arch Surg. 2016;401(1):15–24. https://doi.org/10.1007/s00423-015-1353-4. Epub 2015 Oct 30.
17. Scalea TM, Bochicchio GV, Habashi N, McCunn M, Shih D, McQuillan K, Aarabi B. Increased intra-abdominal, intrathoracic, and intracranial pressure after severe brain injury: multiple compartment syndrome. J Trauma. 2007;62(3):647–56; discussion 656.
18. Balogh ZJ, Martin A, van Wessem KP, King KL, Mackay P, Havill K. Mission to eliminate postinjury abdominal compartment syndrome. Arch Surg. 2011;146(8):938–43. https://doi.org/10.1001/archsurg.2011.73. Epub 2011 Apr 18.
19. Strang SG, Van Imhoff DL, Van Lieshout EM, D'Amours SK, Van Waes OJ. Identifying patients at risk for high-grade intra-abdominal hypertension following trauma laparotomy. Injury. 2015;46(5):843–8. https://doi.org/10.1016/j.injury.2014.12.020. Epub 2015 Jan 15.
20. Khan S, Verma AK, Ahmad SM, Ahmad R. Analyzing intra-abdominal pressures and outcomes in patients undergoing emergency laparotomy. J Emerg Trauma Shock. 2010;3(4):318–25. https://doi.org/10.4103/0974-2700.70747.
21. Scollay JM, de Beaux I, Parks RW. Prospective study of intra-abdominal pressure following major elective abdominal surgery. World J Surg. 2009;33(11):2372–7. https://doi.org/10.1007/s00268-009-0191-3.
22. Yi M, Leng Y, Bai Y, Yao G, Zhu X. The evaluation of the effect of body positioning on intra-abdominal pressure measurement and the effect of intra-abdominal pressure at different body positioning on organ function and prognosis in critically ill patients. J Crit Care. 2012;27(2):222.e1–6. https://doi.org/10.1016/j.jcrc.2011.08.010. Epub 2011 Oct 26.
23. Schachtrupp A, Wetter O, Höer J. Influence of elevated intra-abdominal pressure on suture tension dynamics in a porcine model. J Surg Res. 2019;233:207–12. https://doi.org/10.1016/j.jss.2018.07.043. Epub 2018 Aug 31.
24. Kirkpatrick AW, Roberts DJ, De Waele J, Jaeschke R, Malbrain ML, De Keulenaer B, Duchesne J, Bjorck M, Leppaniemi A, Ejike JC, Sugrue M, Cheatham M, Ivatury R, Ball CG, Reintam Blaser A, Regli A, Balogh ZJ, D'Amours S, Debergh D, Kaplan M, Kimball E, Olvera C,

Pediatric Guidelines Sub-Committee for the World Society of the Abdominal Compartment Syndrome. Intra-abdominal hypertension and the abdominal compartment syndrome: updated consensus definitions and clinical practice guidelines from the World Society of the Abdominal Compartment Syndrome. Intensive Care Med. 2013;39(7):1190–206. https://doi.org/10.1007/s00134-013-2906-z. Epub 2013 May 15.

25. Popescu GA, Bara T, Rad P. Abdominal compartment syndrome as a multidisciplinary challenge. A literature review. J Crit Care Med (Targu Mures). 2018;4(4):114–9. https://doi.org/10.2478/jccm-2018-0024. eCollection 2018 Oct.

26. Roberts DJ, Ball CG, Kirkpatrick AW. Increased pressure within the abdominal compartment: intra-abdominal hypertension and the abdominal compartment syndrome. Curr Opin Crit Care. 2016;22(2):174–85. https://doi.org/10.1097/MCC.0000000000000289.

27. Cheatham ML, Safcsak K. Intra-abdominal hypertension and abdominal compartment syndrome: the journey forward. Am Surg. 2011;77(Suppl 1):S1–5.

28. Muresan M, Muresan S, Brinzaniuc K, Voidazan S, Sala D, Jimborean O, Hussam AH, Bara T Jr, Popescu G, Borz C, Neagoe R. How much does decompressive laparotomy reduce the mortality rate in primary abdominal compartment syndrome?: a single-center prospective study on 66 patients. Medicine (Baltimore). 2017;96(5):e6006. https://doi.org/10.1097/MD.0000000000006006.

29. Wandling MW, An GC. A case report of thoracic compartment syndrome in the setting of penetrating chest trauma and review of the literature. World J Emerg Surg. 2010;5:22. https://doi.org/10.1186/1749-7922-5-22.

30. Smith M. Refractory intracranial hypertension: the role of decompressive craniectomy. Anesth Analg. 2017;125(6):1999–2008. https://doi.org/10.1213/ANE.0000000000002399.

31. Beuriat PA, Javouhey E, Szathmari A, Courtil-Tesseydre S, Desgranges FP, Grassiot B, Hequet O, Mottolese C. Decompressive craniectomy in the treatment of post-traumatic intracranial hypertension in children: our philosophy and indications. J Neurosurg Sci. 2015;59(4):405–28. Epub 2015 Mar 10.

32. Miglietta MA, Salzano LJ, Chiu WC, Scalea TM. Decompressive laparotomy: a novel approach in the management of severe intracranial hypertension. J Trauma. 2003;55(3):551–4; discussion 554–5.

33. Joseph B, Zangbar B, Pandit V, Vercruysse G, Aziz H, Kulvatunyou N, Wynne J, O'Keeffe T, Tang A, Friese RS, Rhee P. The conjoint effect of reduced crystalloid administration and decreased damage-control laparotomy use in the development of abdominal compartment syndrome. J Trauma Acute Care Surg. 2014;76(2):457–61. https://doi.org/10.1097/TA.0b013e3182a9ea44.

Compartment Syndromes: Short-Term Outcomes

17

Andrew Nguyen, Arnold Tabuenca, and Raul Coimbra

17.1 Abdominal Compartment Syndrome

17.1.1 History and Definition

In the 1800s there began to emerge an understanding that elevated intra-abdominal pressure caused physiologic changes in several organ systems. Both Marey in 1863 and Paul Bert in 1870 demonstrated respiratory changes with rising intra-abdominal pressure. In 1890, Haase showed that intra-abdominal pressure increased with inspiratory effort. In 1890 also, Heinricius published that in cats and guinea pigs, intra-abdominal pressures of 27–46 cm of water caused death by interference of respiration [1].

By 1911, Emerson noted that elevated intra-abdominal pressure would "fatigue the diaphragm." Elevated intra-abdominal pressures would also cause "venous stagnation in the abdominal viscera" and thus diminish right-heart venous return. This resulted in "diminished [cardiac] output and fall in arterial pressure" [2].

In the modern era, Kron published in 1983 a series of postoperative patients that developed increased intra-abdominal pressure as well as new-onset renal failure.

A. Nguyen
Loma Linda University School of Medicine, Loma Linda, CA, USA

Division of Acute Care Surgery, Riverside University Health System, Moreno Valley, CA, USA

A. Tabuenca
Department of Surgery, University of California Riverside, Riverside, CA, USA

Riverside University Health System, Moreno Valley, CA, USA

R. Coimbra (✉)
Loma Linda University School of Medicine, Loma Linda, CA, USA

Riverside University Health System Medical Center, Moreno Valley, CA, USA
e-mail: r.coimbra@ruhealth.org, rcoimbra@llu.edu

© Springer Nature Switzerland AG 2021
F. Coccolini et al. (eds.), *Compartment Syndrome*, Hot Topics in Acute Care
Surgery and Trauma, https://doi.org/10.1007/978-3-030-55378-4_17

The patients' renal failure resolved with re-laparotomy and abdominal decompression [3].

We now recognize that abnormal abdominal pressures exist along a continuum, with maladaptive changes occurring at certain lower pressures and more severe ramifications at higher pressures. While pressures at which maladaptive changes can occur may vary from patient to patient, more significant than a single pressure value is the recognition of critical organ failure. Thus, with an improved understanding of intra-abdominal pressure, and standardization to measurements in mmHg instead of cm H_2O, the World Society of the Abdominal Compartment Syndrome (WSACS) has standardized the classification of intra-abdominal hypertension into [4]:

Grade I: IAP 12–15 mmHg
Grade II: IAP 16–20 mmHg
Grade III: IAP 21–25 mmHg
Grade IV: IAP >25 mmHg

Abdominal compartment syndrome itself is now defined as bladder-pressure measurements higher than 20 mmHg with new-organ failure.

17.1.2 Etiology and Pathophysiology

While elevated intra-abdominal pressure can have significant clinical repercussions, there were many direct causes that were quickly recognized to contribute to the phenomenon. Direct intra-abdominal pathologies include intraperitoneal causes, such as trauma, hemorrhage, and retained lap pads from intra-abdominal packing. Nontraumatic causes include malignancy, pancreatitis, ascites, ileus, bowel obstruction, and ruptured abdominal aortic aneurysm. It was quickly recognized that rapidly increasing space-occupying lesions within the abdomen can contribute to elevated intra-abdominal pressure.

It was recognized later that resuscitation can induce a "secondary abdominal compartment syndrome." In 1994, Greenhalgh and Warden published a series involving 30 children with burns [5]. Defining elevated intra-abdominal pressure as more than 30 mmHg, five patients had elevated intra-abdominal pressure during acute resuscitation, two of which required escharotomies. Seven patients developed elevated intra-abdominal pressures from sepsis, one of which required a laparotomy and another required decompression with an intra-abdominal catheter. In 1995, Burrows reported a trauma case in which intra-abdominal compartment syndrome resulted from management of an isolated extremity injury [6]. Fabian et al., in 1999, published the first large series of secondary compartment syndrome, finding that while 46 of 1216 ICU admissions required laparotomy for compartment syndrome, 6 of their patients had no intra-abdominal injuries [7]. Resuscitation in these six patients prior to decompressive laparotomy averaged 19 L of crystalloid and 29 units of packed red blood cells. They concluded that abdominal compartment syndrome could occur without intra-abdominal injury. The World Society on Abdominal Compartment Syndrome recognized Secondary ACS in 2006 as abdominal compartment syndrome arising from conditions that do not originate in the abdomino-pelvic region [8]. Primary ACS, in contrast, was associated with injury or disease in the abdominopelvic region. They also recognized recurrent ACS as arising after previous surgical or medical treatment of primary or secondary abdominal compartment syndrome.

17.1.2.1 Cardiac Effects

The effect of intra-abdominal hypertension on cardiac function is multifactorial. Classically, it is accepted that increased abdominal pressure augments pressure on the inferior vena cava and reduces venous return to the heart; thus, cardiac output drops as predicted by the Starling curve dynamics. However, studies in patients as well as in an animal model have shown that as intra-abdominal pressure rises, central venous and wedge pressures rise [9, 10]. During this time, there is a decline in cardiac output paired with a rise in systemic vascular resistance. This suggests that many of the cardiac derangements and hemodynamic secondary to abdominal hypertension be more related to increased afterload. While decompressive laparotomy improves overall hemodynamics in patients with compartment syndrome, there are reports of hypotension in the immediate post-laparotomy period due to a rapid fall in systemic vascular resistance [11].

17.1.2.2 Renal Effects

As intra-abdominal hypertension progresses, there is decreased urine output and elevation in serum creatinine. Oliguria can be seen at intrabdominal pressures as low as 15 mmHg, while anuria can be seen at pressures of 30 mmHg. Timely decompressive laparotomy often results in rapid improvement in renal function. Several hypotheses have been proposed regarding the underlying pathophysiology for renal failure in this setting. One theory is that direct compression of the kidney causes a decrease in perfusion pressure and glomerular filtration rate. This was proposed in a 1982 study in dogs; intraperitoneal bags were inflated causing a decrease in cardiac output, renal blood flow, and glomerular filtration rate (GFR). Resuscitation improved cardiac output, but renal blood flow and GFR remained low, suggesting that the changes at the level of the kidney were not due to cardiac dysfunction [12]. This concept was challenged by another study showing that direct external renal compression did not affect GFR or renal artery blood flow [13]. Currently, the most commonly suspected mechanism is that compression of the renal vein reduces renal blood flow and induces renal failure. A study in a pig model showed that increasing pressure on the renal vein produced the expected decrease in GFR and renal arterial blood flow [14].

17.1.2.3 Pulmonary Effects

Elevated intra-abdominal pressure places resistance on the diaphragm and results in decreased pulmonary compliance. Elevated peak and plateau pressures are seen in patients undergoing volume-cycled mechanical ventilation. Patients undergoing pressure control ventilation will exhibit decreased tidal volumes. With continued resistance from intra-abdominal pressure, hypercarbia and respiratory acidosis occur. While oxygenation may be better preserved than carbon dioxide exchange, many critically ill patients can also develop worsening hypoxia. Timely decompressive laparotomy results in improvement in lung mechanics, while extended exposure to barotrauma can result in acute respiratory distress syndrome.

17.1.3 Diagnosis

Early investigations into intra-abdominal pressure were confounded by different methods of obtaining an accurate pressure reading. Strictly speaking, true intraperitoneal pressure measurements would utilize intraperitoneal catheters, and such approaches were used by Winkler and Quirin [15]. While surrogate measures for intraperitoneal pressures include stomach, rectum, or IVC pressure, bladder pressure measurement has emerged as an effective, simple, and accurate way of indirectly measuring intra-abdominal pressure. This current methodology centers around the procedure described by Kron in 1983 [3]. After Foley catheter placement and drainage of the bladder, 50–100 mL of saline is instilled. A pressure monitor is then connected to the Foley catheter. Bladder pressure measurement has been validated in an animal study with a rabbit model, with intra-abdominal pressure modulated by a specifically placed intraperitoneal balloon. There was good correlation between intra-abdominal pressure and bladder pressure (correlation factor $>+0.855$ and $p < 0.001$) [16]. Later studies have demonstrated that over-instilling the bladder may produce inaccurate pressure values [17]. Current guidelines recommend instilling no more than 25 mL of saline in the bladder. In an effort to standardize measurements of bladder pressure, the World Society for Abdominal Compartment Syndrome (WSACS) also recommends expressing intra-abdominal pressure in mmHg, measuring at the end of expiration with the patient in the supine position, and zeroing the transducer to the level of the midaxillary line [4].

17.1.4 Current Treatment Recommendations

The World Society for Abdominal Compartment Syndrome recommends several maneuvers to treat intra-abdominal hypertension. Evacuation of intraluminal contents can be done with nasogastric tubes and rectal tubes. Patients with colonic pseudoobstruction can be considered for neostigmine. Patients with ascites as the main driver for their intra-abdominal hypertension can have drainage of their peritoneal fluid to reduce abdominal pressure. Abdominal wall compliance can potentially be improved with adequate sedation and analgesia, and if needed neuromuscular blockade. Optimal fluid balance should be achieved to minimize volume overloading [4].

Patients progressing to abdominal compartment syndrome, however, should be strongly considered for decompressive laparotomy, which remains the mainstay of treatment for patients that develop abdominal compartment syndrome. Kron's 1983 seminal paper noted that all patients that underwent decompressive laparotomy had improvement in renal function. The four patients managed without surgery all continued in renal failure and ultimately died. Patients undergoing laparotomy for abdominal compartment syndrome invariably have improvement in their hemodynamic status and intra-abdominal pressure [3]. Promptness of decompression remains critical. In Fabian's 1999 series, it was noted that time to laparotomy was 3 h in survivors and 25 h in non-survivors. Thus, urgent decompressive laparotomy for abdominal compartment syndrome remains the rule with few exceptions [7].

17.1.5 Outcomes

Before a consensus approach was developed in 2006, the epidemiology of abdominal compartment syndrome was complicated by variable definitions of ACS. Despite a unifying clinical definition, ACS is a heterogenous inciting event, though most studies evaluating the incidence of ACS involve trauma patients. Furthermore, it appears that with changing philosophies and patterns in resuscitation, the incidence of ACS may be decreasing [18]. The prevalence of abdominal compartment syndrome in at-risk patients has ranged from 1 to 14%, with the incidence appearing to be lower in more recent studies [19–22]. It is now clear that when left untreated, abdominal compartment syndrome leads to tissue hypoperfusion, multisystem organ failure, and mortality. While intra-abdominal hypertension alone does not correlate with multiorgan failure, patients that progress to abdominal compartment syndrome can have mortality rates of 36% or more [23, 24]. Malbrain's 2004 multicenter trial showed that non-survivors had higher intrabdominal pressure, were older, and had worse APACHE 2 score [19]. Liver dysfunction and surgical disease process (as opposed to medical admissions) were more likely to be associated with mortality.

Surgical decompression of abdominal compartment syndrome is almost always effective, with improvement in hemodynamics, renal function, and pulmonary pressures. However, surgical decompression also carries a separate metabolic burden [25, 26] as well as reperfusion injury [27].

While many patients overcome these challenges, a recurring clinical goal is successful closure of the abdominal wound. Failure rates to close the abdomen can range from 20 to 78%, and many can develop severe morbidities [28–30]. One recent study showed that 24% of open-abdomen patients had one or more of a variety of complications, ranging from infection, recurrent abdominal compartment syndrome, entero-atmospheric fistula, and hernia [23]. In another multicenter trial from 2011, fistula formation was found in 7% of open-abdomen patients [31].

A concerted effort to close the abdomen as rapidly as possible reduces complications and mortality. In 2010, Cheatham described the change in approach within a single institution regarding the open abdomen [24]. Over the time period of the study, the center saw the adoption of WSACS guidelines and definitions for abdominal compartment syndrome, as well as a reduction in the threshold for laparotomy in accordance with WSACS guidelines. Finding many patients with open abdomens, the institution developed a management algorithm with a focused effort to close the abdomen as early as possible. While severity of illness remained unchanged over the 6-year period, patient survival to hospital discharge increased from 50 to 72% ($p = 0.015$). There was also an improvement in primary fascial closure from 59 to 81%, and improvements in resource utilization. Chen's meta-analysis from 2014 confirmed that early fascial closure (defined as within 2–3 weeks) resulted in a reduction in mortality (12.3% vs. 24.8%, $p < 0.0001$) as well as complications (RR = 0.68, $p < 0.0001$) [32].

Early methods of temporary abdominal closure include sterilized intravenous fluid bags, PTFE sheets, Bogota bags, and gauze dressings [33]. All of these methods can be potentially augmented with negative dynamic retention sutures or Velcro-assisted closure ("artificial burr" or "Wittmann patch").

Since then, negative pressure wound therapy has arisen as a common method of managing the open abdomen. Barker in 2000 published a series of 112 trauma patients with open abdomens; the temporary closure method used a perforated polyethylene sheet as a barrier against the viscera, which was then covered in a moist towel and suction tubing, and finally covered by an iodophor-impregnated adhesive polyethylene sheet [34]. 55.4% of patients had primary closure, while 22.3% had a repair with absorbable mesh. Complication rates included 19.6% who died before abdominal closure was performed, 4.5% with enterocutaneous fistula, and 4.5% with intra-abdominal abscess formation. While the Barker wound closure or a modification of this method is utilized in many centers, now purpose-built commercial wound vacs such as the ABThera are widely available.

There have been many studies seeking to elucidate the best method of temporary abdominal closure. The data, however, are heterogenous. A 2008 meta-analysis suggested that high fascial closure rates were found with Velcro closure (90%), dynamic retention sutures (85%), and wound vac (60%) [35]. A 2012 meta-analysis suggested that the highest fascial closure rate was found with Velcro closure (78%), dynamic retention sutures (71%), and wound vac methods (61%) [36]. Another 2012 meta-analysis with differing methodology suggested that the use of sequential fascial closure to the abdominal wound vac had a higher fascial closure rate [37]. The most recent systematic review published in 2016 compared negative pressure therapy vs. standard temporary closure. There was no difference in fascial closure (63.5% vs. 69.5%, $p = 0.57$) and enterocutaneous fistula rate (2.1% vs. 5.8%, $p = 0.57$). However, the negative pressure wound therapy group did have reduced mortality (28.5% vs. 41.4$, $p = 0.03$) and decreased ICU length of stay [38].

Another technique to augment abdominal negative pressure therapy is direct peritoneal resuscitation (DPR). DPR techniques instill peritoneal dialysate solutions into the abdomen while a negative pressure dressing evacuates excess fluid. Animal studies demonstrated improved visceral blood flow even while visceral edema was reduced [39]. In 2010, Smith et al. published a series of open-abdomen trauma patients, with 20 patients utilizing DPR against 40 control patients (control patients did not have a standardized abdominal wound management technique) [40]. Time to definitive abdominal closure was improved with the DPR group (DPR

4.35 ± 1.6 days versus control 7.05 ± 3.31; $p = 0.003$). The DPR group also had a high rate of primary fascial closure and decreased 6-month ventral hernia rate. While abdominal closure method was not standardized within the control group, subgroup analysis comparing DPR against controls utilizing a Velcro closure technique confirmed decreased time to definitive closure (DPR 4.4 ± 1.7 days versus Velcro 6.4 ± 1.3, $p = 0.003$). While DPR shows promise in improving fascial closure rates and decreasing complications associated with the open abdomen, further prospective studies are needed.

Complications surrounding the open abdomen in abdominal compartment syndrome
 Infection (12%)
 Recurrent abdominal compartment syndrome (6%)
 Bleeding (6%)
 Entero-atmospheric fistula (3%)
 Hernia (15%)
 Mortality (36%)
Efforts to mitigate complications may include
 Protocolized effort to close the abdomen as rapidly as possible
 Use of negative pressure wound therapy
 Velcro closure
 Dynamic retention sutures
 Direct peritoneal resuscitation

Complications adapted from De Waele JJ, Kimball E, Malbrain M, Nesbitt I, Cohen J, Kaloiani V, Ivatury R, Mone M, Debergh D, Björck M. Decompressive laparotomy for abdominal compartment syndrome. Br J Surg. 2016 May;103 (6):709–715. doi: https://doi.org/10.1002/bjs.10097

17.2 Muscle Compartment Syndrome

17.2.1 Pathophysiology and Diagnosis

Compartment syndrome occurs when swelling within a muscle compartment causes tissue ischemia. While commonly associated with bony injury or reperfusion injury after prolonged ischemia, there are a variety of other causes including crush injuries, burns, and electrocution. Many patients present with the syndrome in the lower leg, and in one series this was most associated with the lower leg [41]. However, virtually any muscular compartment of the body can be at risk, including the hands, forearm, upper arm, buttocks, and thighs.

Elevation in compartment pressures exceeds capillary filling pressure, resulting in muscle ischemia. While local muscle ischemia can carry immediate morbid complications, systemic illness can result from compartment syndrome. This includes rhabdomyolysis and renal failure. Renal failure in the critically ill patient is a significant marker for mortality and other complications.

Classically, the diagnosis of compartment syndrome is clinical. The historical six Ps of compartment syndrome are pain, pallor, pulselessness, paresthesia, paralysis, and poikilothermia [42]. While pain out of proportion is an early sign, and paresthesia can result from nerve compression as compartment edema increases, waiting for all the signs to develop can result in irreversible muscle injury and systemic organ failure. Indeed, irreversible muscle ischemia is thought to occur 8 h after loss of perfusion [43].

While there is no consensus for a diagnostic algorithm for muscle compartment syndrome, clinical suspicion based on history and physical exam findings is usually used. To confirm clinical suspicion in borderline cases, compartment pressure measurements can be used. Most typically, a needle connected to a pressure transducer is used, with many considering a compartment pressure between 30 and 50 mmHg as critically high. Others advocate the use of compartment perfusion pressure (MAP—compartment pressure), with a delta-P of less than 30 mmHg thought to be concerning [42]. An adjunct under consideration to improve the rapid diagnosis of extremity compartment syndrome is near-infrared spectroscopy, which measures tissue oxygenation up to 3 cm deep from the skin [44]. Another option is measuring intramuscular glucose concentration, which diminishes as compartment syndrome develops [45]. The role of these adjuncts in the diagnosis of compartment syndrome, however, remains unclear.

17.2.2 Treatment

Treatment of compartment syndrome centers on fasciotomy, the surgical release of the affected muscle compartments. Timing is critical, as worsening time markers allow for increased muscle death and systemic complications.

In patients with rhabdomyolysis, medical therapy includes aggressive hydration to promote renal perfusion and to dilute myoglobin levels, prevention of myoglobin deposition in the renal tubule via alkalization of the urine, and intravenous mannitol for renal vasodilatation and free radical scavenging.

In the past, fluid resuscitation as high as 1.5 L NaCl 0.9% per hour has been advocated [46]. More recently, to prevent complications of overload such as abdominal compartment syndrome or respiratory failure, more modest goals often accepted are 3–6 L in the first 24 h with additional volume dependent on hemodynamic and urinary output parameters [46].

Mannitol is thought to protect against rhabdomyolysis by its free radical scavenging action and may also prevent renal failure by increasing the volume passing through the renal tubule [47]. Another adjunct is bicarbonate. Intravenous bicarbonate results in alkalization of the urine, a goal derived from laboratory data showing that only 4% of myoglobin aggregates at urine pH above 6.5.

17.2.3 Outcomes

Due to the time-critical nature of fasciotomy, one focus on improving outcomes is the rapid identification and rapid surgical decompression of affected muscle compartments. Diagnosis of compartment syndrome still hinges on clinical suspicion; measurement of spot compartment pressures can be used to confirm clinical suspicion, but there is little data to support that it changes outcomes. Indeed, compartment pressures can have false negatives, or an incorrect compartment checked, giving a false sense of clinical stability. Adjuncts to diagnosis, including intramuscular glucose and near-infrared spectroscopy, remain unproven [48].

What is clear, however, is that there are numerous studies confirming that early fasciotomy is effective. In 1984, Rorabeck noted that if fasciotomies were done within 24 h, a good result was "almost always achieved" [49]. In 1976, Sheridan noted that in patients undergoing fasciotomy within 12 h, 68% had normal function compared to only 8% of those undergoing late fasciotomy [50].

More recent data still emphasizes the need for early fasciotomy. Hope noted in 2004 that in patients without fracture, the suspicion for compartment syndrome can be lower and the diagnosis can be delayed. In the setting of patients without fracture, there was greater delay and 20% of these patients had muscle necrosis requiring debridement. In comparison, in patients with a fracture, only 8% needed debridement [51]. In the military population, where medical evacuation can delay fasciotomy, significant morbidities were noted. In 2008, Ritenour noted that soldiers that underwent fasciotomy after medical evacuation (vs. fasciotomy in the combat theatre) had more instances of muscle debridement (25% vs. 11%), higher rates of amputation (31% vs. 15%), and elevated mortality (19% vs. 5%) than patients who had fasciotomies in the combat theatre ($p < 0.01$) [52].

While it is thought to be better to perform an unnecessary fasciotomy than a late fasciotomy, surgical decompression still carries its own risks such as chronic wounds, delayed healing, need for skin graft, pain, nerve injury, and muscle weakness [48]. Dermatotraction techniques such as the "Jacob's ladder" have been demonstrated to assist with wound closure and reduce need for skin grafting [53].

For patients with rhabdomyolysis, modulating outcomes with medical therapy remains unclear. While mannitol is commonly used by many clinicians for rhabdomyolysis in the setting of compartment syndrome, there are no randomized trials involving the use of mannitol. Similarly, the use of intravenous bicarbonate is controversial. In the largest study to date of compartment syndrome in trauma patients, bicarbonate and mannitol together was compared with patients who did not receive combination therapy. The combination did not prevent renal failure or dialysis or reduce mortality [54].

17.2.3.1   Hand

One of the main complications for hand compartment syndrome is the development of hand contracture as ischemic muscle becomes necrotic and eventually fibrotic. There is currently scarce literature regarding functional outcomes in these patients. In a retrospective review by Oulette in 1996, 4 of 19 patients were noted to have poor hand function. Time from diagnosis to treatment for these patients was more than 6 h. Two patients eventually required an amputation. Thirteen had normal function, but some required further surgery to facilitate wound healing and ameliorate nerve compression [55].

17.2.3.2 Forearm and Upper Arm

Forearm compartment syndrome requires a high clinical suspicion. Kalyani's systematic review from 2011 showed a 42% complication rate. Neurologic deficit was the most common complication (20.9%). Other complications were contracture (9.3%), crush syndrome (4.7%), gangrene (2.3%), Volkmann's ischemic contracture (2.3%), and Sudeck's algodystrophy (2.3%) [56]. Outcomes data is less forthcoming in upper arm compartment syndrome due to its exceeding rarity, but the principles of timely fasciotomy remain. A series by Duckworth in 2012 showed that patients with forearm fasciotomies delayed by more than 6 h were more likely to have complications (most commonly neurologic deficit and contractures) [57].

17.2.3.3 Gluteal Region

Gluteal compartment syndrome is exceedingly rare, often creating a delay in diagnosis. In addition to muscle necrosis and complex morbid wounds, sciatic nerve palsy can develop from untreated compartment syndrome in this area [58].

17.2.3.4 Foot

Management of foot compartment syndrome has some controversy, with nine different foot compartments and fasciotomy presenting potential morbidities [59, 60]. There is data that suggest no difference in motor, sensory defects, and pain between patients who undergo fasciotomy versus those that do not [61]. Despite this, fasciotomy remains a mainstay of treatment. Lokiec noted that the most common complications were neurologic defects (52%), toe contractures, (12%), and amputations (12%) [62]. A 2009 systematic review aggregating 39 patients showed that only 10% were able to return to work [63]. More recent data from 2015 showed that 79% were able to return to work [64].

17.2.3.5 Lower Extremity

Due to the relative prevalence of compartment syndrome of the lower extremity in comparison to other compartments, thigh and calf compartment syndrome remains the prototypical example of extremity compartment syndrome [41]. In a 2016 review, acute kidney injury was found in 2.4% of lower extremity compartment syndrome. 12.9% of patients required amputation. 10.2% had lower extremity pain, foot numbness was noted in 20.5%, and a foot drop was found in 1.2%. 69% of patients were able to return to employment [65].

Complications surrounding muscle compartment syndrome
Delay in diagnosis
Rhabdomyolysis with or without renal failure
Contracture
Nerve damage
Tissue necrosis
Mortality
Efforts to mitigate complications may include
Early diagnosis with assistance of pressure monitoring
Near-infrared spectroscopy (experimental)
Intramuscular glucose concentration (experimental)
Early fasciotomy
Adequate resuscitation with possible use of adjuncts such as mannitol and bicarbonate

17.3   Thoracic Compartment Syndrome

17.3.1 Pathophysiology

Thoracic compartment syndrome is an exceedingly rare condition that has been reported after pediatric and adult cardiac surgery, and less commonly seen after trauma. Postoperative myocardial edema or cardiac dilatation, combined with chest wall and mediastinal edema, leads to compression of the heart, diminished diastolic filling, and thus decreasing cardiac output [66]. The condition can occur hours to days after chest closure, and if left untreated can lead to cardiovascular collapse. Diagnosis relies on a high index of suspicion in the setting of cardiac tamponade like physiology.

17.3.2 Management

Temporary closure of the chest can be achieved with a synthetic material, such as polytetrafluoroethylene, which is sutured to the sternal and skin edge [67]. Another option is skin closure without sternal re-approximation [68]. In addition, chest tubes can be used to stent open the sternum and thus elevate the sternum above the heart [69]. In one case report, a sternal traction device was used to maintain the sternum in an open position [70].

In one study in neonates, successful closure of the sternum was still noted to cause some increase in pulmonary arterial pressure, left and right atrial pressure, and peak airway pressure [71].

17.3.3 Outcomes

In the pediatric patient population, a series of 113 patients with prolonged open sternotomy showed a 36.2% mortality rate, versus 5.4% in patients with primary sternal closure. Mortality was higher in patients with low cardiac output after cardiopulmonary bypass, in those that needed a circulatory assist device, and in those that developed postoperative tamponade requiring reopening of the sternum in the ICU. Primary cause of mortality was heart failure, illustrative of the patient population. Other causes of death were pulmonary hypertension, multiorgan failure, and intracranial hemorrhage. Only one patient had mediastinitis [69].

A 1996 series demonstrated a mortality rate of 36.6% in 123 adult patients who underwent cardiac surgery and required prolonged open sternotomy. Need for an intra-aortic balloon pump postoperatively was associated with greater mortality (46.3% vs. 16%, $p < 0.01$). Other reported complications included superficial sternal wound infection (1.6%), mediastinitis (0.8%), and sternal dehiscence (2.4%) [72].

An earlier series in 1992 had a higher rate of mediastinitis in the open chest group (4–6%), but this was still within the range of the overall cardiothoracic patient group (0.15–5%) [73].

Complications surrounding the open chest in thoracic compartment syndrome
  Superficial sternal wound infection (1.6%)
  Mediastinitis (0.8%)
  Sternal dehiscence (2.4%)
  Mortality (36.6%)
Efforts to mitigate complications may include
  Temporary chest closure with synthetic material (such as polytetrafluoroethylene)
  Chest wound skin closure without sternal re-approximation
  Use of chest tube to stent open sternum above the heart

Complication rates adapted from Christenson JT, Maurice J, Simonet F, Velebit V, Schmuziger M. Open chest and delayed sternal closure after cardiac surgery. Eur J Cardiothorac Surg. 1996;10(5):305–11

17.4   Intracranial Hypertension

17.4.1 Pathophysiology

In the 1700s, Scottish physician Alexander Munro and Scottish surgeon George Kellie helped form the hypothesis that models intracranial pressure today. The skull is a fixed volume, and space must be shared by the brain parenchyma, blood, and cerebral spinal fluid. Any increase in any of these components results in elevated intracranial pressure [74]. The underlying disease process is broad, with the phenomenon of increased pressure described as intracranial hypertension. However, we will focus on medical therapies for intracranial hypertension in the setting of trauma.

17.4.2 Outcomes Based on ICP Monitoring

Intracranial pressure monitoring began with Lundberg in 1964, who implanted a ventricular catheter in 30 patients with traumatic brain injury [75]. They proposed that ICP values can be used to guide TBI management. In 1977, Miller's series of 160 patients identified that an ICP of more than 20 mmHg correlated with poor outcomes (defined as severely disabled, persistent vegetative state, or death) [76].

Today, medical options to modulate intracranial pressure include osmotic agents (hypertonic saline, mannitol), traditional sedatives (propofol, midazolam, dexmedetomidine), and barbiturates [77].

Hypertonic saline generates an osmotic gradient across the blood-brain barrier to decrease ICP. The agent demonstrates rapid onset and relatively long-lasting effects, as much as 12 h in some patients. In 2014, Colton showed that patients with ICP decreased for at least 2 h with the use of hypertonic saline had decreased mortality and improved functional outcomes [78]. Mannitol's use as an osmotic diuretic has a long-standing history in reducing ICP, though the agent can also cause hypotension. Studies comparing hypertonic saline to mannitol suggest that hypertonic saline may have a more dramatic and sustained reduction in ICP [77]. However, specific outcomes data is lacking.

Sedatives such as propofol and midazolam appear to decrease ICP similarly. Propofol may have added benefit against cerebral edema, while midazolam has anti-epileptic properties. Dexmedetomidine has been shown to reduce the amount of hypertonic saline or mannitol needed to maintain ICP within normal range [77].

Barbiturates are used as a second-line therapy in patients with refractory ICP. However, need for barbiturate use is associated with poorer outcomes, which is likely a reflection on the disease burden in patients with refractory intracranial hypertension [77].

Despite the ubiquity of ICP-guided management in the setting of TBI, its effectiveness remains unclear. Shafi's 2014 multicenter retrospective study on ICP therapy suggested that adherence to guidelines was associated with reduced mortality (OR 0.88; 95% CI 0.81–0.96, $p < 0.005$) [79]. In contrast, Cremer's 2005 study compared two well-matched trauma centers in the Netherlands: one that utilized ICP measurements, and the other that utilized CT scan and exam findings. The study found that while the ICP-focused center used more sedatives, barbiturates, vasopressors, and mannitol, there was no difference in mortality [80]. The only randomized trial data on ICP management comes from the 2012 Benchmark Evidence from South American Trials: Treatment of Intracranial Pressure (BEST:TRIP). Patients were randomized to ICP-guided management vs. treatment-guided CT imaging in conjunction with physical findings. Ultimately, 6-month mortality was similar in both groups (39% in ICP monitoring vs. 41% in imaging/exam, $p = 0.60$) [81].

It should be noted that these trials are not precisely ICP vs. no-ICP groups, but a comparison of TBI management guided by ICP vs. imaging and findings [74]. Ultimately, additional data are needed to accurately describe the optimal method of TBI management.

References

1. Coombs HC. The mechanism of the regulation of intra-abdominal pressure. Am J Physiol. 1920;61:159–63.
2. Emerson H. Intra-abdominal pressures. Arch Intern Med (Chic). 1911;VII(6):754–84. https://doi.org/10.1001/archinte.1911.00060060036002.
3. Kron IL, Harman PK, Nolan SP. The measurement of intra-abdominal pressure as a criterion for abdominal re-exploration. Ann Surg. 1984;199(1):28–30.
4. Kirkpatrick AW, Roberts DJ, De Waele J, Jaeschke R, Malbrain ML, De Keulenaer B, Duchesne J, Bjorck M, Leppaniemi A, Ejike JC, Sugrue M, Cheatham M, Ivatury R, Ball CG, Reintam Blaser A, Regli A, Balogh ZJ, D'Amours S, Debergh D, Kaplan M, Kimball E, Olvera C, Pediatric Guidelines Sub-Committee for the World Society of the Abdominal Compartment Syndrome. Intra-abdominal hypertension and the abdominal compartment syndrome: updated consensus definitions and clinical practice guidelines from the World Society of the Abdominal Compartment Syndrome. Intensive Care Med. 2013;39(7):1190–206. https://doi.org/10.1007/s00134-013-2906-z.
5. Greenhalgh DG, Warden GD. The importance of intra-abdominal pressure measurements in burned children. J Trauma. 1994;36(5):685–90.
6. Burrows R, Edington J, Robbs JV. A wolf in wolf's clothing—the abdominal compartment syndrome. S Afr Med J. 1995;85(1):46–8.

7. Maxwell RA, Fabian TC, Croce MA, Davis KA. Secondary abdominal compartment syndrome: an underappreciated manifestation of severe hemorrhagic shock. J Trauma. 1999;47(6):995–9.

8. Malbrain ML, Cheatham ML, Kirkpatrick A, Sugrue M, Parr M, De Waele J, Balogh Z, Leppäniemi A, Olvera C, Ivatury R, D'Amours S, Wendon J, Hillman K, Johansson K, Kolkman K, Wilmer A. Results from the international conference of experts on intra-abdominal hypertension and abdominal compartment syndrome. I. Definitions. Intensive Care Med. 2006;32(11):1722–32. Epub 2006 Sep 12.

9. Cullen DJ, Coyle JP, Teplick R, Long MC. Cardiovascular, pulmonary, and renal effects of massively increased intra-abdominal pressure in critically ill patients. Crit Care Med. 1989;17(2):118–21.

10. Ridings PC, Bloomfield GL, Blocher CR, Sugerman HJ. Cardiopulmonary effects of raised intra-abdominal pressure before and after intravascular volume expansion. J Trauma. 1995;39(6):1071–5.

11. Shelly MP, Robinson AA, Hesford JW, Park GR. Haemodynamic effects following surgical release of increased intra-abdominal pressure. Br J Anaesth. 1987;59(6):800–5.

12. Harman PK, Kron IL, McLachlan HD, Freedlender AE, Nolan SP. Elevated intra-abdominal pressure and renal function. Ann Surg. 1982;196(5):594–7.

13. Doty JM, Saggi BH, Blocher CR, Fakhry I, Gehr T, Sica D, Sugerman HJ. Effects of increased renal parenchymal pressure on renal function. J Trauma. 2000;48(5):874–7.

14. Doty JM, Saggi BH, Sugerman HJ, Blocher CR, Pin R, Fakhry I, Gehr TW, Sica DA. Effect of increased renal venous pressure on renal function. J Trauma. 1999;47(6):1000–3.

15. Overholt R. Intraperitoneal pressure. Arch Surg. 1931;22(5):691–703. https://doi.org/10.1001/archsurg.1931.01160050002001.

16. Lacey SR, Bruce J, Brooks SP, Griswald J, Ferguson W, Allen JE, Jewett TC Jr, Karp MP, Cooney DR. The relative merits of various methods of indirect measurement of intraabdominal pressure as a guide to closure of abdominal wall defects. J Pediatr Surg. 1987;22(12):1207–11.

17. Gudmundsson FF, Viste A, Gislason H, Svanes K. Comparison of different methods for measuring intra-abdominal pressure. Intensive Care Med. 2002;28(4):509–14.

18. Rogers WK, Garcia L. Intra-abdominal hypertension, abdominal compartment syndrome, and the open abdomen. Chest. 2018;153(1):238–50. https://doi.org/10.1016/j.chest.2017.07.023.

19. Malbrain ML, Chiumello D, Pelosi P, Wilmer A, Brienza N, Malcangi V, Bihari D, Innes R, Cohen J, Singer P, Japiassu A, Kurtop E, De Keulenaer BL, Daelemans R, Del Turco M, Cosimini P, Ranieri M, Jacquet L, Laterre PF, Gattinoni L. Prevalence of intra-abdominal hypertension in critically ill patients: a multicentre epidemiological study. Intensive Care Med. 2004;30(5):822–9.

20. Hong JJ, Cohn SM, Perez JM, Dolich MO, Brown M, McKenney MG. Prospective study of the incidence and outcome of intra-abdominal hypertension and the abdominal compartment syndrome. Br J Surg. 2002;89(5):591–6.

21. Balogh Z, McKinley BA, Holcomb JB, Miller CC, Cocanour CS, Kozar RA, Valdivia A, Ware DN, Moore FA. Both primary and secondary abdominal compartment syndrome can be predicted early and are harbingers of multiple organ failure. J Trauma. 2003;54(5):848–59; discussion 859–61.

22. Balogh Z, McKinley BA, Cocanour CS, Kozar RA, Holcomb JB, Ware DN, Moore FA. Secondary abdominal compartment syndrome is an elusive early complication of traumatic shock resuscitation. Am J Surg. 2002;184(6):538–43; discussion 543–4.

23. De Waele JJ, Kimball E, Malbrain M, Nesbitt I, Cohen J, Kaloiani V, Ivatury R, Mone M, Debergh D, Björck M. Decompressive laparotomy for abdominal compartment syndrome. Br J Surg. 2016;103(6):709–15. https://doi.org/10.1002/bjs.10097.

24. Cheatham ML, Safcsak K. Is the evolving management of intra-abdominal hypertension and abdominal compartment syndrome improving survival? Crit Care Med. 2010;38(2):402–7.

25. Rotstein OD. Modeling the two-hit hypothesis for evaluating strategies to prevent organ injury after shock/resuscitation. J Trauma. 2003;54(5 Suppl):S203–6.

26. Claridge JA, Weed AC, Enelow R, Young JS. Laparotomy potentiates cytokine release and impairs pulmonary function after hemorrhage and resuscitation in mice. J Trauma. 2001;50(2):244–52.

27. Kaçmaz A, Polat A, User Y, Tilki M, Ozkan S, Sener G. Octreotide improves reperfusion-induced oxidative injury in acute abdominal hypertension in rats. J Gastrointest Surg. 2004;8(1):113–9.
28. Miller PR, Meredith JW, Johnson JC, Chang MC. Prospective evaluation of vacuum-assisted fascial closure after open abdomen: planned ventral hernia rate is substantially reduced. Ann Surg. 2004;239(5):608–14. discussion 614–6.
29. Fabian TC. Damage control in trauma: laparotomy wound management acute to chronic. Surg Clin North Am. 2007;87(1):73–93, vi.
30. Joels CS, Vanderveer AS, Newcomb WL, Lincourt AE, Polhill JL, Jacobs DG, Sing RF, Heniford BT. Abdominal wall reconstruction after temporary abdominal closure: a ten-year review. Surg Innov. 2006;13(4):223–30.
31. Cheatham ML, Demetriades D, Fabian TC, Kaplan MJ, Miles WS, Schreiber MA, Holcomb JB, Bochicchio G, Sarani B, Rotondo MF. Prospective study examining clinical outcomes associated with a negative pressure wound therapy system and Barker's vacuum packing technique. World J Surg. 2013;37(9):2018–30. https://doi.org/10.1007/s00268-013-2080-z.
32. Chen Y, Ye J, Song W, Chen J, Yuan Y, Ren J. Comparison of outcomes between early fascial closure and delayed abdominal closure in patients with open abdomen: a systematic review and meta-analysis. Gastroenterol Res Pract. 2014;2014:784056. https://doi.org/10.1155/2014/784056.
33. Stevens P. Vacuum-assisted closure of laparostomy wounds: a critical review of the literature. Int Wound J. 2009;6(4):259–66. https://doi.org/10.1111/j.1742-481X.2009.00614.x.
34. Barker DE, Kaufman HJ, Smith LA, Ciraulo DL, Richart CL, Burns RP. Vacuum pack technique of temporary abdominal closure: a 7-year experience with 112 patients. J Trauma. 2000;48(2):201–6; discussion 206–7.
35. Boele van Hensbroek P, Wind J, Dijkgraaf MG, Busch OR, Goslings JC. Temporary closure of the open abdomen: a systematic review on delayed primary fascial closure in patients with an open abdomen. World J Surg. 2009;33(2):199–207. https://doi.org/10.1007/s00268-008-9867-3.
36. Quyn AJ, Johnston C, Hall D, Chambers A, Arapova N, Ogston S, Amin AI. The open abdomen and temporary abdominal closure systems—historical evolution and systematic review. Color Dis. 2012;14(8):e429–38. https://doi.org/10.1111/j.1463-1318.2012.03045.x.
37. Roberts DJ, Zygun DA, Grendar J, Ball CG, Robertson HL, Ouellet JF, Cheatham ML, Kirkpatrick AW. Negative-pressure wound therapy for critically ill adults with open abdominal wounds: a systematic review. J Trauma Acute Care Surg. 2012;73(3):629–39.
38. Cirocchi R, Birindelli A, Biffl WL, Mutafchiyski V, Popivanov G, Chiara O, Tugnoli G, Di Saverio S. What is the effectiveness of the negative pressure wound therapy (NPWT) in patients treated with open abdomen technique? A systematic review and meta-analysis. J Trauma Acute Care Surg. 2016;81(3):575–84. https://doi.org/10.1097/TA.0000000000001126.
39. Hurt RT, Zakaria ER, Matheson PJ, Cobb ME, Parker JR, Garrison RN. Hemorrhage-induced hepatic injury and hypoperfusion can be prevented by direct peritoneal resuscitation. J Gastrointest Surg. 2009;13(4):587–94. https://doi.org/10.1007/s11605-008-0796-0.
40. Smith JW, Garrison RN, Matheson PJ, Franklin GA, Harbrecht BG, Richardson JD. Direct peritoneal resuscitation accelerates primary abdominal wall closure after damage control surgery. J Am Coll Surg. 2010;210(5):658–64, 664–7. https://doi.org/10.1016/j.jamcollsurg.2010.01.014.
41. McQueen MM, Gaston P, Court-Brown CM. Acute compartment syndrome. Who is at risk? J Bone Joint Surg Br. 2000;82(2):200–3.
42. Garner MR, Taylor SA, Gausden E, Lyden JP. Compartment syndrome: diagnosis, management, and unique concerns in the twenty-first century. HSS J. 2014;10(2):143–52. https://doi.org/10.1007/s11420-014-9386-8.
43. Heckman MM, Whitesides TE Jr, Grewe SR, Rooks MD. Compartment pressure in association with closed tibial fractures. The relationship between tissue pressure, compartment, and the distance from the site of the fracture. J Bone Joint Surg Am. 1994;76(9):1285–92.

44. Shuler MS, Reisman WM, Kinsey TL, Whitesides TE Jr, Hammerberg EM, Davila MG, Moore TJ. Correlation between muscle oxygenation and compartment pressures in acute compartment syndrome of the leg. J Bone Joint Surg Am. 2010;92(4):863–70. https://doi.org/10.2106/JBJS.I.00816.
45. Doro CJ, Sitzman TJ, O'Toole RV. Can intramuscular glucose levels diagnose compartment syndrome? J Trauma Acute Care Surg. 2014;76(2):474–8. https://doi.org/10.1097/TA.0b013e3182a9ccd1.
46. Harrois A, Libert N, Duranteau J. Acute kidney injury in trauma patients. Curr Opin Crit Care. 2017;23(6):447–56. https://doi.org/10.1097/MCC.0000000000000463.
47. Zager RA. Combined mannitol and deferoxamine therapy for myohemoglobinuric renal injury and oxidant tubular stress. Mechanistic and therapeutic implications. J Clin Invest. 1992;90(3):711–9.
48. Schmidt AH. Acute compartment syndrome. Injury. 2017;48(Suppl 1):S22–5. https://doi.org/10.1016/j.injury.2017.04.024.
49. Rorabeck CH. The treatment of compartment syndromes of the leg. J Bone Joint Surg Br. 1984;66(1):93–7.
50. Sheridan GW, Matsen FA 3rd. Fasciotomy in the treatment of the acute compartment syndrome. J Bone Joint Surg Am. 1976;58(1):112–5.
51. Hope MJ, McQueen MM. Acute compartment syndrome in the absence of fracture. J Orthop Trauma. 2004;18(4):220–4.
52. Ritenour AE, Dorlac WC, Fang R, Woods T, Jenkins DH, Flaherty SF, Wade CE, Holcomb JB. Complications after fasciotomy revision and delayed compartment release in combat patients. J Trauma. 2008;64(2 Suppl):S153–61. ; discussion S161–2. https://doi.org/10.1097/TA.0b013e3181607750.
53. Janzing HM, Broos PL. Dermatotraction: an effective technique for the closure of fasciotomy wounds: a preliminary report of fifteen patients. J Orthop Trauma. 2001;15(6):438–41.
54. Brown CV, Rhee P, Chan L, Evans K, Demetriades D, Velmahos GC. Preventing renal failure in patients with rhabdomyolysis: do bicarbonate and mannitol make a difference? J Trauma. 2004;56(6):1191–6.
55. Ouellette EA, Kelly R. Compartment syndromes of the hand. J Bone Joint Surg Am. 1996;78(10):1515–22.
56. Kalyani BS, Fisher BE, Roberts CS, Giannoudis PV. Compartment syndrome of the forearm: a systematic review. J Hand Surg Am. 2011;36(3):535–43. https://doi.org/10.1016/j.jhsa.2010.12.007.
57. Duckworth AD, Mitchell SE, Molyneux SG, White TO, Court-Brown CM, McQueen MM. Acute compartment syndrome of the forearm. J Bone Joint Surg Am. 2012;94(10):e63. https://doi.org/10.2106/JBJS.K.00837.
58. Elkbuli A, Sanchez C, Hai S, McKenney M, Boneva D. Gluteal compartment syndrome following alcohol intoxication: case report and literature review. Ann Med Surg (Lond). 2019;44:98–101. https://doi.org/10.1016/j.amsu.2019.07.010.
59. Lutter C, Schöffl V, Hotfiel T, Simon M, Maffulli N. Compartment syndrome of the foot: an evidence-based review. J Foot Ankle Surg. 2019;58(4):632–40. https://doi.org/10.1053/j.jfas.2018.12.026.
60. Manoli A 2nd, Weber TG. Fasciotomy of the foot: an anatomical study with special reference to release of the calcaneal compartment. Foot Ankle. 1990;10(5):267–75.
61. Bedigrew KM, Stinner DJ, Kragh JF Jr, Potter BK, Shawen SB, Hsu JR. Effectiveness of foot fasciotomies in foot and ankle trauma. J R Army Med Corps. 2017;163(5):324–8. https://doi.org/10.1136/jramc-2016-000734.
62. Lokiec F, Siev-Ner I, Pritsch M. Chronic compartment syndrome of both feet. J Bone Joint Surg Br. 1991;73(1):178–9.
63. Ojike NI, Roberts CS, Giannoudis PV. Foot compartment syndrome: a systematic review of the literature. Acta Orthop Belg. 2009;75(5):573–80.

64. Han F, Daruwalla ZJ, Shen L, Kumar VP. A prospective study of surgical outcomes and quality of life in severe foot trauma and associated compartment syndrome after fasciotomy. J Foot Ankle Surg. 2015;54(3):417–23. https://doi.org/10.1053/j.jfas.2014.09.015.
65. Lollo L, Grabinsky A. Clinical and functional outcomes of acute lower extremity compartment syndrome at a Major Trauma Hospital. Int J Crit Illn Inj Sci. 2016;6(3):133–42.
66. Wandling MW, An GC. A case report of thoracic compartment syndrome in the setting of penetrating chest trauma and review of the literature. World J Emerg Surg. 2010;5:22. https://doi.org/10.1186/1749-7922-5-22.
67. Mestres CA, Pomar JL, Acosta M, Ninot S, Barriuso C, Abad C, Mulet J. Delayed sternal closure for life-threatening complications in cardiac operations: an update. Ann Thorac Surg. 1991;51(5):773–6.
68. Rizzo AG, Sample GA. Thoracic compartment syndrome secondary to a thoracic procedure: a case report. Chest. 2003;124(3):1164–8.
69. Alexi-Meskishvili V, Weng Y, Uhlemann F, Lange PE, Hetzer R. Prolonged open sternotomy after pediatric open heart operation: experience with 113 patients. Ann Thorac Surg. 1995;59(2):379–83.
70. Riahi M, Tomatis LA, Schlosser RJ, Bertolozzi E, Johnston DW. Cardiac compression due to closure of the median sternotomy in open heart surgery. Chest. 1975;67(1):113–4.
71. McElhinney DB, Reddy VM, Parry AJ, Johnson L, Fineman JR, Hanley FL. Management and outcomes of delayed sternal closure after cardiac surgery in neonates and infants. Crit Care Med. 2000;28(4):1180–4.
72. Christenson JT, Maurice J, Simonet F, Velebit V, Schmuziger M. Open chest and delayed sternal closure after cardiac surgery. Eur J Cardiothorac Surg. 1996;10(5):305–11.
73. Furnary AP, Magovern JA, Simpson KA, Magovern GJ. Prolonged open sternotomy and delayed sternal closure after cardiac operations. Ann Thorac Surg. 1992;54(2):233–9.
74. Adams CA, Stein DM, Morrison JJ, Scalea TM. Does intracranial pressure management hurt more than it helps in traumatic brain injury? Trauma Surg Acute Care Open. 2018;3(1):e000142. https://doi.org/10.1136/tsaco-2017-000142.
75. Lundberg N, Troupp H, Lorin H. Continuous recording of the ventricular-fluid pressure in patients with severe acute traumatic brain injury. A preliminary report. J Neurosurg. 1965;22(6):581–90.
76. Miller JD, Becker DP, Ward JD, Sullivan HG, Adams WE, Rosner MJ. Significance of intracranial hypertension in severe head injury. J Neurosurg. 1977;47(4):503–16.
77. Alnemari AM, Krafcik BM, Mansour TR, Gaudin D. A comparison of pharmacologic therapeutic agents used for the reduction of intracranial pressure after traumatic brain injury. World Neurosurg. 2017;106:509–28. https://doi.org/10.1016/j.wneu.2017.07.009.
78. Colton K, Yang S, Hu PF, Chen HH, Stansbury LG, Scalea TM, Stein DM. Responsiveness to therapy for increased intracranial pressure in traumatic brain injury is associated with neurological outcome. Injury. 2014;45(12):2084–8. https://doi.org/10.1016/j.injury.2014.08.041.
79. Shafi S, Barnes SA, Millar D, Sobrino J, Kudyakov R, Berryman C, Rayan N, Dubiel R, Coimbra R, Magnotti LJ, Vercruysse G, Scherer LA, Jurkovich GJ, Nirula R. Suboptimal compliance with evidence-based guidelines in patients with traumatic brain injuries. J Neurosurg. 2014;120(3):773–7. https://doi.org/10.3171/2013.12.JNS132151.
80. Cremer OL, van Dijk GW, van Wensen E, Brekelmans GJ, Moons KG, Leenen LP, Kalkman CJ. Effect of intracranial pressure monitoring and targeted intensive care on functional outcome after severe head injury. Crit Care Med. 2005;33(10):2207–13.
81. Chesnut RM, Temkin N, Carney N, Dikmen S, Rondina C, Videtta W, Petroni G, Lujan S, Pridgeon J, Barber J, Machamer J, Chaddock K, Celix JM, Cherner M, Hendrix T, Global Neurotrauma Research Group. A trial of intracranial-pressure monitoring in traumatic brain injury. N Engl J Med. 2012;367(26):2471–81. https://doi.org/10.1056/NEJMoa1207363.

Long-Term Outcomes After Open Abdomen for ACS: Complex Abdominal Wall Reconstructions and Entero-Atmospheric Fistulas

18

Fausto Catena, Belinda De Simone, Federico Coccolini, Gennaro Perrone, Antonio Tarasconi, Vittoria Pattonieri, Harishine Abongwa, Salomone Di Saverio, Massimo Sartelli, and Luca Ansaloni

Abbreviations

ACS	Abdominal compartment syndrome
AW	Abdominal wall
EAF	Entero-atmospheric fistula
LOD	Loss of domain
OA	Open abdomen
VH	Ventral hernia

F. Catena (✉) · G. Perrone · A. Tarasconi · V. Pattonieri · H. Abongwa
Emergency Surgery Department, Parma University Hospital, Parma, Italy

B. De Simone
Département de Chirurgie Viscérale (Bariatrique and Métabolique, Oncologique, et d'Urgence), Centre Hospitalier Poissy/Saint-Germain, Saint-Germain-en-Laye, France

F. Coccolini
General, Emergency and Trauma Surgery Department, Pisa University Hospital, Pisa, Italy

S. Di Saverio
General and Trauma Surgery, Addenbrooke's Hospital, Cambridge University Hospitals NHS Foundation Trust, Cambridge, UK

Department of General Surgery, University of Insubria, University Hospital of Varese, ASST Sette Laghi, Regione Lombardia, Varese, Italy

M. Sartelli
General and Emergency Surgery, Macerata Hospital, Macerata, Italy

L. Ansaloni
General, Emergency and Trauma Surgery Department, Bufalini Hospital, Cesena, Italy

© Springer Nature Switzerland AG 2021
F. Coccolini et al. (eds.), *Compartment Syndrome*, Hot Topics in Acute Care Surgery and Trauma, https://doi.org/10.1007/978-3-030-55378-4_18

In some cases, abdominal compartment syndrome (ACS) has to be treated using an open abdomen (OA). In particular decompressive laparotomy and OA are indicated in ACS if medical treatment has failed after repeated and reliable intra-abdominal pressure measurements both in trauma and nontrauma patients.

Moreover, OA is an option for emergency surgery patients with severe peritonitis and sepsis/septic shock under the following circumstances: abbreviated laparotomy due to severe physiological derangement, the need for a deferred intestinal anastomosis, a planned second look for intestinal ischemia, persistent source of peritonitis (failure of source control), or extensive visceral edema with the concern for development of abdominal compartment syndrome.

The abdomen should be maintained open if requirements for ongoing resuscitation and/or the source of contamination persists, if a deferred intestinal anastomosis is needed, if there is the necessity for a planned second look for ischemic intestine, and lastly if there are concerns about abdominal compartment syndrome development.

Early fascial and/or abdominal definitive closure should be the strategy for management of the open abdomen once any requirements for ongoing resuscitation have ceased, the source control has been definitively reached, no concern regarding intestinal viability persists, no further surgical reexploration is needed and there are no concerns for ACS.

Primary fascia closure is the ideal solution to restore early the abdominal closure. Component separation is an effective technique. The use of synthetic mesh (polypropylene, polytetrafluoruroethylene, and polyester products) as a fascial bridge should not be recommended in definitive closure interventions after OA and should be placed only in patients without other alternatives. Biologic meshes are reliable for definitive abdominal wall reconstruction in the presence of a large wall defect, bacterial contamination, comorbidities, and difficult wound healing. Non–cross-linked biologic meshes seem to be preferred in sublay position when the linea alba can be reconstructed.

Cross-linked biologic meshes in fascial-bridge position (no linea alba closure) may be associated with less ventral hernia recurrence.

In Figs. 18.1 and 18.2, you can find the score proposed by the "Italian Biological Prosthesis Work-Group (IBPWG)" to achieve information about the best biological mesh choice. This decisional model combines the infection grade with tissue lost grade [1].

Planned ventral hernia (VH) (skin graft or skin closure only) remains an option for the complicated OA (i.e., in the presence of entero-atmospheric fistula or in cases with a protracted OA due to underlying diseases) or in those settings where no other alternatives are viable.

In case of present entero-atmospheric fistula, effluent isolation is essential for proper wound healing. Separating the wound into different compartments to facilitate the collection of fistula output is of paramount importance: negative pressure wound therapy makes effluent isolation feasible and wound healing achievable. Definitive management of entero-atmospheric fistula should be delayed to after the patient has recovered and the wound completely healed [2].

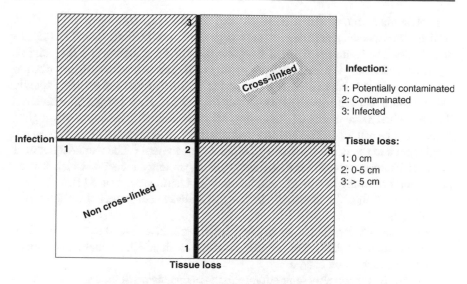

Fig. 18.1 Decisional model diagram: the product of the infection and the loss of tissue scores gives as a result the value which indicates the kind of biological prosthesis to use

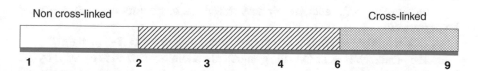

Fig. 18.2 Decisional line: the different results indicate the kind of biological prosthesis to use

So VH repair and entero-atmospheric fistula are the most significant long-term complications after OA.

VH can be planned ventral hernia after skin graft or skin closure only or they can be recurrences after early fascial and/or abdominal definitive closure especially in difficult cases when it is necessary to use biological prostheses.

In the majority of cases, these abdominal wall (AW) defects are huge and patients need permanent incisional hernia belts with a significant impact in their quality of life (self-body image disturbance to the patient).

On the other hand, these large defects very rarely become complicated hernias, precisely because of the big dimensions of the defect and it is practically impossible a bowel strangulation.

For this reason, high-risk patients must be informed that this hernia repair is not absolutely necessary and their VH will change their quality but not their quantity of life.

In particular, if there is a previous respiratory insufficiency, AW repair will affect negatively the respiratory dynamics because of the loss of domain (LOD).

Moreover, it was reported that the impact of the defect size, BMI, hernia volume (HV), subcutaneous volume, intra-abdominal volume, and the ratio of hernia to intra-abdominal volume (IAV) on respiratory insufficiency after open VH repair is collinear. Patients with large defects and a large ratio of HV:IAV (greater than 0.5) are also at significantly increased risk of respiratory insufficiency after open VH repair [3].

"Loss of domain" is a term used commonly in the hernia literature to describe the distribution of abdominal content between the hernia and residual abdominopelvic cavity. After repairing hernias with significant LOD (i.e., large hernias with much of the abdominal viscera outside the abdominal compartment), serious physiological complications can arise. The increase in intra-abdominal pressure pushes up on the diaphragm and can cause respiratory failure and pneumonia. The rise in abdominal pressure increases also the tension along the laparotomy incision, which can be pulled apart resulting in wound complications and hernia recurrence [4].

A patient with a VH after and OA has to be always considered a complex AW reconstruction.

Mesh implantation should be advised during definitive fascial closure: the final decision to use a mesh, the type of mesh, and the mesh position should be balanced by an expert surgeon in charge.

The use of component separation/relaxing incisions/myoplasties can be techniques of utmost importance to apply in these difficult cases [5].

First, it is fundamental to analyze to AW defect and bowel adhesions performing an MR scan.

If there are concerns about respiratory dynamics, respiratory function tests must be performed.

A salient clinical test during the patient abdominal exam is the "pich test."

In the planned VH after OA, the granulated abdominal wound is covered by the skin: this is achieved by creating subcutaneous flaps on both sides of the wound and closing the released skin in the midline. If the gap was too large to allow this technique, the wound could be covered with split thickness skin graft.

Reconstruction should be delayed until complete separation of the skin graft from the underlying tissue is evident (positive pinch test), usually after at least 6–12 months.

The underlying tissue is in the majority of cases bowel loops that can be harmed if the surgical reconstruction is performed too early [6].

Laparoscopic approach to these complex AW hernias is practically impossible for three reasons: (1) dimensions of the defect, (2) adhesions, and (3) closeness to bony prominences. Hopefully in the near future, with new mini-invasive techniques, also for these patients this kind of solutions will be found [7].

As general surgeons are increasingly adopting robotic surgery, there is substantial interest in harnessing the potential advantages of the robotic platform for ventral hernia repair, in particular for complex cases. Since then, the application of robotics in ventral hernia repair has grown steadily. As of 2018, more than 6000 robotic ventral hernia repairs have been reported in the medical literature. Henriksen et al. carried out a meta-analysis and stated that for ventral hernias that would normally require an open procedure, a robot-assisted repair may be a good option, as the use of a minimally invasive approach for these procedures decreases length of stay significantly [8].

The problem related to robotic surgery is the limited availability; therefore, the standard preferred technique is with an open approach.

The incision has to be chosen to gain the best visualization of residual AW but not to interfere or devascularize possible skin grafts.

The second step is adhesiolysis that has to be limited to the achievement of an effective surgical exposure.

Caution must be used to avoid bowel tears with consequent bacterial contamination and increased prostheses infection risk precluding the use of a synthetic mesh.

If possible a Rives–Stoppa technique utilizing a polypropylene mesh has to be carried out (if there is a direct contact with bowel loops a double-layer mesh is mandatory): in case of bacterial contamination, the same technique with a cross-linked or not cross-linked biological prostheses has to be employed. In the majority of cases, a component separation approach has to be added.

In brief, if midline tissue cannot be easily approximated, then separation of lateral components or some sort of tissue transposition needs to be done.

Component separation results in medial advancement of intact rectus myofascial units bilaterally, closing defects of up to 10 cm in the upper abdomen, of up to 20 cm in the mid-abdomen, and 6–8 cm in the lower abdomen.

In extreme cases, when Rives–Stoppa technique is not feasible, a Chevrel approach should be employed. It is important to underline that the latter technique has higher prostheses infections and recurrence rates so it is absolutely not equivalent to Rives–Stoppa technique.

The effectiveness of mesh reinforcement has been demonstrated in several studies which have shown that both short-term and long-term recurrence rates decrease by up to 50% when the fascial closure is reinforced with mesh. Although most studies suggest at least 5 cm of overlap or underlap, this requires further study, as there is some evidence that the amount of under/overlap depends on the size of the defect itself.

In general, mesh should be placed under adequate tension to avoid ripples or folds in the mesh. It should be taut, flat, and planar to promote increased contact with vascularized tissue and promote better integration. The ideal mesh location would insulate the viscera from the mesh, while protecting the mesh from exposure in case of wound-healing complications. The retrorectus/retromuscular plane (Rives–Stoppa technique) satisfies these criteria because the mesh is located in a well-vascularized plane between the underlying posterior rectus sheath and the overlying rectus abdominis muscle. Indeed, mesh placement in the retro-rectus plane has been shown to have excellent outcomes. Another excellent option for mesh placement is the wide intraperitoneal underlay position, although synthetic mesh used in this position should be coated with a barrier layer to protect the viscera, and should be appropriately fixated so as to prevent internal herniation. Again the highest rate of hernia recurrence, bulge, and surgical site infections (SSI) occurs with interpositional bridge mesh placement, where the fascia cannot be closed primarily.

The preservation of skin and soft tissue vascularity is essential to reducing the risk of SSI. This vascularity is derived, on each side, largely from two rows of perforators, which themselves originate from the superior and deep inferior epigastric vessels. Techniques that preserve as many of those vessels as possible have been shown to result in significantly fewer SSI than techniques that involve wide undermining.

The presence of skin undermining greater than 2 cm has been found to more than double the risk of SSI If possible, marginal and undermined skin and subcutaneous tissue should be excised before closure.

One of the enemies is dead space, which can result in seroma/abscess formation, leading to wound breakdown. Every effort must be made to obliterate any potential dead space. Closed suction drains should be used wherever dead space is present and should be maintained until the output is less than 20 mL a day for two consecutive days with the patient ambulatory [9].

Another long-term complication after OA is entero-atmospheric fistula.

Entero-atmospheric fistula (EAF) is an enteric fistula occurring in the setting of an open abdomen, thus creating a communication between the GI tract and the external atmosphere.

The onset of an EAF within open abdomen represents a surgical nightmare, carrying several extremely challenging issues in the field of critical care and nutritional management; EAF is therefore associated with significant morbidity and mortality.

Despite the advances in OA management and the subsequent decrease of the initial reported mortality rates of 70%, EAF's mortality is nowadays still as high as up to 40%.

EAF has unique features, therefore, making its spontaneous closure almost impossible to achieve; for this reason, the management of the fistula should be aimed to completely divert the fistula output, thus allowing a clean granulation of the exposed bowel and promoting the fistula to become a chronic but well-controlled fistula.

This result is hard to achieve, that, and before placing any dressing over the OA, a proper thorough irrigation of the abdominal cavity should be performed to reduce peritoneal contamination and limit the ongoing sepsis.

A large spectrum of techniques and surgical devices is described in literature; every surgeon usually develops his own technique, and none of those can perfectly fit well in every kind of clinical situation.

It is easy to figure out that EAFs being single, small, distal, superficial, and of low output are more likely to close spontaneously; in this group of fistulas, it may be worth an initial attempt of primary closure with sutures and different types of sealants (fibrin glue and cyanoacrylates). In contrast, when dealing with large, deep, proximal, and high-output fistulas, or with multiple openings, primary closure is absolutely unlikely to be successful; furthermore, the fistula should be exteriorized as much as possible outside the abdominal cavity, thus creating a flat surface where a diversion device can be applied more easily.

All different management options are aimed to bridge the patient to a delayed definitive treatment when the sepsis and the peritonitis are resolved and the surrounding bowel has granulated enough to allow the definitive closure of the wound either by skin grafting or use of any other biological materials.

Definitive surgery for fistula resection and abdominal wall reconstruction should be delayed for at least 8–12 months, to allow proper loosening of the visceral adhesions, and should be performed only when the patient is well nourished and has reached a well-balanced physiological homeostasis. Multiple surgical approaches for definitive fistula takedown and abdominal bowel reconstruction may be required in a multistep fashion, and several strategies are described in literature [10].

Fistula location, demonstration of any other intra-abdominal abscesses or associated collections, and exclusion of any distal gastrointestinal obstruction can be demonstrated with a wide variety of imaging diagnostic methods, that is, methylene blue test, upper and lower GI series with water-soluble contrasts, fistulography, computed tomography, and magnetic resonance imaging [11].

When possible, the surgeon should avoid going through the same incision used in prior operations. Instead, attempts should be made to enter the abdomen from non-violated areas of the AW. Some authors have suggested alternative methods of entering the abdomen through a transverse incision.

Some authors suggest that surgeons should mobilize and identify the entire gastrointestinal tract, from the gastroesophageal junction to the rectosigmoid junction but this is not absolutely demonstrated to be useful. Identifying all of the fistulas and the entire GI tract is pivotal. Resecting multiple fistulas as one segment en masse is preferable, but this may not be possible if the fistulas are located at a distance from one another. Thus, difficult decisions must often be made during the course of the operation: should more than two or three anastomoses be created, running the risk of a leak? Or, should the number of anastomoses be minimized? Should large segments of small bowel be resected, potentially creating GI-crippled patients with possible short gut syndrome? Or should one create more anastomoses? Only an expert operating surgeon can make that judgment. It is important to recognize that intestines look shorter than they in fact are in the abdomen that has been operated previously. If at least 20–25 cm of bowel can be left between anastomoses, a hand-sewn or stapled technique can be used. To avoid resecting a large amount of bowel, adjunct procedures (such as a modified strictureplasty) can be used in certain fistulas.

If the integrity of anastomoses or anastomosis is questionable, revision is reasonable, as is the creation of a proximal diverting ostomy. Surgeons should not promise their patients that they will not have a stoma, temporary or otherwise.

These operations can take a long time, so surgeons should consider stopping and returning the next day to complete the anastomosis or to reconstruct the abdominal wall.

During the interim period, patients can be resuscitated, coagulation and acidosis can be corrected, and the surgeon and surgical team can get some much-needed rest before performing the definitive surgery. Intraoperatively, these patients need adequate oxygen delivery and maintenance of normal tissue perfusion and adequate body temperature are mandatory. Fluid status should be monitored. Hypotension should be avoided, especially if the patient underwent preoperative bowel preparation.

Definitive AW reconstruction at the time of hernia repair or at the time of takedown of EAF, even in contaminated fields, should be attempted.

Stoma or fistula takedown at the time of complex hernia repair has been reported to be associated with significant complications. These studies suggest that biologic mesh implantation is a valid option for complex AW reconstruction in high-risk trauma and acute care surgery patients. The three most common techniques used to place mesh during AW reconstruction are again onlay placement, interposition, or bridge, underlay placement with the criticisms already described.

Different techniques for AW reconstruction include the use of tissue expanders or other highly sophisticated plastic surgery tools and operations have been described.

In comparison with prosthetic mesh repairs, autologous vascularized tissue flaps have the advantage of not implanting foreign material into the body thus reducing the risk of infection when applied to a contaminated field. They can also be used when there is a large skin defect. Furthermore, they can be combined with other methods, such as components separation of mesh, to reduce the size of the flap needed. The disadvantages include the complex techniques required as well as the morbidity associated with the donor site. Although pedicled flaps can be used in small- and mid-sized defects within the arch of the rotation of the flap, the size and location of the defect usually preclude the use of a rotational flap.

The main indication for using a microvascular flap is a large, full-thickness tissue defect (with grafted skin) extending into the upper abdomen. The tensor fascia latae (TFL) myocutaneous free flap use has been reported in more than 100 patients in the world.

The advantages of the TFL flap compared with an anterolateral thigh flap are the more constant anatomy of the TFL pedicle and larger vessel caliber matching the vessel size of the great saphenous vein loop. In addition, the size of the flap can be quite large although in very wide flaps the relative thinness of the anteromedial portion of the fascia, especially in women, sometimes requires mesh enforcement. Furthermore, the location of the donor site in the thigh has no effect on postoperative respiratory function and usually heals well [12].

In conclusion, surgical treatment of patients with EAF-hostile abdomen and other complex abdominal defects is challenging and expensive; it requires significant resources, both surgical and financial. Careful planning and advanced surgical techniques are required, often involving the use (alone or combined) of biologic mesh and composite tissue transfer. With careful planning and proper surgical techniques, using biologic mesh may be the only viable choice and could offer excellent results. Furthermore, while abdominal reconstruction in patients with or without fistulas and abdominal defects is challenging and complex, and is associated with significant morbidity and potential mortality, AW reconstruction offers the only possible option to significantly improve the quality of life of this group of patients [13, 14].

References

1. Coccolini F, Agresta F, Bassi A, et al. Italian Biological Prosthesis Work-Group (IBPWG): proposal for a decisional model in using biological prosthesis. World J Emerg Surg. 2012;7:34.

2. Coccolini F, Roberts D, Ansaloni L, Ivatury R, Gamberini E, Kluger Y, Moore EE, Coimbra R, Kirkpatrick AW, Pereira BM, Montori G, Ceresoli M, Abu-Zidan FM, Sartelli M, Velmahos G, Fraga GP, Leppaniemi A, Tolonen M, Galante J, Razek T, Maier R, Bala M, Sakakushev B, Khokha V, Malbrain M, Agnoletti V, Peitzman A, Demetrashvili Z, Sugrue M, Di Saverio S, Martzi I, Soreide K, Biffl W, Ferrada P, Parry N, Montravers P, Melotti RM, Salvetti F, Valetti TM, Scalea T, Chiara O, Cimbanassi S, Kashuk JL, Larrea M, Hernandez JAM, Lin HF, Chirica M, Arvieux C, Bing C, Horer T, De Simone B, Masiakos P, Reva V, De Angelis N, Kike K, Balogh ZJ, Fugazzola P, Tomasoni M, Latifi R, Naidoo N, Weber D, Handolin L, Inaba K, Hecker A, Kuo-Ching Y, Ordoñez CA, Rizoli S, Gomes CA, De Moya M, Wani I, Mefire AC, Boffard K, Napolitano L, Catena F. The open abdomen in trauma and non-trauma patients: WSES guidelines. World J Emerg Surg. 2018;13:7.
3. Schlosser KA, Maloney SR, Prasad T, et al. Too big to breathe: predictors of respiratory failure and insufficiency after open ventral hernia repair. Surg Endosc. 2019. https://doi.org/10.1007/s00464-019-07181-3.
4. Parker SG, Halligan S, Blackburn S, Plumb AAO, Archer L, Mallett S, Windsor ACJ. What exactly is meant by "loss of domain" for ventral hernia? Systematic review of definitions. World J Surg. 2019;43(2):396–404.
5. López-Cano M, García-Alamino JM, Antoniou SA, Bennet D, Dietz UA, Ferreira F, Fortelny RH, Hernandez-Granados P, Miserez M, Montgomery A, Morales-Conde S, Muysoms F, Pereira JA, Schwab R, Slater N, Vanlander A, Van Ramshorst GH, Berrevoet F. EHS clinical guidelines on the management of the abdominal wall in the context of the open or burst abdomen. Hernia. 2018;22(6):921–39.
6. Klein Y. Closure of the open abdomen: a practical approach. Curr Trauma Rep. 2016;2:196–201.
7. Belyansky I, Weltz AS, Sibia US, Turcotte JJ, Taylor H, Zahiri HR, Turner TR, Park A. The trend toward minimally invasive complex abdominal wall reconstruction: is it worth it? Surg Endosc. 2018;32(4):1701–7.
8. Henriksen NA, Jensen KK, Muysoms F. Robot-assisted abdominal wall surgery: a systematic review of the literature and meta-analysis. Hernia. 2019;23:17–27.
9. Khansa I, Janis JE. The 4 principles of complex abdominal wall reconstruction. Plast Reconstr Surg Glob Open. 2019;7(12):e2549.
10. Di Saverio S, Tarasconi A, Walczak DA, Cirocchi R, Mandrioli M, Birindelli A, Tugnoli G. Classification, prevention and management of entero-atmospheric fistula: a state-of-the-art review. Langenbecks Arch Surg. 2016;401(1):1–13.
11. Marinis A, Gkiokas G, Argyra E, Fragulidis G, Polymeneas G, Voros D. "Enteroatmospheric fistulae"—gastrointestinal openings in the open abdomen: a review and recent proposal of a surgical technique. Scand J Surg. 2013;102(2):61–8.
12. Leppäniemi A, Tukiainen E. Reconstruction of complex abdominal wall defects. Scand J Surg. 2013;102(1):14–9.
13. Latifi R, Joseph B, Kulvatunyou N, Wynne JL, O'Keeffe T, Tang A, Friese R, Rhee PM. Enterocutaneous fistulas and a hostile abdomen: reoperative surgical approaches. World J Surg. 2012;36(3):516–23.
14. De Simone B, Birindelli A, Ansaloni L, Sartelli M, Coccolini F, Di Saverio S, Annessi V, Amico F, Catena F. Emergency repair of complicated abdominal wall hernias: WSES guidelines. Hernia. 2020;24(2):359–68.

Future Directions

19

Alcir Escocia Dorigatti and Gustavo Pereira Fraga

19.1 Briefing

Decision-making in treatment of an acute compartment syndrome is based on clinical assessment, supported by invasive monitoring. Thus, evolving compartment syndrome may require repeated pressure measurements. In suspected cases of potential compartment syndromes clinical assessment alone seems to be unreliable.

Point-of-care ultrasound (POCUS) is a propaedeutic modality more often used in daily practice. Since the establishment of sonography bases for lung ultrasound, it has become a valuable extension of physical examination, providing new information about lungs, pleural structures, and volume status.

POCUS has become an indispensable tool in the management of critically ill patients including echocardiography; fluid assessment; lung, optic nerve, abdominal, and venous thromboembolism evaluation, as examples [1, 2].

The possibility of obtaining responses with potential to direct the patient treatment instantly changed the modern approach in the intensive care. Following you can learn examples of how the POCUS can help in the early diagnosis and treatment of the main compartmental syndromes shown in the previous chapters.

19.2 Abdominal Compartment Syndrome

The World Society of the Abdominal Compartment (WSACS) guidelines were updated in 2013 and included the medical management algorithm [3]. These guidelines recommend either continuous or intermittent intra-abdominal pressure (IAP)

A. E. Dorigatti
School of Medical Sciences (SMS), University of Campinas (Unicamp), Campinas, SP, Brazil

G. P. Fraga (✉)
Division of Trauma Surgery, School of Medical Sciences (SMS), University of Campinas (Unicamp), Campinas, SP, Brazil

© Springer Nature Switzerland AG 2021
F. Coccolini et al. (eds.), *Compartment Syndrome*, Hot Topics in Acute Care Surgery and Trauma, https://doi.org/10.1007/978-3-030-55378-4_19

monitoring. Medical management for intra-abdominal hypertension (IAH) and abdominal compartment syndrome (ACS) is divided into five categories: evacuation of intraluminal contents; evacuation of intraluminal occupying lesions; extraluminal (intra-abdominal) contents; improvement of abdominal wall compliance; optimization of fluid administration; and optimization of systemic and regional perfusion.

Pereira et al. [4] studied a group of 50 critically ill patients who developed IAH, in whom POCUS proved to be extremely useful in evaluation of bowel activity, identification of large intestinal contents, the identification of patients who would benefit from bowel evacuation as an adjuvant to lower IAP and the diagnosis of moderate to large amounts of free intra-abdominal fluid.

Following first step of the WSACS medical management algorithm, ultrasound was used for nasogastric tube placement, confirmation of correct positioning, and to check stomach contents. In the second step that addresses intraluminal evacuation through the administration of enemas, POCUS allowed assessment of bowel activity (movements); allowed identification of large bowel contents (right and left colon) and identified patients that may benefit from continued enema-treatment to lower IAP. Also, during the second stage of the WSACS medical management algorithm, it was a useful adjuvant tool for diagnosing moderate to large amounts of free intra-abdominal fluid.

POCUS echocardiography also can detect indirect but nonspecific signs of ACS, decreased preload as well as dysfunctions of systolic and diastolic ventricular functions [5].

In 2017, International Fluid Academy (IFA) published the Critical and Acute Care Ultrasound Book (CACU) including the use of POCUS as a tool for intra-abdominal hypertension management.

19.3 Extremity Compartment Syndrome

Acute compartment syndrome of the lower extremity is a condition of rapidly increased pressure leading to reduced perfusion below a vital level for muscles and nerves within limited anatomic space [6]. Without immediate surgical decompression, nerve lesions, muscle contracture, amputation, or even sepsis may occur [7].

Invasive pressure measurement is recommended as an adjunct to clinical examination [8, 9]. Noninvasive alternatives such as near-field spectroscopy, microvascular blood flow, muscle oxygenation and pH, laser Doppler flowmeter, quantitative hardness measurements, or compression sonography have been examined but were not feasible for routine diagnosis of acute compartment syndrome [10–12]. Ultrasound examination is noninvasive, easy to perform, painless, and could be used in addition to invasive pressure measurement [13, 14].

A study found that intra-compartmental pressure of the anterior compartment of the calf can be well estimated by ultrasound-based tibia–fascia angle difference between legs [13]. Another study showed the volume of anterior tibial compartment had relation with intra-compartmental pressure [14].

19.4   Intracranial Compartment Syndrome

The patient's assessment with trauma brain injury with intracranial pressure (ICP) increase is a challenge in the emergency service. Many of these patients display serious complications and an early diagnosis might settle therapeutic measures that could contribute to a better survival. The physical examination is not enough in the emergency services to assess the ICP increase in patients with traumatic brain injury.

The optic nerve sheath ultrasonography measure seems to be a valid alternative method with several advantages like the accessibility, opportunity, cheapness, monitoring (since it can be repeated), and not being invasive in critical patient context since morbidity and mortality can increase especially in the emergency services and intensive care unit [15].

A prospective study showed the ocular ultrasonography benefit in neurosurgical patients, it proved a positive correlation between the diameter of the optic nerve sheath and the ICP measurements. 95% sensitivity and 80% specificity were the most specific in those patients with a history of traumatic brain injury [16].

In 2015, a study case in children was checked and it confirmed that ocular ultrasonography was an examination that might provide two signs related to papilledema; the optic disc elevation (elevation of one or more mm above the retina of entry of the optic nerve) and the crescent sign using point-of-care as the fluid that surrounds the optic nerve when it is seen in transverse windows with vertical orientation that demonstrated its relationship with an increase in ICP [16, 17]. Optic nerve sheath diameter also may be useful for predicting neurologic outcomes in post-cardiac arrest patients according to a recent study [18].

When comparing ICP measurements in an invasive way with the optic nerve sheath measure through ultrasonography, the results show a good correlation among the values and the ICP estimated. Same results were achieved with the computed axial tomography measuring the negative predictive value and sensibility.

19.5   What Next?

So far, we have not intended to carry out a comprehensive review regarding the use of POCUS in compartmental syndromes, but to present some of the most recent lines of research in order to assist in the early diagnosis and treatment of compartment syndromes.

It is quite difficult to predict what will happen to the treatment of compartmental syndromes, but it is possible to observe the current trends where we are going. More important than this is to create awareness about these conditions.

We already know how to solve the issue of compartmental syndromes in our patients, but often we come too late. When diagnosed, definitive lesions are often already present or even multiple organ dysfunctions, which cause morbidity and mortality related to the syndrome to increase dramatically.

These studies above had many methodological limitations that do not allow coming up with a recommendation about it. However, they all have something in common: the search for a simpler, less-invasive method for the patient, and cheaper for the health system or health care provider.

We need to Keep It Stupid Simple (KISS). When we KISS, things have gone easier. It is impossible to have emergency physicians possess the ability to perform invasive monitoring of intracerebral pressure, for example, but by allowing them to perform their screening, or to be able to act directly on intra-abdominal hypertension through POCUS, the possibilities to act directly on time-response and change in mortality of these diseases could increase.

A study demonstrated that although most of the physicians who answered the questionnaire stated that they were familiar with IAH and ACS, knowledge is incoherent and inadequate about the definitions published in the consensus of the WSACS, the clinical measurement, and the treatment techniques [19]. This makes it clear that the next move is toward education.

We need to strive for concepts about compartmental syndromes to be part of the clinical curriculum in medical school, while societies such as WSACS, IFA, and World Society of Emergency Surgery (WSES) struggle for continuing education initiatives to reach the greatest number of physicians around the world, familiarizing them with this pathology.

Just reading this book already puts you in a select group of physicians who continue in the incessant search for the best way to take care of our patients. But more is needed, only those who already have an interest in the subject will be here unless you disseminate what you already know and make more people curious to get to the end of this reading.

The future belongs to those who learn more skills and combine them in creative ways.
—*Robert Greene, Mastery*

References

1. Ha YR, Toh HC. Clinically integrated multi-organ point-of-care ultrasound for undifferentiated respiratory difficulty, chest pain, or shock: a critical analytic review. J Intensive Care. 2016;4:54.
2. Kameda T, Taniguchi N. Overview of point-of-care abdominal ultrasound in emergency and critical care. J Intensive Care. 2016;4:53.
3. Kirkpatrick AW, Roberts DJ, De Waele J, Jaeschke R, Malbrain ML, De Keulenaer B, et al. Intra-abdominal hypertension and the abdominal compartment syndrome: updated consensus definitions and clinical practice guidelines from the World Society of the Abdominal Compartment Syndrome. Intensive Care Med. 2013;39(7):1190–206.
4. Pereira BM, Pereira RG, Wise R, Surgrue G, Zakrison TL, Dorigatti AE, et al. The role of point-of-care ultrasound in intra-abdominal hypertension management. Anaesthesiol Intensive Ther. 2017;49(5):373–81.
5. Mahjoub Y, Plantefeve G. Cardiac ultrasound and abdominal compartment syndrome. Acta Clin Belg. 2007;62(Suppl 1):183–9.
6. Matsen FA 3rd, Winquist RA, Krugmire RB Jr. Diagnosis and management of compartmental syndromes. J Bone Joint Surg Am. 1980;62:286–91.
7. Sheridan GW, Matsen FA 3rd. Fasciotomy in the treatment of the acute compartment syndrome. J Bone Joint Surg Am. 1976;58:112–5.

8. Rorabeck CH, Castle GS, Hardie R, Logan J. Compartmental pressure measurements: an experimental investigation using the slit catheter. J Trauma. 1981;21(6):446–9.
9. Mubarak SJ, Owen CA, Hargens AR, Garetto LP, Akeson WH. Acute compartment syndromes: diagnosis and treatment with the aid of the wick catheter. J Bone Joint Surg Am. 1978;60:1091–5.
10. Shadgan B, Menon M, O'Brien PJ, Reid WD. Diagnostic techniques in acute compartment syndrome of the leg. J Orthop Trauma. 2008;22:581–7.
11. Sellei RM, Hingmann SJ, Weber C, Jeromin S, Zimmermann F, Turner J, et al. Assessment of elevated compartment pressures by pressure-related ultrasound: a cadaveric model. Eur J Trauma Emerg Surg. 2015;41:639–45.
12. Bloch A, Tomaschett C, Jakob SM, Schwinghammer A, Schmid T. Compression sonography for non-invasive measurement of lower leg compartment pressure in an animal model. Injury. 2018;49:532–7.
13. Mühlbacher J, Pauzenberger R, Asenbaum U, Gauster T, Kapral S, Herkner H, et al. Feasibility of ultrasound measurement in a human model of acute compartment syndrome. World J Emerg Surg. 2019;14:4.
14. Gershuni DH, Gosink BB, Hargens AR, Gould RN, Forsythe JR, Mubarak SJ, et al. Ultrasound evaluation of the anterior musculofascial compartment of the leg following exercise. Clin Orthop Relat Res. 1982;(167):185–90.
15. Goel RS, Goyal NK, Dharap SB, Kumar M, Gore MA. Utility of optic nerve ultrasonography in head injury. Injury. 2008;39(5):519–24.
16. Raffiz M, Abdullah JM. Optic nerve sheath diameter measurement: a means of detecting raised ICP in adult traumatic and non-traumatic neurosurgical patients. Am J Emerg Med. 2017;35(1):150–3.
17. Marchese RF, Mistry RD, Scarfone RJ, Chen AE. Identification of optic disc elevation and the crescent sign using point-of-care ocular ultrasound in children. Pediatr Emerg Care. 2015;31(4):304–7.
18. Lee SH, Jong Yun S. Diagnostic performance of optic nerve sheath diameter for predicting neurologic outcome in post-cardiac arrest patients: a systematic review and meta-analysis. Resuscitation. 2019;138:59–67.
19. Wise R, Roberts DJ, Vandervelden S, Debergh D, De Wacle JJ, De Laet I, et al. Awareness and knowledge of intra-abdominal hypertension and abdominal compartment syndrome: results of an international survey. Anaesthesiol Intensive Ther. 2015;47(1):14–29.

Printed in the United States
by Baker & Taylor Publisher Services